The Veterinarian's Son

My Seventy-Five Years in Veterinary Medicine

by John W. Merrick, DVM

Iatro Publishing Company
Post Office Box 895281
Leesburg, Florida 34789

The Veterinarian's Son
My Seventy-Five Years in Veterinary Medicine
Copyright © 2012 by John W. Merrick, DVM

All rights reserved, including the right to reproduce this
book or portions of this book in any form whatsoever.

Web site: TheVeterinariansSon.com

The author is available to speak at your live event.
For more information, or to book Dr. Merrick for your event,
contact him at: DrMerrick@TheVeterinariansSon.com

For information about special discounts for bulk purchases,
contact Dr. Merrick via e-mail at the address shown above.
100% of all profits will be donated to charity.

Book design by Randy Drake
Cover design by KC Pollak
Cover portrait by Jim Pollard (p. 179)

The Veterinarian's Son
First edition • April, 2012
ISBN-13: 978-0-9852-5800-9
ISBN-10: 0-9852-5800-4

Printed in the United States of America
Last digit is print number: 9 8 7 6 5 4 3 2

To my father and mother, Andrew C. Merrick and Dorothy Santee Merrick, for their example of what can be possible in life.

To my wife, Carol Hough Merrick, for her wisdom, friendship, and love over 60 years.

To my children, Dorothy, William, David, Byron, Ginger, Peggy, and their offspring for the constant reminder of the glorious future ahead.

To my colleagues, clients, friends, and animals I've encountered on my journey.

Contents

Preface	ix
The Veterinarian's Son	1
Life on the Farm in Iowa	7
Bookkeeping, Then and Now	21
Early City Life	27
The Great Walrus Race	31
Andy's Taj Mahal	33
The Testing Box Mystery	37
Small Animal Practice in the '40s and '50s	43
The Mob Vet	49
Dr. Merrick's Sulfodene	55
How to Own a Dog and Like It!	59
"Topper"	63
Halloween	65
Why I Became a Vet	69
Quiz Kid? Margaret, Not Me!	71
The "O House"	77
Wedding Day	81
Peppermint Schnapps & Timing Gears	87
Associate Vets	91
Technical Knockout	99
Short Order Cooks & College Jobs	101
Take Two and Hit to Right	105
The Men's Old Gym	109
Large Animal Practice	111
Explosions in Vet Med	117
Wives' Revenge	121
Senior Trips	123
State Boards	127
Uncle Russ, Chicago Bears, and Golf	131
And Baby Makes 3, 4, 5, 6, 7, 8, 9, and 10	137
Dog Whisperer	141
Private Zoo Vet	145
Carol Hough Merrick	149
City Girl	155
Dyna Mite, Canine Variety	159

Mrs. Doherty—Compliments 163
The Music Box Vet 167
Dinner Guests and Visitors 173
The Art of Bartering 177
Sweet Georgia Brown—Globetrotters 181
Barry Z—Hidden Talents 185
The Corral Story 189
The Night Before Christmas 193
Carroll Rikli and Immanuel Magomolla 197
Leblanc, Cailliet, & KSL 201
Oscar Zerk Story 205
Back on the Farm 207
What Cheer, Dr. Maxwell, and Corn 213
DMSO—Wonder Drug??? 217
AAHA Conventions 225
Madeline Reynolds Hough 229
Dorothy Santee Merrick 233
Carol Merrick's Special Deliveries 241
Mrs. Charles Roberts 247
Vet Aid 251
Minneapolis to Tuskegee 257
Super Family—Pfarr Excellence 261
Irish Wolfhounds, Gentle Giants 265
Majestic Hills and Checker Limos 269
Homer the Hospital Cat 273
Celebrities 277
Elephant Man 281
Ping Pong to Acupuncture 285
Admissions—Then & Now 289
Women in Vet Med—The Title 9 Effect 293
The '70s: Great Books, Protests, Sensitivity,
  & Dress Codes 297
Ray Robertson, MD 301
Drugs—Legal and Illegal 307
Remembering Sensei 317
Lucky Friday the 13th 323
Herschel and Dominique 325
Carol in Kindergarten 329
Torn Toenails at Midnight—Emergency Clinics ... 333

Pet Spas 337
Seminars: Greyhounds, Behavior, and Cardio 341
Norm Abplanalp 345
Shant Harootunian 351
Elective Surgery & Animal Cruelty 355
Specialists & Pet Insurance 361
Itch, Itch, Lick, and Scratch 365
Petco & Animal Hospital of Oshkosh 369
Noah's Ark—Lion, Tiger, and Bear 375
St. Andrews and Mr. James Herriot 379
Masters 2009-2011 383
New Zealand—Animals and Gardens Down Under 389
Cardiac Surgery—Dogs, Pigs, and daVinci 399
Five-Finger Discount 407
Corporate Vets 413
Lake Shore Animal Hospital 423
The Chef's Sons—Taste of Kenosha 427
The Marvelous Mahones 433
What's in a Name? 437
Remembering Jesse Payne 441
Jerry Banicki 445
War Stories 449
Second Time Around 457
A Bell for Crabapple Elementary School 459
250 and Counting 463
That's a Wrap! 469

Preface

Despite our impression that events just "happen," nothing evolves without previous thought, leading to action. Serendipity also plays its part. Conditions must be appropriate for the action to take place, as in the events leading up to this book.

In 1990 I received a nicely printed letter from my grandson, Adam Robinson, asking me to describe what life was like when I was his age living on my grandparents farm in Iowa.

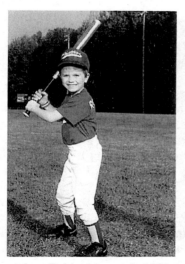
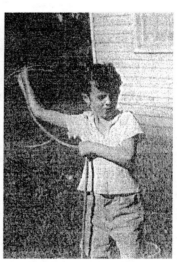

Adam Robinson, age 8, 1990   John Merrick, age 7, 1936

This was a class assignment by Adam's teacher to encourage communication with relatives. He was surprised to learn how primitive life was just sixty years ago. Adam related to his classmates that in the 1930s, most Americans in rural areas lived in homes with no electricity, indoor plumbing, central heat, air conditioning, or paved roads. They were also surprised to learn television, cell phones, and computers were not available. Younger readers will be assured that Facebook, Google, and Twitter were in the distant future.

This experience motivated me to begin to write stories of my youth. I had spent two years on that Iowa farm, attending first and third grade classes in a one-room schoolhouse. Many happy summers afterward were spent on the farm. I wanted to record what history I could remember for my children and beyond.

I retired from small animal veterinary practice in 2001, moving from Kenosha, Wisconsin to Peachtree City, Georgia to be near our three daughters.

In 2006 I received a letter from the Wisconsin Veterinary Medical Association (WVMA) honoring me and a few other older vets for our 50 years of membership in the WVMA. I was invited to speak after the presentation at the WVMA's state convention in Madison that fall. Carol, my wife of 56 years, had recently died, and I was not able to attend the meeting. I called the WVMA director to ask if my son, David, who lives in Madison, could pick up my plaque and deliver my response. She replied, "Yes, of course, we'll be delighted to have David attend the luncheon."

I composed a short speech reminding the group of mostly young veterinarians—now nearly one half of whom are female—of the efforts of men like Dr. Frank Gentile of Milwaukee, Dr. Ray Pahle of West Allis, and especially my good friend, Dr. Art Skewes of Union Grove, in promoting veterinary medicine. David also mentioned the work these veterinarians and vet school dean, Dr. Bernard Easterday, had been instrumental in finally getting a vet school in Wisconsin. I talked about of how times have changed over the fifty years since I started practice in Wisconsin. To illustrate my point, I related the story of how I got my license to practice fifty years ago. (I'll tell the story later in the book.)

Art Skewes, my good friend and colleague, had died the previous year. In 1975 Art had left his mixed animal practice in Union Grove, 10 miles west of Kenosha, and relocated to Lexington, Kentucky to join the practice of his brother in law, Dr. Arthur H. Davidson. Art became the president of the American Equine Veterinary Medical Association in 1985 and traveled the country to advance the vet horse practice. "Horse doctors" now routinely treat million dollar thoroughbred horses in addition to regular equines. Someone sent Art's wife, Helen, a copy of my speech. She called me to express her gratitude for remembering Art and urged me to continue my story writing. She thought they would appeal to a wide audience.

The result is the following manuscript.

Besides Adam Robinson and Helen Skewes, there are many others who contributed to this collection of memories. My six children, Dorothy, Bill, David, Buzz, Ginger, and Peggy, each contributed their recollection of how the various family stories took place. Buzz was especially helpful in proofing and editing, as was Robert Haslam for preliminary expert editing and advice. Thanks also to Dr. W. A. Merrick and Cc Robinson for editing the final proof.

Friends and classmates suggested and clarified stories, and Randy Drake was invaluable for his editing and publishing help. KC Pollak designed the elegant front and back covers.

This series of stories is dedicated to sharing some of the people I've met, successes, failures, challenges, tall tales, and anecdotes I have found along the way. I am fortunate to bear witness to three generations of veterinary practice, from the times when we argued the relative merits of wearing gloves during surgery, to the proliferation of specialty practices, and the ever-present saga of extracting money from clients for services rendered. I hope you will enjoy them.

> John W. Merrick, DVM
> Spring, 2012

The Veterinarian's Son

I may not have been "born in a barn," but I was delivered near one by a midwife. As a young veterinarian in the winter of 1929, my father couldn't afford the doctor or hospital fees. The stock market crash of '29 left farmers with little cash for veterinary bills. My life dawned in one generation's Great Depression. My life's dusk finds me in another generation's financial upheaval. Through it I experienced the remarkable life and adventures of an animal doctor. I saw the profession I seemed destined to follow adjust and refine, adapt and change, grow and mature. If there's a romanticized picture of life as a vet, I've lived it.

I was a veterinarian's son. I went on to become one myself, and I retired proud, humble, and forever grateful to be associated with a profession so widely respected and esteemed. The success of James Herriot's *All Creatures Great and Small* is no coincidence. Throughout my life and travels I have found people everywhere to hold a universal respect and admiration for position of the "vetnary," as the British call it. It has opened many a closed door. It has broken many a night's sleep. But that, as they say, is an occupational hazard. This is my story.

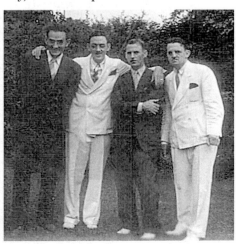

Russ, Ruffy, Buzz, and Andy • 1950s

To say that being a vet "runs in the family" is an understatement. My father and three of his seven brothers graduated from Ohio State Veterinary School: James (Russ), 1920; Byron (Buzz), 1922; Andrew (Andy, my father), 1924; and Gerard (Ruffy), 1930. Family folklore—of doubtful veracity—was that the boys really wanted to be architects, not vets. Their home in Columbus, Ohio was over a mile from the architecture school, but

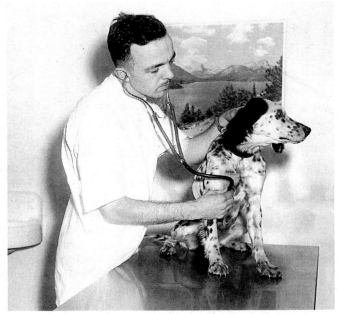

John W. Merrick, DVM • Merrick Animal Hospital
Kenosha, Wisconsin • November, 1956

only two blocks from the vet school. "Easy decision," they said, tongue in cheek. They each started in large animal practice, then switched to small animals in the late 30s. At one time, three brothers practiced within 15 miles of each other in west suburban Chicago.

In 1927 my Dad, Andy, married a farm girl from Iowa, Dorothy Santee, and eventually took a job with Swift and Company as a meat inspector in the Chicago Stockyards. His salary of $32.50/week was enough to rent a two-bedroom flat near the Midway on Chicago's south side, buy a car, and support our growing family of three children. Back then, furnished apartments rented for $12–$15/month, eggs sold for 15¢/ dozen, and hogs brought $3.00/cwt (hundredweight). Andy eventually went on to operate a very successful small animal practice, write a book, *How To Own A Dog And Like It!*, develop a number of animal care products (Scratch-X and Sulfodene, for example), and have a weekly "15 minutes of fame" time slot on a Chicago-based children's television program on WTTW-TV.

As for me, I got my veterinary degree from the University of Illinois in 1954 at the ripe old age of 24 and joined my father's practice in Brookfield, Illinois, 15 miles west of Chicago. In 1956 my wife, Carol, and I moved to Kenosha, Wisconsin, where I began my practice and my life as a small town animal doctor.

I had been practicing with my father in Brookfield, Illinois for two years when Dad let me know that a partnership was not likely, so Carol and I started exploring opportunities in neighboring suburbs. The rental house behind the animal hospital was getting crowded since the arrival of my third child, David, which made three kids under five. A few months after graduation I had purchased my first new car, a 1954 Chevy 4-door, for $1,640—which would be about $15,000 in 2010 dollars. We drove all over the northwestern suburbs of Chicago, looking for a good location to build a clinic. We explored commercial buildings that could be remodeled and vacant lots to build on. Nothing looked promising until I answered an ad in the AVMA Journal listing a practice for sale in Kenosha, Wisconsin, just over the state line, 60 miles north of Chicago on Lake Michigan. Dr. A. J. Fortmann had died from an undiagnosed brain cancer. Lacking the benefits of CAT scans, the cause for his migraine headaches was diagnosed only at autopsy. Carol and I visited the animal hospital and were very

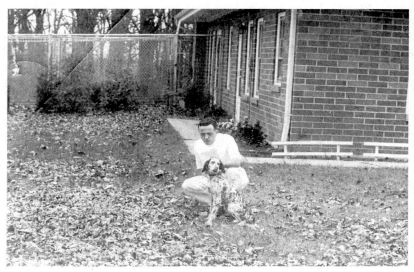

John W. Merrick, DVM, and "Rover"
Merrick Animal Hospital • Kenosha, Wisconsin

favorably impressed with the building and the town. Kenosha's population at the time was 60,000. In the fall of 1956 I bought the practice from his widow, with the help of a loan from my uncle, Dr. Byron Merrick.

The Wisconsin State Veterinary Board Exam was held in January and July, which meant that my arrival in October put me three months away from state licensing. The State Licensing Board told me to see Dr. T. H. Ferguson, chair of the Wisconsin State Board of Veterinary Examiners, who practiced in Lake Geneva, 30 miles west of Kenosha. (Most students now take the National Veterinary Exam at the end of their second year in vet school, but in those days, there were no National Boards given.) Dr. Ferguson was known for his expertise in dairy cattle management, so I tried to recollect what little I knew about dairy practice. I was sure most of my classmates who were raised on a farm would have had an easier time. I was confident, however, because I had already passed the Illinois and Minnesota licensing exams.

I called Dr. Ferguson's office and made an appointment to see him, explaining to his wife/receptionist the purpose of my visit. While driving the 80 miles through the farm country of northern Illinois with its many dairy farms, I tried to imagine what I would need to know to impress the great man. Lake Geneva has long been the close vacation spot for Chicagoans, so he also saw a few pets, especially in summers. Upon arriving at his house/veterinary hospital, Mrs. Ferguson greeted me in what used to be the parlor, now the reception room. I was ushered into the dining room, now converted into his exam/laboratory/surgery/treatment room, where the good doctor was in the middle of a spay (Ovariohysterectomy) of a large mixed bred shepherd—sans gloves or gown. The young dog was suspended head-down in the then-common vertical surgical position. (The practice is not recommended now because elevating the rear quarters of an animal for an extended time puts pressure on the diaphragm and may restrict breathing.) During surgery, Dr. Ferguson grilled me about my intentions—large animal, small animal or both; my married life and children; my wife's involvement in the practice; etc. Very little if any questions pertained to my knowledge of disease, diagnosis, and treatment protocols.

When I mentioned I had practiced with my dad, Andrew C. Merrick, Dr. Ferguson stopped short and said words to the effect of, "I remember your dad very well when he attended UW, working on his master's in '25 or maybe '26. Any son of Andy's will be a fine vet. Go ahead and practice until January when you can take the State Boards. If anybody asks, just send them to me."

Life was simpler then...

The drive back to Brookfield was delightful. The alfalfa hay fields were fragrant from recent mowing. The corn was as high as an "elephant's eye," and all was right with my world.

Sentimental romanticism aside, it was a good life, worthy of sharing with those who are blessed to continue the tradition.

Life on the Farm in Iowa

Times were tough in the early 1930s for 90% of the families in America. I had always been told that Mom and Dad were very poor when I was young. That is now open to question. By the summer of 1932 Dad was working as a federal meat inspector at Swift and Company in the Chicago stockyards.

Dad tells of moving the entire family from Iowa in his old Model A. Instead of driving directly to our apartment on Chicago's Southside, Dad took us on a tour of downtown. Driving slowly down Michigan Boulevard, all of us gawking at the tall buildings, Dad was passed by a honking cab. The driver leaned out his window and shouted, "Hayseed, keep driving like that and you'll get killed." Dad learned later that his Iowa license plates gave him away as a "hick." He also found out big city drivers stay in their lane until they want to change, then immediately change—don't dawdle.

The 1933 Chicago World's Fair was about to open. Wikipedia reports the following:

> The site selected was new parkland being created along the Lake Michigan shoreline between 12th and 39th streets. Held on a 427 acre (1.7 km^2) portion of Burnham Park the Century of Progress opened on May 27, 1933. The fair was opened when the lights were automatically activated when light from the rays of the star Arcturus was detected. The star was chosen as its light had started its journey at about the time of the previous Chicago world's fair—the World's Columbian Exposition—in 1893. The rays were focused on photo-electric cells in a series of astronomical observatories and then transformed into electrical energy which was transmitted to Chicago.

Our apartment was just over a mile south of the fairgrounds.

Within a year, my big sister, Marg, was sent to live with Uncle Byron and Aunt Jo in Berlin Heights, Ohio. It's possible that internal family problems were the cause for the family split up.

Dr. Clarence Pals, DVM, wrote to me in a letter dated February 4, 1991, "When I reported to Chicago as a junior veterinarian in the meat inspection division, my salary was $35/week.

This would be about $700/wk in today's dollars." Dr. Pals mentions that Andy took him around to purchase his first work clothes, knives, hook, steel, and knife pouch. He remarked what good children Phil and I were. By then, Margaret was already living in Ohio with Uncle Byron and Aunt Jo. Sometime in 1933, Mom went to visit in Iowa and took me along. Dr. and Mrs. Pals kept Phil in their apartment. Lacking a baby bed, they put Phil to sleep in the bathtub. One time they heard the water running and found Phil washing his feet in the tub. At the time of his letter, Dr. Pals had been retired from the government for 20 years. When he left, he was Director of Meat Inspection in the entire USA.

In any event, we three kids were parceled out to relatives who had no children of their own and could provide care for an extended period of time—Phil to Uncle Ruffy and Aunt Manon in Forreston, Illinois and me to the farm in Iowa to stay with Grandma and Grandpa Santee and Uncle Wendell. Both of Dad's brothers were practicing large animal vets.

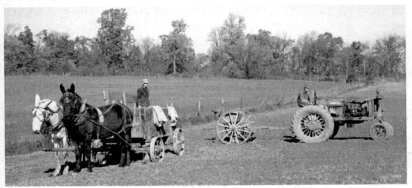

My grandparent's farm in Iowa • 1930s

In 1934, the summer before I turned five, I went to live with my grandparents on their farm in Iowa. Too young for "chores," I would sometimes play "Cowboys and Indians" in the apple orchard behind the farmhouse, chasing the chickens (Indians). Cows were often allowed in the orchard to keep the grass down.

Grandmother Santee had strung a length of barbwire across one corner of the orchard fence to keep the cattle from chewing her hollyhocks and iris in the back yard next to the orchard fence. I ducked under the wire going in, but forgot to duck coming out. The barbwire caught me just below my right eye, laying a piece of flesh 2 inches long hanging wide open on my cheek . I screamed and ran to the house. Grandma washed the wound and Grandpa had to hurry to the "south 40," one mile away where my Uncle Wendell, the only automobile driver in the household, was plowing a field with horse power. He ran home, cutting across neighboring fields on the way. I was taken to the nearest—and only—doctor within 20 miles, Dr. John Maxwell, MD, in What Cheer, some 5 miles away. He cleaned the laceration, sutured and bandaged it, with the admonition to "watch where you're was going when chasing bad guys in the future." Due to my young age and the doctor's skill, the large scar disappeared within a few years. In 1972, the Chicago Tribune published a story about What Cheer featuring Dr. Maxwell – now, both physician and pharmacist.

Some of my earliest memories are of the small church 200 yards south of Grandpa's farm. My grandparents were Quakers. As I recall, the service was somber. It was followed by singing then "settling," a Quaker meditation practice. I still remember the words to "Brighten the Corner Where You Are"; it has fit right in with my philosophy of life ever since. I'm told I learned to whistle in church, to the dismay of my grandparents.

Returning to Chicago was usually done by train on the "Burlington" from Ottumwa, Iowa to downtown Chicago's Union Station. I was around ten when I was assigned a seat next to a distinguished-looking gentleman dressed in suit and tie—unusual in those days of train travel. After introductions by the conductor, he asked where I was headed and did I belong to any church? I announced proudly, "I'm a Quaker." He replied, "Well, so

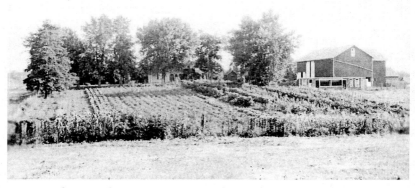

Santee farm, circa 1940 • View from the church

am I. I teach college at William Penn in Oskaloosa." Although I didn't know it at the time, Mom had attended Penn ten years earlier. She might have taken some of his classes.

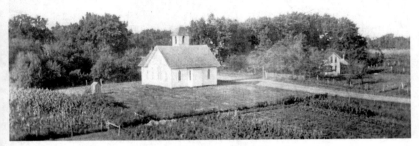

Quaker Church • Coal Creek
Grandma's garden in right foreground.

The following year was an entirely different experience. Grandpa was sending some cattle to market to the Stockyards in Chicago. The time was early September, 1942, and I was due back home to start the eighth grade. The truck driver, Ernst Weaver, lived a mile north of our farm. Uncle Wendell arranged for him to carry me along with the cows—in the front seat, of course. We left as night approached and the weather cooled. At a truck stop near the Mississippi River, Ernst bought me a Coke to go with the sandwich Grandma had sent along. Ernst then directed me to the sleeping area above and behind the driver. The next thing I heard was the whoosh of the air brakes as Ernst stopped on Highway #34, five blocks north of our home in Western Springs, Illinois. The time was 4:15 am. It was pitch black except for street lights. I didn't encounter a single person, only a couple of barking dogs alerting the neighborhood of the stranger in their territory.

Uncle Wendell tells of the Halloween when he was about 16—probably 1916 or 1917. The common prank at that time was tipping over outhouses. Most families were onto that caper, so Wendell and a few of his friends decided to dream up a new "trick." His grandfather (my great-grandfather), Isaac, was living with my grandparents at the time. "Old Grandpa" had a prize "Sunday Buggy," which he rarely let anyone drive. Wendell and his high school friends managed to take the buggy apart and reassemble it on the church roof on Halloween night. By the time Grandpa noticed, the boys were home in bed. They finally had to confess, as they were the only ones who could get the buggy off the roof without any damage.

Fourth of July on the Farm

My brother, Phil, came to the farm for the month of July in the summer of 1938. Rummaging through one of Grandma Santee's dresser drawers, Phil and I discovered a hidden prize—a box of 12 Roman candles Dad had sent for the family to celebrate Independence Day. Grandma had carefully hidden them, as the family did not believe in anything that involved "fun." The devout Quakers did not drink, dance, or use foul language. The only cuss word Grandma would allow was "Gosh!"—and even that could only be uttered if you stepped in a "CowPie" while barefoot. Even though we were two weeks late, we decided to celebrate anyway. That evening, as dusk approached, Phil and I snuck out the back door and headed for the pasture, some 200 yards behind the house. We'd watched Dad light fireworks the previous year, so we felt like we could easily do the same. The pasture was not easily seen from the farmhouse, but we hadn't counted on the neighbors. Harvey Molyneaux and his dad were doing late chores when they spotted this strange light coming from our pasture. It didn't take but two or three candle eruptions for them to figure what was going on. A phone call to our house sent Wendell and Grandpa out to spoil our fun. Their timing was perfect; we had just exploded the last candle when they arrived.

Farm life, besides being very hard work, is extremely dangerous. Soon after coming out to visit in the summer of 1938, Phil was made aware of the hazards. Jumping over the freshly sharpened disk (a contrivance consisting of 12 to 16 upright 24" diameter sharp metal plates pulled behind horse or tractor to break up and even out a plowed field), Phil slipped and fell, lacerating his chest with three deep cuts 6 inches in length. Antiseptics and TLC were the standard treatment. Fortunately, the wounds healed within two weeks.

Grandpa convinced Grandma that playing cribbage and dominoes were not gambling, but rather educational tools to teach a five year to count, add, and subtract. Fifteen two, fifteen four, a pair for two is six and a run of three gives a total of nine. I believe that started my love of numbers and math. Another "trick" my Grandpa Santee used was to offer me a penny if I could sit still with my eyes closed for 20 minutes after supper. I never collected the penny.

Life on the Farm in the 1930s

Imagine living as most Americans did just 100 years ago. Over 90% of us lived on a farm. All water came from a well, either pumped by hand or a windmill. There was no electricity, so light came from candles or kerosene lamps. There were no yard or street lights, of course. When the sun went down it was dark, unless the moon provided a little illumination.

Our phone was a party line with 20 other neighbors sharing a single wire connected to a central operator. Our ring was "two longs and a short." You could hear other people pick up to listen, then drop off if you were not discussing any gossip.

The road in front of our farmhouse was dirt covered with a thin layer of shale—not nearly enough hard surface to provide for good water runoff after a heavy rain. As a rule, no one wanted to be the first one driving on the road after a rainstorm. The wheels sunk into the mud up to the hubcaps. Many cars had to be rescued from the mud by real horse power. After the first driver created ruts, the excess water had a place to drain and the road was soon drivable, if you avoided the deep ruts. All farm houses were built 100 to 200 feet back from the road. This was due in part to protect the freshly hung damp clothes from picking up dust from the road. It also provided a little privacy, as if that was really needed. Most farm houses were one quarter mile apart. I've always thought it strange that most farmhouses have a front door facing the road. Our front door opened into the parlor. In all my time spent on the farm, I never saw anyone use that door. Everyone came and went through a side porch or back door into the kitchen.

Gibson, the small town two miles north of Granddad's farm, was two blocks long. Across from the Bank of Gibson was a general store, half groceries and half hardware. Next door, the post office connected to a small restaurant, then to a vacant store, and finally to a garage/service station. Gibson also had a large grain elevator beside the single track railroad. The population was less than 100 people. On Saturday nights during the warm weather, a sheet was hung on the west wall of the garage. A cartoon always preceded the feature movie. The field behind the garage could accommodate perhaps 50 or 60 people. This was well before the TV age, as most the farms had no electricity in their homes in the thirties. The regular movie house in What Cheer charged 25 cents for adults and 10 cents for kids, but the outdoor movies in Gibson cost 15 cents and a nickel. Another draw was the raffle after the show. Everyone—including kids—got a ticket with a number. The first number drawn won twenty cents; the second got a dime. I won a dime once and promptly invested in a handful of candy.

Donkey baseball involved nine donkeys and eighteen players. The rules of donkey baseball are relatively simple. Everyone in the outfield has a donkey that they can't let go of. This means that fielding a ball requires taking the donkey along. Players other than the pitcher or catcher have to jump on their donkey's back to throw the ball.

If a player lets go of his donkey, or forgets to mount before throwing, the opposing team gets a free base. After hitting the ball, the batter has to jump on a donkey and ride it around the bases. After the second strike, batters replaced the bat with a barn shovel to ensure they hit the ball.

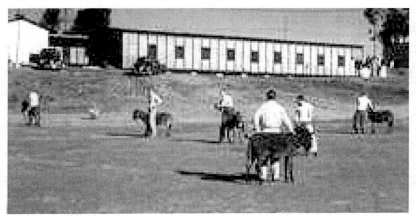

The well-behaved donkeys may have been the favorites of the players, but the crowd of more than 400 people at the Saturday night church fundraiser spent much of the time laughing uproariously at the problems caused by donkeys more interested in eating grass. "It's absolutely ridiculous," said Gibson resident Jeremy Green, "I've never seen anything like it." Green was referring to the spectacle of watching grown men and women strain against their donkey's lead rope trying to reach the base with a ball while the donkey, completely unaffected, calmly chomped away at grass.

The most crowd-pleasing moments were when members of the outfield tried to mount their donkeys to throw the ball. Players fell off, ended face down over the withers or, in one case, mounted facing almost backward.

Everyone works on a farm. Grandma Santee would say, "The Devil finds work for the idle and lazy." My chores as a seven year old were appropriate for my age. During the summer months, pigs, chickens and cattle were allowed to graze in the orchard behind our farmhouse. My job was to supply water to the animals. This required pumping water from the well by the house into two five-gallon buckets and carrying them 50 yards to the water tank in the orchard. Filling the "chicken/ hog waterer" was a tedious but necessary chore and took about 40 trips—often twice a day.

Digging Dandelions and Plantains. This was a real "job"—not a chore. I would fill a two-gallon bucket and receive 5¢. Sometimes I managed to sneak a couple of pine cones on the bottom of the pail before showing the group to Grandmother, Viola, and dumping it in the roadside culvert.

Killing Chickens. Chop the head off of the chicken on stump with an axe—then throw it into a gunny sack to avoid blood all over the yard and us. Some would escape the sack and run or flop around headless for a minute or two. Life magazine had a story at the time about a chicken who survived beheading. The farmer had aimed too high, leaving part of the brain. After the bleeding stopped, the chicken was able to walk around almost normally. The farmer's wife convinced him to spare the rooster, like the Thanksgiving turkey at the White House. They were able to feed the animal and show him at county fairs and carnivals for the next few months.

Tonsillectomy. Ether dripped into a mask covering my face. It went too fast and I got liquid ether on my mouth. I tried to tell them—to no avail—as my hands were restrained and I was soon sound asleep. At least I got an ice cream cone afterwards. The practice was common until the 1950s. Wikipedia reports:

> The effectiveness of the tonsillectomy has been questioned in a 2009 systematic review of 7765 papers published in the journal *Otolaryngology—Head and Neck*

Surgery. The review found that it was most likely not effective all the time, but rather was modestly effective, and that "not a single paper reported that tonsillectomy is invariably effective in eliminating sore throats.
I rarely performed the procedure in my practice, relying on medical treatment instead.

County Fair in late August. There were traveling side shows, rides, buildings full of home-raised 4H pigs, calves, steers, etc., buildings with prize cooking, quilts, vegetables etc., and lots of barkers advertising sideshows. I was too young to be allowed in to watch. Harness racing was a weekend attraction in the grandstand. This usually took place a week or two before the grand Iowa State Fair in Des Moines.

Age 7—too young to help "Make Hay." I helped walk the horse hooked up to the rope pulling the hay up from the wagon into the mow. After the load of hay was dropped into the mow, the rope released to return rapidly to its original spot. I made the mistake of holding the rope in my left hand. The subsequent rope burn removed half the skin from my palm. Even after 75 years, my left hand is still one size smaller than my right, probably due to scar tissue formation in healing.

Homemade toys and playthings.

Arrows from pieces of shingle, shot with a stick with a string knot.

Horse shoe pitching with real horse shoes

Home made tops

Homemade reed or willow whistles. (Grandpa was good at cutting holes for the whistles.)

John and Phil rope a calf? Not as easy as it looks. The cowboys make it look so simple; throw a lariat over the calf's head and pull. We forgot that in the movies there is usually a horse on the other end of the rope. In our case, the calf ran, we pulled, and both fell in the barn lot. Not in any cow piles, thankfully. There was no catching the calf again or hiding our mischief as the 20-foot rope dragged behind the calf the rest of the day.

Phil and I had spent the summer of 1940 on the farm. Mom, Dorothy, drove out with Margaret and Sue to pick us up. The Iowa family had not seen Sue since she was born one year earlier. Marg had not been on the farm recently as she spent vacations with Byron and Jo in Ohio.

Dousing. I recall Grandpa Frank and Wendell dousing in the pasture, 100 yards east and a little south of the windmill. I con-

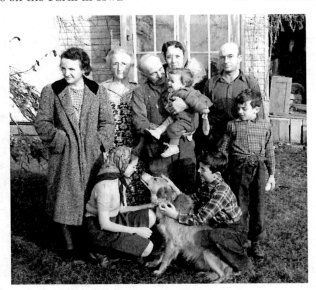

Dorothy, Viola, Frank, Grayce, Wendell
Margaret, Shep, Susan, Phil, John

tacted my cousin, Les Santee, who was born and raised on the farm to ask him about the "dousing" incident. Do you recall your dad or Frank ever mentioning dousing? I remember one cut the branch and the other doused. It pointed to the spot where Wendell dug. As I recall, they found water within 20 feet. His email follows:

> I remember it well. It was also called water witching or "divining." They used a forked branch from a fruit tree. I remember the ones I saw were from a plum tree. I saw them do it, and it worked, but I couldn't get it to work. I can do the divining with No. 9 wires or coat hangers bent in an "L" shape. You hold gently the short end of the "L," letting the 18 to 24 inches of the long side stick straight out in front of you parallel. As you move toward a water pipe, tile, or underground pipe of some kind, they will move from parallel to horizontal if you hold them loosely and level. Try walking toward a sink in your kitchen and see if they don't move. I used them to find tile lines that were plugged that I had to dig out. Hope this helps. — Les

I tried it using a coat hanger—no luck. Maybe it takes more skill than I possess.

Ice Cream in Summer. Cracking ice with a small sledge to put around the ice cream bucket, Uncle Wendell gave me a glancing blow to head which almost killed me when I darted for a piece of ice. Fortunately, I was only momentarily stunned and sustained only a small bruise. The ice cream was especially rich because of the pure cream used in the process. The good part was being able to lick the paddle of the churn. The bad part was the two hour wait for the ice cream to set.

Once in a while a sow would refuse to nurse her offspring. These "Orphan" pigs were kept in a bedded box in the dining room bay window during day and the sitting room by the stove during the evening. Wendell could usually convince another sow to take over the nursing duties within a few days.

Of course, a lack of rain can cause even worse problems. Farmers have forever depended upon adequate rainfall to grow their crops and provide water for their livestock and themselves. Some will remember 1936 as the year of the "Dust Bowl"—the *Grapes of Wrath* saga and all that implies. Iowa, like the rest of the Midwest, was experiencing a severe draught—less than one half the normal rainfall. Farmers were selling their hogs for $5.00 per hundredweight, about one quarter of the usual price. I recall riding on a wagon with Uncle Wendell to the abandoned coal mine a half mile south of the farm to fill large barrels of water from a deep well. It was one of the few places in the area with any available water during the drought of 1936.

One Room Schoolhouse

The school was located on the outskirts of Coal Creek. It was hardly a town—more like a community extending from a crossroads. There were perhaps 12 to 14 houses, a church, and the school. One quarter mile from the crossroads, there were farms in every direction—no stores, no service stations, etc. For those services you went to two miles north to Gibson (population 85) or four miles south to the metropolis of What Cheer, with nearly 800 residents at that time.

The schoolhouse was set on five acres donated by a local farmer. It was one room, perhaps 24' X 24'. The front door faced east, with a small enclosed porch to provide shelter form the prevailing winter blasts. The prerequisite bell was ensconced on the roof inside a small cupola. If you were especially fortunate, or a teacher's pet, you were allowed to ring the bell to announce the start of classes. There was adequate room for 30 desks, but the school only had 23 students in all eight grades in 1934. Three were enrolled in my first grade. Older students were expected to help the younger ones and perform chores such as bringing in coal or wood for the stove and general housecleaning. Younger kids were assigned tasks appropriate for their age. I doubt that the teacher had more than a high school education. Before she had children, my grandmother, Viola, had taught school after leaving school in the eighth grade.

After a year at home in Brookfield, Illinois, I was back on the farm in 1936 to attend the third grade in that same one room schoolhouse. The total enrollment had dropped to 13 for all eight grades. I had one other student in my grade. Unlike today, if you were brought to school by grandparents, you were admitted. No questions asked about residency requirements.

A Franklin stove was the only source of heat, and you were either too warm or too cold, depending upon where you sat. The school year was determined by the time for planting and harvest. The so-called vacation was a work time for farm children, both boys and girls. Two outhouses were situated behind school. There was an area for softball practice, a swing set with two small and two large swings, and a slide. My favorite was the maypole swing, a central 10-foot steel pole and eight to ten ropes hanging down with a steel bar at the end to hang on to. By winding the chains around one another, two strong boys could run in a circle and, by pulling their chains, cause the last couple of kids to fly four to six feet off the ground—round and round at great speed. What fun!! Today, school board attorneys would not allow anything like that on school grounds. Too bad. If someone had broken their arm at school in 1934, par-

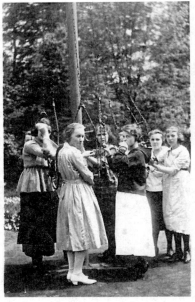

Dorothy Santee • 7th Grade
Coal Creek School • 1916

ents would have admonished the child to be more careful and learn a lesson from his mistake.

The school was closed the next summer in 1937 for lack of enrollment, and the play yard was planted with corn.

unday, March 19, 1972 — CHICAGO TRIBUNE

In What Cheer, Future's Bleak; Few Seem to Care

BY DAVID THOMPSON AND DAVID YOUNG
[Chicago Tribune Press Service]

WHAT CHEER, Ia.—The name seems more and more of a misnomer as What Cheer, a tiny Iowa community of 877 persons, slowly erodes.

Nobody seems to care.

Every morning, many local residents gather in small groups around a large round table in the rear of the Chuck Wagon Cafe, sip owner Audrey Smith's coffee, and discuss corn and the weather, seemingly oblivious to the deteriorating main street outside with its score of boarded-up stores.

Vacant Houses, Stores

Abandoned railroad spurs protrude from What Cheer. South of town, beyond the shuttered Little Chicago Club and adjacent abandoned live stock pens, are the crumbling ruins of the kilns and factory that were once the What Cheer Clay Products Co. The town is dotted with vacant houses, and the nicest looking business in town is the recently remodeled funeral home.

"We just talk about day-to-day topics," said Mrs. Dorothy Baylor, head of the one-room First State Bank of What Cheer, housed on the first floor of a turreted brick Victorian building along the main drag. "We are all happy the hog prices are up.

"It seems like you make a lot of money each year, but you seem to spend it all.

"So that takes care of everything but the weather," she concluded.

"Business has really been bad," said Mrs. Raymond Newcomb, who with her husband puts out the What Cheer Chronicle [circulation 1,700]. "There's only one large grocery store left in town. There's no lady's shop; so when women want something to wear, they have to go to Oskaloosa, Ottumwa, or Sigourney."

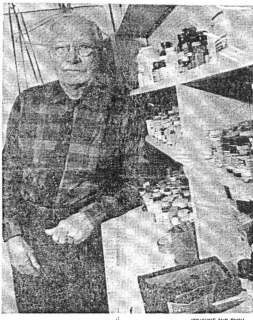

[TRIBUNE Staff Photo]
Dr. John Maxwell, 81, the only doctor in What Cheer. There is no drug store so he also acts as pharmacist.

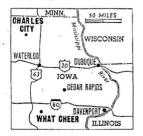

Few Young People Left

She said the town has many residents on pensions and welfare, and most young people leave town to find jobs elsewhere.

Dr. John Maxwell, 81, who is the town's only physician and who figures he will be its last, guessed he had delivered 2,500 babies since he came to town just after World War I. Last year he delivered only two.

"The rarity of a baby born around here indicates the absence of young people, who have left What Cheer in search of jobs," he said. His own two sons entered medical professions but practice elsewhere.

Dr. Maxwell, by the way, charges $1 for an office call.

Another town pillar is Carl G. Draegert, What Cheer's only lawyer and the municipal attorney. He dismissed any idea of What Cheer's getting an infusion of state or federal money to help revive it.

Attempts Made, but Failed

"They [the city fathers] would be glad to have some help from somewhere if they knew where to get it and what to do with it if they got it.

"Two or three development groups have been established from time to time, but they never got very far. After a while, they just gave up."

The white-maned Draegert likes to lean back in a chair in his modern but unpretentious office and reminisce about the historical What Cheer—a bustling coal mining town of an estimated 8,000 persons served by two railroads with daily passenger trains.

"But the coal mines played out, and the railroads eventually left," he said with a sigh.

The future? He sighed again. "All I can see at the moment is just a small community accommodating the needs of the local farm trade."

Have Opera House

The apparent rigor mortis is not complete, however. The town recently built, with a federal loan, a four-unit low-income housing project for the elderly, and many residents have high hopes for the town's civic icon, the What Cheer Opera House, Inc., a 600-seat theater within an overaged, former Masthall astride the main street.

The opera house, since its creation in 1965, has featured the likes of Fred Waring, Guy Lombardo, Wayne King and Stan Kenton. Kenton was considered too loud for local tastes, according to Mrs. Wanda Burriss, wife of the president of the opera association.

Her husband, Thomas, who raises 500 market hogs each year on his nearby farm, believes the opera house can continue to subsist on a diet of bands and country and western shows and may even draw attention to What Cheer. He is also contemplating luring a resident straw hat company made up of students from an Iowa college performing for credit.

Aside from Burriss, few people have any plans for What Cheer's destiny.

"It's a friendly, close little town," Mrs. Newcomb said. " I guess people like it that way."

Those were the "Good Old Days." It is difficult for children of today with their computers, smart boards, busing and frequently locked-down schools to appreciate what was commonplace just 75 years ago. I feel privileged to share these stories with them.

Bookkeeping, Then and Now

I've always liked numbers. For that I credit my grandfather, Frank Santee. When I stayed on the farm as a five year old, Grandpa taught me how to play cribbage and dominoes. Grandma Santee, being a good Quaker, thought card playing was the Devil's work. Dominoes involved matching like numbers and counting the tiles at game's end.

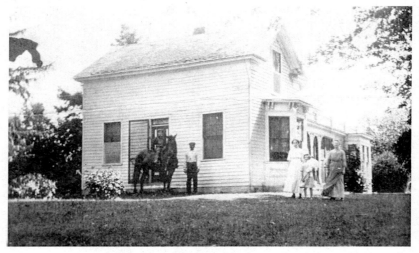

Wendell Santee (13), Frank Santee, Unknown Lady, Dorothy Santee (9), Viola Santee • Circa 1914

Grandpa Santee kept meticulous records. He recorded every cash transaction. The years from 1918 to 1928 were recorded in a large bound journal. His balance sheet for Jan. 1, 1928 listed the following:

Resources

Real Estate 169 acres including 2 barns and farmhouse	$26,453.00

Livestock
   1 team + mare: $120; 3 mules: $400;
   4 cows, 1 calf: $395; 33 ewes, 1 buck: $350;
   64 hogs: $900; 16 steers (on feed): $1,800
	$3,965.00

Poultry
   8 red hens, 10 rocks: $22; 1 red pullet, 124 rocks:
   $185; 2 cocks, 77 adult rocks: $275
	$482.00

Vehicles + Harness
   4 sets work harness: $105; 2 wagons: $70;
   sled: $2.50; 1 spring wagon: $40; 2 sets light
   harness: $10; saddle, bridles, collars, halters:
   $25; 1 Chevrolet Landau: $600; 1 Ford: $15
	$867.50

Grain + Seed	$1,602.00
Pasture and R. Feed	$640.00

Fruit + Vegetables
   Canned Fruit + Butters: $125; Potatoes: $20;
   Beets: $5
	$150.00

Tools + Implements
   Hay Loader: $70; Side Delivery Rake: $45;
   Hay Rake: $10; Sulky Plow: $10; Disk: $33.50;
   Corn Planter: $37.50; Cultivators (2): $30;
   3-Section Harrow: $7.50; Sprayer&Tank: $5; Cider
   Mill: $5.00, 1/2 interest in Spreader: $25; 14" Plow +
   Garden Harrow: $10; End Gate Grain Spreader:
   $7.50; Carpenter Tools + Chest: $25; Lard Press +
   Sausage Grinder: $7.50; Hay Rack + Tools: $35;
   Corn Sheller + 3 Feed Bunks: $45; Gas Engine +
   Pump Jack: $45; Corn Slicer + Belt: $34; 250
   Bushel Baskets + Lids: $35; Water Tank: $15
	$551.50

Furniture + Fixtures	$500.00

F. N. Bank	$850.98
Cash	$20.00
H. H. Sant	$50.75
J. P. Carlson (for tile sent)	$100.00
Total Assets	**$19,360.75**

Liabilities

Mortgage Payable — $10,900.00
    48½ acres, due Mar 1, 1928, favor L. S. Cory: $4,000
    40 acres, due Jun, 22, 1928, favor Thos. Geneva: $4,000
    48½ acres, due Apr 4, 1928, favor W. C. Legoe: $1,300
    ½ int. 80 acres, due Mar 1, 1928, favor Thos. Geneva: $1,600

Bills Payable — $5,448.00
    Notes, favor F. N. Bank: $3,800
    Notes, favor Viola Santee: $500
    Due to I. P. Santee: $1,148

Interest — $526.50
    Int. due to date on Mortgages: $459.50
    Int. due to date on Notes: $67.00

Total Liabilities — **$16,874.50**

Net Worth — **$1,036.55**

To put the preceding prices in perspective, a $1.00 bill in 1930 is worth 7.7 cents today. In other words, multiply all 1930 prices by 13 to get an approximate of the price in 2011 dollars. Modern farmers can spend hundreds of thousands of dollars on equipment today. Grandpa Frank didn't have, or need, a corn dryer. Today's farmer/entrepreneur couldn't be without one. The cost can be well over $100,000. Farming is big business today. Farmers can no longer survive on 169 acres.

Analysis of Grandpa's Balance Sheet reveals the fact that he had no outstanding debt except four mortgages on land and three bills—one to a bank and two to individuals. I. P. Santee was my great-grandfather (Frank's dad), and Viola was my grandmother (Frank's wife). I never dreamed she had any money of her own. Maybe she got to keep the egg money.

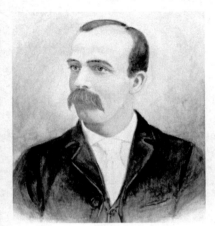
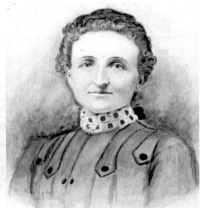

Frank Santee • Circa 1905 • Viola Santee

Every penny counted in those days. The great depression of 1929 was about to start, and it lasted ten years until the start of World War II. I recall Grandpa Santee complaining about having to pay income tax of $10.00 in 1943 or '44. He had never paid any federal tax before.

My dad, Andy Merrick, was just the opposite of Frank Santee. He seemed oblivious to the need to keep track of income or expenses. He would put all bills in a desk drawer and pay them once or twice a month, in no special time or order. Fortunately, in those days companies were not as quick to add on extra fees for missed or late payments. Dad never balanced his checkbook. Once every month or so, Bob Williams, President of the LaGrange Bank would call to say, "Andy you're overdrawn. I need you to put some money in your account." Where he got the money, I don't know. Maybe from a safety deposit box. His bookkeeper, Harold, came in three or four times a year. Harold spent the first few hours balancing Dad's checkbook, then a couple of hours determining exactly what items were deductible. No matter what Harold said was the final amount owed to Uncle Sam, Dad complained. Dad was audited by the IRS at least a couple of times. One agent finally threw up hands and said something to the effect, "Give me a check for $200.00, payable to Uncle Sam. I've got to have something to show for the two days I spent here." Another agent ended up adopting a puppy from Dad's giveaways.

Dad carried a "wad"— probably four or five hundred dollars – rolled up in his pants pocket. Hundred dollar bills were on the outside. I'm not sure if it was a gambler's habit or an attempt to impress people. One morning I had accompanied Dad on his morning break to the post office for mail pickup, the bank for yesterday's deposit, then to Walgreen's for coffee and gossip. Lloyd Hebert, owner of the Walgreen's pharmacy in LaGrange, was a good friend and client. After a cordial greeting, he reminded Dad he hadn't paid his bill in three months. "How much is it?" Dad asked. "Almost $500.00," Lloyd responded. Without any hesitation, Dad pulled out his bankroll and put it on the counter. "Double or nothing." Just as quickly, Lloyd said, "Sure." Lloyd flipped a fifty cent piece, Dad called "Heads," and heads it was. Lloyd looked unhappy but said, "Damn, Andy, you win this time." They both laughed as if they'd been betting for nickels or dimes. Ah, the life of a gambler—easy come, easy go.

As Dad approached retirement age he was introduced to the stock market. Ira Fash was a long time neighbor and stock broker. During a front yard visit, Ira talked Dad into investing in stocks. The time was the mid fifties. The Dow was around 300. With Ira's advice, Dad doubled, then tripled his investments over the next few years. He had a number of shares of "Oxy"— Occidental Petroleum—that benefited from the rise in oil prices. Dad tried to convince me to enter the market and invest in Oxy. I still regarded it as gambling. He said, "Johnny, this is better than craps or playing the ponies, and it's legal." With a new practice and kids to feed, I didn't have any spare investment money. By the time of Dad's death in the fall of 1976, the market was flirting with 1,000. Only later did I learn the idea of saving for retirement and kids college—put a little money into a good mutual fund each month and watch it grow.

Living with a "city girl," it was a challenge to make sure we spent less than I took in each month. Carol was a great shopper, but the "bargains" she found in upscale Women's Shoppes' could be costly. The $500.00 dresses reduced to $70.00 still cost double the price of clothes in other local stores.

There could not have been two more contrasting life styles—Grandpa Santee and Dad. I'm much more comfortable in the slow and steady pace; however, I do enjoy playing poker with the boys. At least I know what the odds are and can limit my risk.

Farmers must be gamblers at heart. I can't imagine the risk they take every year—commodity price fluctuations, depending upon rain, risking wind and hail storms. On a farm call as a senior vet student, Dr. Hatch, our professor in large animal medicine, asked the farmer client, "Amos, what are you going to do if this drought continues and we don't get any rain?" Without hesitation, Amos replied, "It always has." That seems to be the difference—faith triumphs over luck.

Early City Life

Dad took us to see the Stockyards soon after moving to the big city. Phew!!! He had been working as a government meat inspector for a few weeks when we got to see where Dad earned his living. I was used to farm odors, but the stench in the stockyards was overwhelming. It all looked too brutal to watch—noise, blood, excrement everywhere. Dad showed us what sausage was made of—leftovers.

We lived behind Dad's first animal hospital, 8908 Ogden Avenue, Brookfield, Illinois. It was a storefront with a two-bedroom apartment behind. Not much signage in 1934.

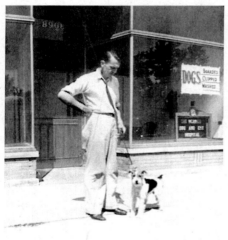

Playing with matches one afternoon, we three kids managed to set the adjacent vacant lot's weed patch on fire. In the excitement, I neglected to retrieve my only warm coat. I've forgotten what punishment was forthcoming.

My sex education began early thanks to the two sisters across the street. Phil and I weren't especially interested in girls at the age of 6 and 8, but that didn't apply to these girls. The 12- and 13-year-olds taught us a lot about the difference between the sexes by playing "doctor" when their folks were absent. Farm kids learn about sex from a very early age as they witness breeding of livestock. I probably knew about the birds and bees, but instruction from older girls is much more educational.

Within a year we moved from the back of Dad's first animal hospital. We lived in three different homes in La Grange, two miles east of the hospital. The new animal hospital, one half mile west of the original, was completed in 1936–37.

Three kids with no bike, we borrowed a neighbor kid's bike to learn how to ride. We came up with creative ways to beg, borrow, or occasionally steal one of our more fortunate playmates' ride. After moving into our new house in Western Springs, Marg, Phil and I calculated how long it would take us to save 25 cents from our weekly allowances to afford to buy a community bike. It was the Christmas in 1940 when the folks presented us with our first wheels.

By 1939, Dad had purchased our permanent residence in Western Springs. The price for the five bedroom, 2½ bath house was $7,500. This also featured a lot and a half, 75 feet wide. Mom sold it in 1982 for $125,000. Today it is appraised at over $550,000.

The large bachelor quarters on the third floor are not shown in this south-facing photo. They contained two large bedrooms, a full bath, and a 30′ storage space under the slanted roof.

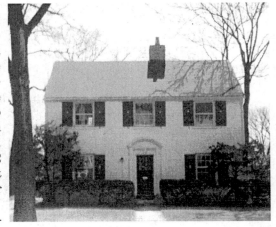

1237 Walnut Sreet, Western Springs, Illinois

Our new furniture was shipped from Des Moines, Iowa. The prices seem amazingly low until one compares it with the house which went from $7,000 to $550,000 in 70 years. At that rate, the furniture would cost $18,000 today. My oldest son, Bill, reports it's still in very good condition. He's getting ready to pass it on to his children. With the abuse Phil and I gave the beds, I'm surprised they've survived.

Our family wasn't big on birthdays or holidays. We attributed it to Dad's seven-day-a-week job. I got my first ever birthday gift when I turned eleven. I had joined the cub scouts and needed a knife to go with my new uniform. Phil reports he got his first birthday gift about the same year. The following Christmas we got the gift of our lifetime—a Red Ryder BB Gun. The joy lasted about two weeks. From our third floor vantage, Phil and I could control the neighborhood. Shooting at birds, bad guys, and whatever target was presented. Our garage had a small, round win-

FRANK F. BLACK   ELMER ECKBURG

FURNITURE SALES CO.
120 S. 5TH STREET
2ND. FLOOR WHITE LINE TRANSFER & STORAGE CO.
DES MOINES, IOWA

February 23rd 1939

Dr.A.C.Merrick
9115 Ogden Avenue
Brookfield, Ill

Qty	Item #	Description		Price
1	#3722	Cherry Chest		19.50
1	#3723	Cherry Vanity		27.00
2	#3722	Cherry Beds 3/3	@ 15.50	31.00
1	#3722	Cherry Bench		5.75
1	#3642	Mahogany Vanity		27.50
1	#3642	Mahogany Hiboy		23.75
1	#3640	Mahogany Bed 4/6		17.75
1	#3640	Mahogany Bench		5.25
1	#3813	Cherry Vanity		24.75
1	#3814	Chest, Cherry		18.75
1	#3814	Cherry Bed 4/6		15.50
1	#3812	Cherry Bench		5.00
1	#3812	Cherry Nite Table		6.50
1	#3722	Cherry Nite Table		7.00
			$	235.00
	Plus 10 %			23.50
			$	258.50
				200.00
				58.50

Duplicate of the invoice covering merchndise shipped to
you last October direct from Springfield factory.

dow divided by eight panes. Our fatal mistake was to hit this target and shatter two of the windows. We never saw the Red Ryder again. I suspect Mom was waiting for any chance to show her Quaker pacifism.

Dad joined AA in 1939. I mention elsewhere how active he became in "Twelve Stepping," sponsoring and assisting other alcoholics. One of Dad's recruits turned out to be a problem for me. Dr. Larry Gordon (not his real name) might have been a great dentist when he was sober, but he was a terrible one when under the influence. Dr. Gordon had come to a couple of AA meetings at our house. He seemed like a very nice guy. Soon afterwards I developed a toothache so naturally Dad recommended Dr. Gordon. I don't recall all the details concerning the incident, but the baby tooth I needed treated was untouched and two permanent molars were extracted. This was the last time any of the family visited Dr. Gordon. I'm thankful the two bridges I've had for 70 years were installed by excellent dentists.

Our family joined St. Francis Catholic Church in La Grange. I spent the seventh and eighth grades in St. Francis School. Dad would drop us three kids on his way to Sunday office hours. We were expected to walk or bum a ride home, two miles away. In those days the church had a "pew rent" policy. Every adult was expected to pay at least a dime upon entering the church, with no charge for kids. Originally, a substantial source of income for the church came from pew rent, which was paid by seatholders. The payment entitled seatholders to sit in a specific pew (with their names on it). This practice assured everyone would contribute as they entered for worship. Later, when general seating was established in the 1960s, the practice was discontinued.

When older sister Margaret was not along, Phil and I would enter the front door, walk down the side aisle, genuflect, and leave thru the rear door. This led to the side entrance of the main alter and a door to freedom. We could pretend, if stopped, that we were going to prepare for alter boy duties. We were really headed for our ten o'clock "Pool Mass" at the local bowling alley/pool hall, four blocks south of St. Francis. Both Phil and I "set pins" in the establishment, so we were well acquainted with the staff and crowd. One hour later—about the time for church to be over—we headed for home. I don't believe we were ever found out.

Harold Johnson had ten acres of sweet corn planted a few blocks from our house in Western Springs. In the summers of 1943 and '44 Phil, a half dozen other teenagers, and I picked the fields every few days. Neighbor and classmate, Dick Crawford, who later became a vet in Milwaukee, was also a picker. It meant getting up before sunrise, walking down to Mr. Johnson's house, and riding his truck to the field. We picked two rows at a time, all of us starting at one end and slowly progressing thru the field. There were 40 ears to the bag. We'd inspect every 3rd or 4th ear for worms by pulling down the husk—this was in the days before pesticides were routinely used on edible vegetables—then leave the bag for the pickup guy to load on the truck, and begin again. The sun would be up for an hour or two before we completed our task. Now the fun part. Two of the older boys were chosen to ride "shotgun" on the corn piled on the truck. One more rode with Mr. Johnson up front.

We delivered to the best Chicago restaurants—The Palmer House, Drake, Edgewater Beach, and more—always through the back alleys. We were often met by the chefs, who personally inspected the produce and occasionally engaged in a shouting match with Mr. Johnson about the quality. There was never an argument about the freshness.

The Great Walrus Race

It would have made a great YouTube video—maybe have gone viral. Two young boys "riding" walruses in the Brookfield Zoo. The headline read, "HOLD 'EM, WALRUS." The caption under the photograph which appeared in a Chicago newspaper stated, "Here's a race that will be won by a whisker—a walrus whisker."

In the fall of 1937, the Brookfield Zoo acquired two walruses, Fibber and Molly. For those under the age of 60, "Fibber McGee and Molly" was a popular Radio show in the '30s, a precursor to "All in the Family" and "The Honeymooners" on television in the '70s. The zoo was looking for a way to publicize the arrival of their new prized acquisitions. How about a human interest story involving animals and kids? It was a natural.

The walrus (*Odobenus rosmarus*) is a large, flippered marine animal weighing up to 3,700 pounds. Male sea lions are distinguished from walruses by having ears, no tusks, and weighting around 2,000 pounds.

My dad, Dr. A. C. Merrick, had recently opened the first small animal hospital on the west side of Chicago in Brookfield, Illinois. The hospital occupied the front half of a typical mom-and-pop business building on Highway #34. The back half was our living quarters, consisting of a two bedroom flat. Marg, 9, Phil, 6, and I, 7, shared one bedroom. We had recently returned that summer from staying with relatives for the previous year. Mom enrolled us in the nearby St. Barbara's Catholic Grade School.

We had no bicycles, so walking was our only means of transportation. There were no close neighborhood parks in those days, but the Brookfield Zoo offered distraction and entertainment for young and old alike. Admission for kids under 12 was free. My brother, Phil, and I walked the mile trek over to the zoo one Saturday. We were approached by two men asking if we would like to have our pictures taken with a walrus. We readily agreed. The first photos showed us next to the animals rubbing their tummies like they were overweight canines. The photographer suggested a more interesting shot—two jockeys on walruses in a mock race. That's the one that ended up in the Sunday issue of the *Chicago Herald Examiner*, October 17, 1937. The photo shows us racing in opposite directions, getting the walruses to line up for a photo shoot is easier said than done.

We did manage to get Dad's name and refer to his animal hospital in the story. He forgave us for going alone to the zoo in the first place.

The search for the original story and photos is another story. I had a copy of the photo and the story from my Uncle Russ. Unfortunately, the page was torn and the exact date and newspaper name were missing. Contacting Brookfield Zoo revealed information about the walruses but no trace of the story. The *Chicago Tribune* related they were not the source of the story. Other Chicago newspapers stopped publishing long ago. The search goes on.

The letter from Brookfield Zoo contained the sad news of the passing of Fibber and Molly in 1938.

Wikipedia reports that the Brookfield Zoo, also known as Chicago Zoological Park, opened on July 1, 1934, and quickly gained international recognition for using moats.

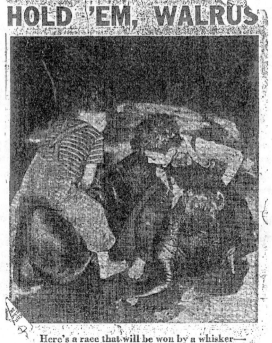

Here's a race that will be won by a whisker—
 us whisker—and probably the first of its
 be world. Urging the walruses on are
 errick, 6 (left), and his brother, John,

Andy's Taj Mahal

The building stood out from the rest of the commercial storefronts on Ogden Ave, Route 34, in Brookfield, Illinois. Dr. A. C. Merrick, Andy, was building one of the largest, most modern animal hospitals in the United States. Taking up the entire 50'×100' lot, the buildings curved glass brick and porcelain enamel front was modeled after Frank Lloyd Wright's creation for Johnson Wax in Racine, Wisconsin. No shingle hanging above the front door to announce the business name and owner was good enough for Dad. Instead he had "ANIMAL HOSPITAL" baked into the porcelain panels extending the length of the front of the building just below the roof line. Next to the double door entrance was the more modest declaration:

A. C. Merrick, DVM
Director

The design included a spacious private office, reception area, waiting room, kitchen, exam room, laboratory, surgery, three dog boarding rooms to accommodate 40 animals, a feline room for 20 cats, isolation ward, attendants' quarters, storage rooms, and outside kennels. The structure was twice the size of most small ani-

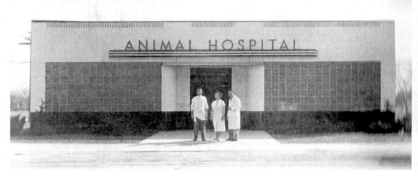

The Merrick Animal Hospital shortly after opening in 1937.
Joe Wylie, DVM; Dorothy S. Merrick; A.C. Merrick, DVM, Director

mal hospitals built in the '30s. Vets were still considered "horse doctors" by most of the general public, only for treating farm animals. Many treated pets' problems as a sideline and inconvenience. Colleagues of Dad scoffed at the money he wasted on what they called "Andy's Taj Mahal." Dad, as it turned out, was 50 years ahead of his time.

There were no manufactured stainless steel cages in 1935. Dad's were made on-the-spot out of cement with a center drain in each. I asked him how he determined the size. He replied, "I told the masons to make them as wide as the unfolded Chicago Tribune newspaper and tall enough for a collie or German Shepherd to stand up." That turned out to be the standard size for large manufactured stainless steel dog cages even today—36" wide × 30" deep × 36" high. A few were even wider, made to fit the extra length in a kennel room. Old newspapers are still used today to give the animal a little cushion from the hard floor and soak up any accidents.

The original hospital had eight outside runs. This made it difficult to exercise animals in rainy or cold weather. Soon after World War II, Dad enclosed the runs and added a grooming and bathing room behind them. He complained that the six cement cages, built to the same specs as the original, cost $600.00, the same price as the 60 cages built in 1935.

When brother Phil and I worked together during the summer boarding season as kennel boys, mischief was often the rule. Water fights with hoses at 20 feet were common. Dad would have fired us on the spot if he thought he could find any replacements. World War II had taken all able-bodied men into the service, so he could put up with a little horseplay from two teenagers.

In 1940 Dad bought the small "Bohemian Bungalow" across the alley, behind the animal hospital. This avoided a noise complaint from nearby neighbors and provided an office for the Brookfield Laboratories. Dr. Merrick's Sulfodene, marketed under the company name, Brookfield Laboratories, was selling well around the country. There was no room in the animal hospital for the Brookfield Laboratories staff. Fourteen years later, in 1954, after Dad had sold the patent medicine business and I had graduated, Carol and I moved our family into the home. Thus began my lifetime of very short commutes to work. l never had to travel more than three city blocks.

Until Dad sold the practice, it was first come, first served. Appointments were not a common practice in veterinary

Former Iowa Veterinarian Talks Here
$50,000 DOG HOSPITAL
Once Paid in Hickory Nuts

Dog lovers have elevated Dr. A. C. Merrick, former Oskaloosa, Ia., veterinarian, from hickory nuts to a $50,000 dog hospital at Brookfield, Ill.

Dr. Merrick, in Des Moines to address the Iowa Veterinary Medical association convention at Hotel Fort Des Moines, left Oskaloosa five years ago.

Hickory Nuts.

"The last case I had there, a farmer paid me in hickory nuts for treatment of his dog. I've been paid in canned goods, cord wood, butter and eggs and other foodstuffs," said Dr. Merrick.

"Often people think more of their dog than they do of their children. I had a case last week in which a couple with two children brought their pet to the hospital. The dog needed a shot for distemper—which would cost $3.

"The parents looked at each other a minute and then said, 'go ahead.' I found out they only had $4 and were on their way to have the children vaccinated against diphtheria. And they decided to let the children go, but treat the dog," said the veterinarian. "I took care of the dog, but sent them on their way to the doctor."

"Modern dog hospitals, Dr. Merrick said, compare favorably with hospitals for humans. In his own hospital, in a suburb of Chicago, Ill., he has two assistant veterinarians, a nurse-receptionist, and two hospital attendants.

Equipment.

The Merrick Dog hospital itself has waiting room, reception room, x-ray laboratories, kitten and puppy wards, isolation quarters for contagious diseases, and all-glass walls between divisions. The place is air-conditioned and has kennels for 97 "patients."

"I'm planning to add private rooms to the hospital," said Dr. Merrick.

Refugee Dogs.

The veterinarian, author of "How to Own a Dog and Like It," now has 12 British refugee dogs at his kennels. These dogs are suffering largely from malnutrition and tape-worms. The tape-worms are caused largely from eating rabbit meat.

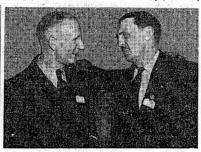

Dr. C. C. Franks (left) of Grimes, Ia., secretary of the Iowa Veterinary Medical association, chats with Dr. A. C. Merrick, former Oskaloosa, Ia., veterinarian who now operates a $50,000 dog hospital at Brookfield, Ill.

The veterinarians' convention which opened Tuesday, will close Thursday evening.

---

medicine until the '80s, corresponding with the advent of computers. During the daytime there was rarely anyone waiting more than a few minutes for service. Evening hours were different. Regular evening office hours were 7:00 to 8:00 PM. By 6:30 there was often a number of clients with their pets in line. Our waiting room had ten chairs, and when they were full, people waited outside. Many times I would get home around 9:30 to 10:00 PM. Dad would stop at the La Grange News Agency, located in the Norland Hotel, across the street from the Burlington train station. He would get the late edition of the *Chicago Daily News* (now long gone), the *Daily Racing Form* to calculate tomorrows picks, and left over papers to take to the hospital for papering the cages.

The average office visit today requires 20 to 30 minutes. Most practices operate with an appointment schedule. Clients today consider their time as valuable as the professional they are consulting. Vaccinations are preceded by a full examination of the animal. In the '40s to the '70s we were much quicker—lax, actually. If the owner did not mention a problem, or it was not noticed with a cursory exam, the entire visit for a routine vaccination usually took five to ten minutes.

Dad said his only regret was failing to provide for off-street parking. At first everyone parked along the highway, even though it was an "interstate." The four lane highway #34 was rarely busy enough to cause any problems. Dad did not open until 9 AM, which avoided most of the morning rush. There was a small narrow lot next to the animal hospital which Dad thought was overpriced. The owner wanted $2,000. "Way too high," Dad said. "Bedsides, they'll never be able to build anything on that narrow piece of property." For years I mowed the lot and planted flowers, as if it was part of our property. As the years went by, the price of the property increased. About the time that Dad sold the practice and retired in 1968, disaster struck. Someone bought the land and established a used car sales business, complete with a small garage-like building for auto repair. Dad was heartbroken to see this piece of "$*#%" next to his Taj Mahal.

Over time, parking was restricted on the highway. Fortunately, the hospital was only 25 feet from a side street which did allow parking for clients. Staff parking was provided by utilizing the backyard of my old house, across the alley from the back door of the hospital.

Dad sold the practice in 1968 to Dr. Ted Fitch, who operated a very successful practice until his retirement in 1995. Dr. Fitch sold the practice to Dr. Jeff Weiser, and he in turn sold it to Dr. James Hosek in 2007, but the name remains Merrick Animal Hospital.

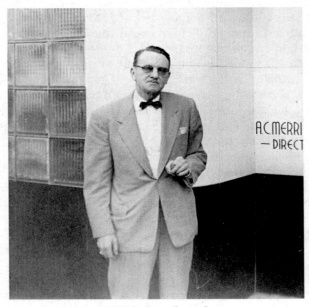

Andy in 1965, before the sale
of Merrick Animal Hospital.

The Testing Box Mystery

The letter written on December 20, 1940, by attorney Harold J. Fleck of Oskaloosa, Iowa, stated: "Dr. Killips of our city has employed me in connection with the collection of royalties on a certain testing cabinet patented by you." I vaguely recall Dad mentioning working for or with a Dr. Killips about the time he met my mother in Oskaloosa. I had always assumed he was working as a large animal vet. Now it seems he may have been employed in the Killips Laboratories.

LAW OFFICES
HAROLD J. FLECK
123½ HIGH AVENUE WEST
OSKALOOSA, IOWA

COLLECTION DEPARTMENT
FLOYD T. REUTER, MANAGER

TELEPHONE 52

December 20, 1940

Dr. Andrew Merrick
9115 Ogden Avenue
Brookfield, Illinois

Dear Dr. Merrick:

Dr. Killips of our city has employed me in connection with the collection of royalties on a certain testing cabinet patented by you.

I have examined the patent papers, and, in my opinion, the patent is good, and the collection of royalties can be made.

Also, I have examined a contract between you and Dr. Killips with reference to this patent, in which you employed Dr. Killips for the period of this patent or patents to prosecute and collect all royalties and damages, the expense of the same to be born equally by both parties.

In view of this provision with reference to your liability for one-half of the expenses and the anticipated large expenses which will be necessary in conducting numerous lawsuits, I am interested in knowing about the collection of my fees. It is my usual practice to make an investigation first from ones who would be liable, as to their ability to pay: what property they own, whether there are mortgages, and with what bank they do business. I would appreciate a letter from you with reference to these facts. It is my understanding that you own a hospital, a home, and personal property in connection therewith. Will you please indicate the value, whether they are mortgaged, and give me the name of your bank which you desire for reference.

In view of the fact that we are ready to start proceedings, an early reply from you will be greatly appreciated. You will find an addressed, stamped envelope inclosed for your convenience.

Yours very truly,

Harold J. Fleck

HJF:md

I was cataloging boxes of mementos—pictures, letters, newspaper articles and keepsakes that my mother had squirreled away during her lifetime. After her death in 1987, the boxes traveled from our home in Western Springs, Illinois, to my sister's home in Houston, Texas. After her passing in 2009, they ended up in my attic. As anyone who has gone through a lifetime of a loved one's stuff—treasures or junk, depending on your viewpoint—can attest, it's a monumental task. My first inclination was to toss the entire lot in the garbage. Instead, I asked my five kids to plan on spending a long weekend in Peachtree City to sort, catalog, and divide the loot. All readily agreed in the spring. Labor Day came and went, and still no one was able to work the event into their busy schedule. So I began, piece by piece, picture by picture, to divide the items into seven boxes—one for each child and brother Phil, and one for me. After three months, I was less than half way through. An added benefit was being able to add many period photos to the stories in this book.

Personal letters to Dad from Dr. Killips listed Herbert Killips, DVM, as president of the Killips Laboratories, manufacturer of poultry vaccines and various other animal medical products. From the general tone of the correspondence, it seems someone was selling the "Testing Box" and not paying royalties. Dr. Killips thought Dad may have been receiving money and not giving Dr. Killips his share. He wanted Dad to either join in lawsuits against the accused parties or drop out.

Dad had developed a number of patent medicines for dogs and cats in the early forties, but I never heard a mention of any patents while he was in Oskaloosa. The question became how to search for a patent from 1927–29, not knowing exactly when or the purpose of the item. The attorney's letter had mentioned a "testing bench." In my years in the vet field, I've never encountered a testing bench.

Google came up with a couple of 1928 newspaper ads for Killips poultry products. Calls to Oskaloosa Public Library were unsuccessful. They could find no record of Dad or Dr. Killips, as the records from 1925–29 were lost. My niece, Katie Todd, suggested contacting the patent office directly. They were eager to help but said they needed a patent number for records prior to 1973. They did mention I could contact the regional office located in the Georgia Tech library.

A phone call connected me to Lisha Li, Patent and Trademark Coordinator. I hoped she would have some insider's way of solv-

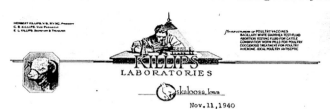

Nov. 11, 1940

Dr. A. C. Merrick
9115 Coden Ave.
Brookfield, Ill.

Dear Andy,

I was very much surprised at your answer to my letters.

I am not trying to involve you in law suits nor in the unfavorable comments and criticisms which will follow them. You understand that as things now stand I will have to bring suit under your name - since that is the way you INSISTED it be when the patent was applied for.

I wish to make it clear to you once and for all - I am not setting you in or out - you, are making your own choice.

Now that you are making money and able to hold up your end, I would prefer to have you in. You know Andy that I have always been square with you - or have you forgotten that I gave you money out of my own pocket when you left Oskaloosa? (This I have never mentioned before.)

In my letter of Sept. 20, 1940 I made you a proposition, this is your way out.

I have had an attorney working on these cases for several months, and we are about ready to start our suits. Therefore, an early reply will be appreciated.

Your old friend Charley is down in Florida fishing and having a grand time. I still play handball and can beat most of the young crop of players. Kindest regards to your wife and family.

Respectfully,

Hubert Killips

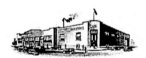

ing my mystery. I explained my dilemma of being unable to find anything in 1928–29 under Dad's name. Lisha was also unsuccessful, but she took my name and number and promised to contact me after further searching.

In less than 24 hours I received an email from Lisha with the patent attached. Lisha had simply expanded her search to the early thirties. Sure enough, Dad's "Testing Box" patent was approved on January 8, 1932. The patent application process had taken over three years. By then, Dad and the family were long gone from Oskaloosa, Iowa.

Accompanying the design page were detailed instructions as to how to construct and use the invention.

The application stated: "The object of my invention is to provide a method and apparatus for testing the blood of the poultry and other animals or beings for discovering the existence of certain disease conditions in the blood.

More particularly, it is my object to provide a method of relatively simple and brief technique, whereby tests may be quickly, conveniently and accurately made. It is also my purpose to provide a simple and inexpensive and convenient apparatus for making such tests.

Almost every television story today about some scientific breakthrough shows a handsome lab technician in a starched white coat pipetting a liquid into a series of vials

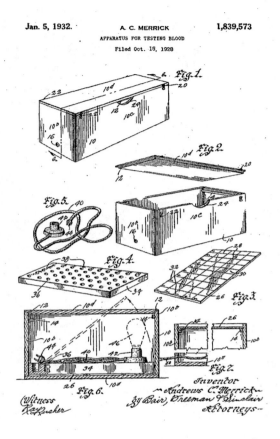

contained in a "testing box." What goes around, comes around.

Dad had no interest in pursuing a lawsuit to recover monies for patent infringement. He had several patent medicines selling

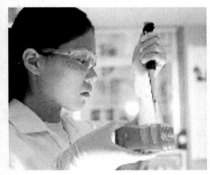

every day to all corners of the USA. He wrote Dr. Killips a letter, giving him the full authority to act on Dad's behalf and keep all the income he received for himself. Dad had much bigger fish to fry.

Here again, there are so many questions but so few answers. One benefit of writing stories about bygone days is the reaction they elicit from my children and friends. "Did you *really* do this or that? Are you sure this or that happened? Or, "Dad, let me tell you what really happened."

I encourage my readers to jot down stories as they come to mind. Your reward will be in the delight elicited from family and friends.

State of Illinois)
) ss.
County of Cook   )

REVOCATION OF POWER OF ATTORNEY

WHEREAS the undersigned did, in, to wit, the year 1928, give and grant unto one M. Killips, a doctor, of Oskaloosa, Iowa, by a document in writing, a certain power of attorney for the purpose and to the end that the aforesaid Dr. Killips might do certain acts on behalf of and as the agent for the undersigned in connection with certain letters patent granted to the undersigned, and

WHEREAS the undersigned wishes to terminate all and any agency created by the aforesaid power of attorney,

NOW THEREFORE the undersigned does by this document revoke any and all powers purported to have been granted by the undersigned as aforesaid, or otherwise in connection with the letters patent above referred to.

Andrew C. Ulwick

Given under my notarial seal
this 6th day of January, 1941.

Blanche Jelinek

Dated at Brookfield, Illinois, this 6th day of January, A. D. 1941.

Small Animal Practice in the '40s and '50s

Sixty hours a week! It seems incredible now, but Merrick Animal Hospital, in suburban Brookfield, Illinois, kept those hours from 1935 to 1955.

Mon–Fri: 9 to 5 and 7 to 9
Sat: 9 to 5
Sun: 9 to 12

Appointments were unheard of; it was always first come, first served. Our waiting room had ten chairs. The overflow waited outside in good weather and stood inside in winter. It was the rare family who had two cars, so evening and weekend hours allowed for working families to bring their pets in for treatment and routine vaccinations. Most animal hospitals were built on or near a bus route to help "carless" pet owners.

Office calls were $3.00, plus injections and meds dispensed. Other practices would often advertise, "No Charge for Exams," but somehow there was always a need for one or two injections and medicine sent home. Total client visit charges averaged around $8.00 to $10.00.

Cat castration, including an overnight hospitalization, was $5.00. Dog spay, including one or two nights hospitalization was $15.00. A series of three vaccinations for distemper totaled $10.00. (We tried to get the money up front in case they did not show up for later visits.)

Computers were still a distant dream. Or a nightmare, depending upon your point of view. All records were hand written. I remember learning to write what would now be a page of notes on three lines of our 5×8 file cards. Reminder cards were making their appearance. At first it was just a note in next year's appointment book to send Mrs. Jones a card that Buffy was due for her distemper or rabies booster. This led to complicated file systems with coded and flagged cards showing which animals were due each month.

The computer eliminated all the guesswork. Once a month it spits out a preprinted card to alert owners of their animal's next recommended visit. Most veterinarians now put greater emphasis on a yearly or biyearly exam rather than repeated vaccinations. This is similar to the yearly dental exam. As with humans, preventive medicine is cheaper in the long run and more beneficial to the pet.

Dad kept accurate records of all charge accounts to be billed at the end of the month. Cash receipts sometimes were another matter. My guess is that some unrecorded money ended up in Dad's pocket. As the junior associate, I wasn't about to complain.

I had started as a kennel boy at the age of 14 making 40 cents an hour, which gradually increased to 60 cents per hour over the next two years. During the summer when Dad might have as many as 60 dogs and cats boarding, my younger brother, Phil, was recruited to help clean kennels. Tom Drije was also kennel help until he was accepted in vet school in 1952. Tom bought my Uncle Gerard's practice in Elmhurst after he died in 1958.

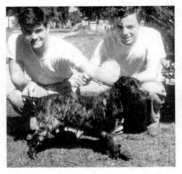

Tom Drije and John • 1951

Dad had custom-made cement cages with a drain in each cage. The width of the cage had been determined by the length of an unfolded *Chicago Tribune* newspaper. It worked out very well. I'm sure any one of us who has "papered cages" has had the experience of reading an amazing story, only to discover the paper was two or three years old. What goes around, comes around.

Water fights with the many hoses were an occasional hazard to employees and animals alike. Dad would remark, "One boy = one boy working; two boys = one half boy working; three boys = no boy working at all." How true.

I remember promising to give up cigarettes if they ever got to more than 20 cents a pack—a penny apiece. I hate to think of the money I would have saved over the next 20 years if I'd kept my word. Fortunately, in January, 1964, the day of the first Surgeon General's report on the dangers of smoking, my wife, Carol, and I both quit cold turkey.

After graduation from the University of Illinois in 1954, I was hired by Dad. My salary was the grand sum of $500 a month plus rent-free housing in a bungalow Dad owned behind the animal hospital. Depending upon who's calculating, 1950 prices can be multiplied by 10 to 12 to see how they compare to today. As usual,

I thought I was underpaid, and Dad thought the opposite. I lived next door to the hospital, so I was the delegated emergency vet. I got to keep one half of the fees, so I didn't mind getting up at night or making Sunday afternoon calls. Some months it meant an extra $100 income.

I had been employed in Dad's animal hospital since I was 14—ten years by the time I graduated—so most clients knew me as the kennel boy/tech, not as the associate veterinarian. I got used to people asking to see the "regular doctor" or the "senior vet." I took little offense, but it bothered Carol a lot. That was one of the major reasons we started looking to branch out on our own.

General anesthesia was Nembutal (sodium pentobarbital), administered intravenously. The drug usually allowed good surgical sleep for an hour, with the animal awake, but groggy, in 3 to 4 hours. Occasionally a patient would sleep or be very groggy for 24 hours or more.

We did almost no pre-op blood work or EKGs. Instruments were boiled on the stove—I've forgotten for how long. Gloves were optional—major surgery, usually; minor surgery, occasionally. Strict 3 to 4 minute hand washing was routine. I still recall a debate in the '60s with a colleague in Kenosha about his refusal to wear gloves to perform a spay. This fellow was an excellent orthopedic surgeon. He would don gown, gloves, and mask—the whole nine yards—when performing bone surgery, but not even gloves to perform a spay. He swore he never had a problem. I doubt it.

Radiographs were taken with a 20-amp machine. You needed one-half to one second to get good picture contrast of extremities. Thicker soft tissue X-rays of the belly or chest were poor quality due to the need for longer exposure time. Modern machines with much higher amperage (measured in milliamps, or mA) and peak kilovolts (KVP) have reduced

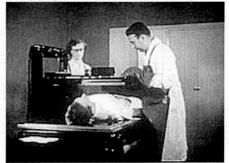

Dr. Joe Wylie and his nurse

the time to a fraction of a second. I still believe I obtained better extremity radiographs with my old 20-amp machine.

Ignorance of the harmful effects of x-rays resulted in the absence of standard radiation safety procedures which are employed today. Wikipedia reports:

> Scientists and physicians would often place their hands directly in the x-ray beam, resulting in radiation burns. Edison's assistant, Clarence Madison Dally (1865–1904), died as a result of exposure to radiation from fluoroscopes, and in 1903, Edison abandoned his work on fluoroscopes, saying "Don't talk to me about x-rays, I am afraid of them." Trivial uses for the technology also resulted, including the shoe-fitting fluoroscope used by shoe stores in the 1930s–1950s. The placement of the radiologist behind the screen resulted in significant radiation doses to the radiologist.

Sadly, Dad used the machine as a fluoroscope for ten years before he became aware of the warnings posted about the cumulative effect of radiation. He developed extensive fingernail damage due to neglecting to wear protective lead gloves.

On one occasion, we were presented with a deaf Boxer. Duke was a 8-year-old male. He was a wonderful sample of the breed, with both excellent conformation and mellow temperament. Over the previous year the owner had noticed Duke showing signs of hearing loss. An external ear exam did not reveal any problems. An EENT (ear, eye, nose, and throat) physician friend agreed to make a hearing aid for Duke. One evening after hours, Dr. Arnold made a mold of Duke's left external ear canal. He attached an elastic band to go around Duke's neck to hold the device in place. So far, so good. Duke seemed to be more attentive when wearing the unit. The owner seemed very happy with the results. Try as we might, we could not come up with a good method of keeping the hearing aid in place. One good head shake and out it came. Duke gradually got used to the device, leaving it in place as long as someone was close by to monitor.

Many years later, after selling his practice in 1968 to Dr. Ted Fitch, Dad continued to go to the office almost every day. It was a good excuse to get out the house, stop at the post office for the mail, and meet friends for coffee. I'm sure many clients were unaware the practice had been sold. Dad, of course, never charged for his services.

The Veterinarian's Son Small Animal Practice in the '40s and '50s

The Mob Vet

What's a nice vet like Dr. A. C. Merrick, my dad, doing getting involved with the mob?

Dad had been in small animal practice in Brookfield, Illinois for a couple of years, circa 1936. A big, black Packard drove up to the hospital one afternoon. Out stepped a gorgeous, young blonde gal drenched in furs—definitely not your average suburban housewife type.

While the chauffeur waited in the car, she came into the office and explained to Dad that her dog, Sweetie, was having breathing problems. She requested Sweetie be examined to determine the cause and instructed her driver to bring in the animal. The chauffeur brought in a large collie who was aptly named—very sweet indeed. Examination revealed a circular, puss-filled wound extending completely around the neck. Dad requested that she leave Sweetie for a few days so he could treat the infection.

When she returned in three days, Sweetie ran and almost knocked her owner backward, head over spike heels. Someone had put a rubber band around Sweetie's neck. Over the course of time, it had cut through the skin. The cause, and the ensuing infection, had been covered by her long hair. Blondie thanked dad, told the driver to pay the bill, and literally skipped to her car.

Over the next few days and weeks, more big black limos pulled up to the animal hospital with a pet to treat. Asked who sent them, they all said Sally recommended them. Next obvious query, "Who is Sally?" The lady answered, "Big Tony's gal." That's Tony, as in Tony "Big Tuna"Accardo, the unchallenged Boss of the Chicago La Cosa Nostra. Actually, "Sally" was the code name for Clarice Pordzany, a Polish-American chorus girl. They later married and had four children. In fact, Accardo had two grandsons, one of whom was Eric Kumerow, who was drafted by the Miami Dolphins of the National Football League. Unlike the majority of his colleagues, Accardo had a strong marriage and was never known to be unfaithful to his wife. Clarice Accardo died on November 15, 2002, at the age of 91, of natural causes. It is estimated that in 1929, organized crime brought in $109 million in untaxed profits.

Over the ensuing years, Mob pets were often brought to the hospital when the "wise guys" made their daily "house calls." They would pick up Dad's horse bets for that day and pay off his winnings, if any. Typically these were low level "punks," but occasionally Dad would be graced by the presence of more famous ones, such as Frank Fascitti or Tony Accardo. Often, these higher-ups would tag along, bringing their wives' or girlfriends' pets. As you could imagine, these fellows got speedy, first-class treatment. There was never any mention of fees. No matter what the procedure—vaccination, x-rays, medicines, toenail trims—the payment was in $100 dollar bills. Usually one, but occasionally two or three for exceptional service. No one ever expected or received change.

Upon learning I was compiling stories of vet practice in the '40s, my cousin, Mike Merrick, sent me the following email.

> To: Dr. John
> Re: Big Tuna
>
> My Dad, Gerard, also known as Ruffy, and his brother, Andy, had similar small animal practices. Andy was in Brookfield, Illinois and Dad was in Elmhurst. They were both suburbs of Chicago, not far apart.
>
> Back in those days, small animal vets were few and far between. Because of this you not only had clients who were local, but also clients from surrounding towns. Most were average hardworking people who had pets that needed care. I say "most," because there was one exception.
>
> He had two Doberman Pinchers that he just loved. His name was Tony "Big Tuna" Accardo, the head of the Chicago Mafia from 1943 to 1957. He was said to be one of the most brutal mob bosses in the country. Tony lived in River Forest, a very affluent suburb of Chicago, in a huge mansion on a large corner lot surrounded by a tall wrought iron fence and electronic gate. Dad said it was like getting into Fort Knox.
>
> Dad's car was searched, and they went through his vet bag before letting him in to the house. He only saw Tony once, and all Tony said was "take good care of my babies." The dogs and Tony lived the good life in a huge home with bowling alleys on the lower level.
>
> Mom did not like Dad going to the Accardo home. Once she asked him why he treated that terrible man's

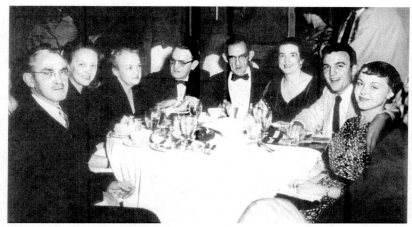

Gerard, Manon, Dorothy, Andy, Russ, Bess, Phil, and Francine
The Palmer House • Chicago • 1954

dogs? His reply, "Because they don't know who he is or what he does for a living." As it turned out, taking care of the Mob's animals was a family affair.

In the 1950s, Chicago mobsters or their assistants controlled gambling. One would call in bets before noon or give them to runners who came daily to deliver yesterday's winnings or collect the losses. It was the way gambling worked around the country—"House Call Vegas."

The "Bible" was the Daily Racing Form. Since beginning in 1894, this thick newspaper is available in the evenings, 364 days a year—not on Christmas—containing yesterday's results and tomorrow's entries for every major track in the country.

The DRF publishes over two dozen stats on every horse entered on tomorrow's race card. These include, but are not limited to, each horse's name, weight, color, DOB, breeding, analysis of performance over the last two years, track conditions, weight carried, speed the horse ran, winners, and the number of horses entered. One could spend a few minutes calculating today's results (wins and losses), and a few hours figuring tomorrow's bets. Today's picks and cash were placed in an envelope to be picked up by the courier. Yesterday's winnings were delivered in a similar fashion. Individuals could also run a tab, depending upon your credit history.

Before the era of Native American casinos and Las Vegas, the Mob had a few gambling dens situated around the Chicago suburbs to accommodate Vegas-style gambling—mostly craps, poker, blackjack, and slots. These areas were secluded, heavily guarded buildings, typically located in industrial districts surrounded by tall fences, heavy gates, and armed guards.

The year was 1949, one year before my marriage to Carol Hough. We had been out for a nice dinner with my parents when Dad decided he was feeling lucky and would like to stop by the "Fort" for a little action. My future bride looked a little apprehensive, but I was all for it. Maybe I could con Dad out of $10 to try my luck also.

The "Fort" was aptly named. A bunker-like squat brick building surrounded by a eight-foot wooden fence topped with razor wire in an old industrial region of Melrose Park, Illinois, run by the Mob's political stooges. Good cops were in very short supply. Rumor was that the Mob controlled the town—the mayor, police, city council, etc. I had never been to Vegas or any other gambling casino, but I'm sure Melrose Park was no Vegas. It was a typical lower middle class Chicago suburb, immediately east of what would become O'Hare Airport.

We approached the front gate and flashed our lights to draw the attention of two dark-suited guys carrying very big guns. As Dad rolled down the window, one of the fellows recognized him with, "Hi Doc, where have you been?" We drove to the side door for valet parking. The people ahead were getting body frisked by two other wise guys. Carol was now more than a little nervous. Fortunately, one of these two also recognized Dad and said, "It's okay guys, they're with Doc." We got in with no more than a glance. Without a doubt, I'd never seen so much money in one place at one time. Stacks of bills of all denominations were lined up on every craps table. There was a general buzz as gamblers pleaded with the dice to perform miracles. The whir of slots added to the ruckus. This was before the advent of computerized slots where the old type machines really were "One Arm Bandits." Drinks and munchies were "on the house." The Mob could well afford it. Gambling and prostitution brought in millions of tax-free dollars every year.

Dad immediately headed for the craps tables. He was a shooter, usually wanting to control the dice. He was much more animated than usual when shooting craps—talking, cajoling, and pleading with the dice to have Lady Luck smile on him.

As a rule, gamblers exaggerate their winnings and minimize their loses. After an hour or so, Dad said he'd had enough. He said he was about even, but I didn't believe a word. I'd managed to lose $10 in the first 10 minutes. Mom and Carol sat at a table and watched the action. Mom seemed resigned to the wait. Carol was happy just to be back in the car and headed for home. "Once is enough for me," she said.

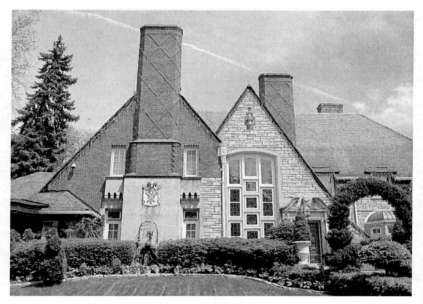

Tony Accardo House
915 Franklin Ave., River Forest, IL

Accardo rose from small-time hoodlum (and Al Capone's bodyguard) to the position of day-to-day boss of the Chicago Outfit from 1943 to 1957 and again in 1972 until his death in 1992. Considering he was posing as a beer salesman, the 22-room Tudor mansion caught the attention of the IRS, so Accardo moved into a small ranch house a few blocks away.

The 24,000-square-foot mansion was built in 1929 by radio pioneer William Grunow, manufacturer of "Majestic" brand radios. It was home to Accardo from 1953–61 and was the site of many mob gatherings. Among its lavish features are a regulation-size bowling alley, an English pub with beamed ceiling and seating for 50, and an indoor swimming pool with blue-glazed Mexican tiles.

Dr. Merrick's Sulfodene

My dad, Dr. A. C. Merrick, was to be installed as the 1941 president of the Chicago Veterinary Medical Association (CVMA) until the "S" hit the fan. In this case, the "S" was Sulfodene.

Dad had developed a medication to treat "hot spots" and "summer itch" in dogs. He tried to patent it under the name "Sulfadene." The U.S. Patent Office refused. Sulfa drugs (containing a sulfonamide) were just coming on the market, and the feds thought the public would assume Sulfadene contained sulfa. Dad assured them the name was to indicate the active ingredients was sulfur, not sulfa, but to no avail. So the name was changed to Sulfodene. Dad thought the product would sell better if his name was on the bottle with a 100% guarantee.

Now it was the AVMA's turn to complain. A professional's name on medications for public sale violated the AVMA code of ethics concerning advertising. Dad was given the choice of dropping his name from the bottle or being kicked out of the AVMA. He countered by offering the AVMA 10% of the profits for whatever they wanted to do with the funds. They refused; therefore, Dad was no longer a member in good standing with the group.

In 1946 the drug company Sharp and Dhome sued Dad because they insisted the name Sulfodene infringed on one of their drugs. The suit was thrown out in the Supreme Court in March of 1951. Years later, the Supreme Court overturned the ban on professional advertising. What a boon for the Yellow Page people!

The following year, Dad developed and marketed Scratchex Flea Powder for Dogs and Cats. This product sold twice as well as Sulfodene. It contained the new insecticide, lindane, which has since been banned in the United States.

Surprisingly, later research discovered that this new product killed more fleas by suffocation than the poison did systemically. Dad's chemist, Jack Verblan, had recommended a new micro-pulverizing technique to prepare the powder. The microsize particles plugged the fleas spiracles—breathing holes along the abdomen—and effectively deprived them of oxygen. Either way, Scratchex sold well all over the country, especially in the South. Dad developed other dermatitis medicines—Ear Canker ointment and shampoos. He received a copyright in 1947 for Dr. Merrick's Dog Food. The dog food venture never fully materialized.

In a few years, as Dad approached retirement, he sold the products to Combe, Inc., the makers of Clearasil and other skin remedies. The sale price would be over two million in today's dollars. The AVMA would be also be a lot richer, too, had they accepted Dad's offer. Sulfodene and Scratchex continue to be widely available in drug stores and pet shops.

In 1993 I received a Christmas card from my cousin, Jerry Menge. He enclosed a full bottle of Sulfodene with the following note: "I opened a box of things I brought back from Ohio and on the bottom was a bottle of Sulfodene. My dad told the story about reading Life Magazine during the war and seeing your dad's ad with a testimony by Edward Menge citing how Sulfodene cured his dog. Then Dad said, 'You know, we did not ever have a pet.' " So much for "Truth in Advertising."

Since his days in Madison when he was starting on a Master's in Bacteriology and Chemistry, Dad was interested in how medications worked. He was especially excited by the effect of phospholipids and fatty acids on the skin. Compounding various ointments, he convinced five bald clients to apply the salve to their pate twice daily. The first month was exciting. Each of the men grew hair—small patchy strands, but real hair. They were convinced they would soon have Sampson's locks. Dad hired professional photographers to track the weekly progress. Alas, despite rubbing and praying, none of the subjects were able to generate more than a few follicles—lonely skaters on the icy domes. A modification of the formula proved equally disappointing.

Dr. Merrick's Sulfodene

By this time Andy had become even more well-known as a veterinarian—and as a veterinary scientist as well, for he developed a number of products for dogs and cats first on his own, and then through his partnership in Brookfield Laboratories. He developed "Dr. Merrick's Sulfodene," a treatment for dog and cat eczema as well as other products such as a scratch powder called "Scratchex" and a flea and fungus soap for dogs. Combe (the makers of products such as Aqua Velva, Grecian Formula, and Brylcreem) bought and further marketed some of Andy's products.

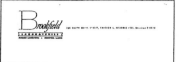

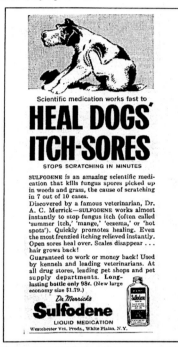

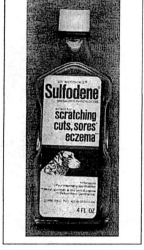

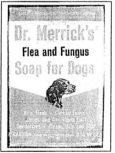

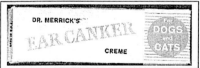

This page is taken from Mari Scheffelin Yamamoto's book, *Margaret Merrick Scheffelin.*

How to Own a Dog and Like It!

I can't believe he did it all. In a matter of eight years Dad went from a large animal practitioner in Iowa, to inspecting meat for Swift and Company in Chicago, to small animal hospital owner and builder. In addition, he found time to invent and market a very successful line of skin medicines for dogs and—believe it or not—to write a book.

Published in 1940, *How to Own a Dog and Like It!* was a huge success and a best seller, partly—maybe mostly—due to the marketing of Swift. Swift had started making canned dog food to appeal to a growing upscale market. They began an advertising campaign in newspapers and magazines like *Life*. The ad promised a copy of Dad's book to everyone mailing in three Pard can labels.

It was during the period of the Napoleonic wars that the Frenchman Nicolas Appert found that food could be preserved against spoilage by first sealing it in an airtight glass jar and then heating it. After many years of careful trials and experiments, he published a book on his process in 1810, which became a great success in many countries. By this time, Appert had set up his own factory to produce and distribute his preserved foods. The French government was so impressed by his discovery that they gave him an award of 12,000 francs.

Although Appert's method clearly worked, nobody knew exactly why at the time. It wasn't until the end of the 19th century that it was found that bacteria were the cause of food spoilage, and that these were destroyed by heating.

Canned horse meat was cheap after World War I, as huge numbers of horses and mules were being replaced by cars and tractors. The growth in canned dog food really shot up in the 1930s, and by 1941, canned dog food represented 91% of the dog food market in the U.S. Swift thought they could convince the public to buy their new "Pard" made with pure beef byproducts—no horse meat. Within a year, Pard was the best selling canned dog food in America.

Canned dog food fell out of favor (and supply) during World War II when a shortage of tin made canning difficult and expensive, and because the horse surplus dried up. By 1946, dry dog food was king once again, and it has remained so to this day.

I remember dad saying he got a lot of help from Chuck Goodall, a good friend and client who raised field Springer Spaniels.

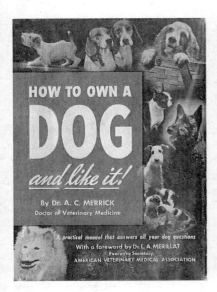

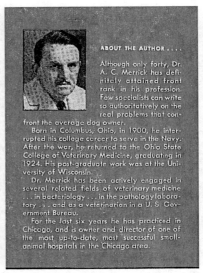

Even by today's standards, *How to Own a Dog and Like It!* is full of very useful information. It contains chapters on selection, training, feeding, home medical treatment, diseases, breeding, and dog laws.

The last paragraph of the book states, "If you make certain that your dog is well mannered and well behaved and follow the laws of your particular section, it will be a welcome member of the community."

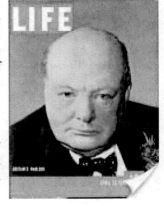

An ad for *How to Own a Dog and Like It!* is on page 6 of the April 29, 1940 issue of *Life*. (Winston Churchill is on the cover.)

How to Own a Dog and Like It!

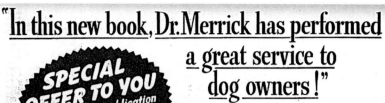

I have a couple of the original books and have purchased them on line for my kids and grandchildren over the years. One of my books was given to me by a client, Mrs. Elaine Tabbert, with this note...

Written inside the jacket were the names of her pet cat, Soot, and her new puppy, Topper. She marked the dates when Topper learned to shake hands and sit.

I wonder if Swift and Company has any more products they would like to promote? Maybe it's time for an update. I can already see my next project on the horizon.

Dr. Merrick,

Thank you for many years of kindness.

You look like your father! I hope your family enjoys the book — I was 13 when I received it. The last paragraph says it all — too bad more people don't realize it.

Thank you again
Elaine Tabbert

"Topper"

Running away from home seems to be a common occurrence in our family. I tried it at the age of eleven. Bill, my son, was only seven when he left for the wild blue yonder. I imagine most kids try it at some time in their youth. Carol had refused to allow Bill to go and visit a neighbor because he had neglected to clean his room and complete his other chores. A loud argument ensued, with Bill threatening to leave home. Carol told him to go to his room and take a nap. Instead, Bill packed a few clothes into a small suitcase and slipped out the front door while Carol was in the kitchen. Thirty minutes later, a neighbor, Helen Estill, found Bill sitting on the curb at the street corner one half block from our house, crying. Helen asked Bill what was the matter. Bill replied, "I'm running away from home." Helen asked, "Then why are you sitting on the street corner?" Bill said, "My mom won't let me cross the street."

My experience with running away was a little different. One year after we moved into our new house in Western Springs, Illinois, Dad brought home a two year old Skye/Cairn Terrier mix, "Topper."

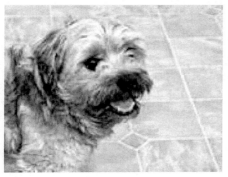

Topper was dropped off at Dad's animal hospital and given up for adoption. In the days before animal shelters were commonplace, veterinarians often served that purpose.

Topper was a wonderful pet. He had many good qualities—affectionate, obedient and relatively short haired. He had only one bad behavior—he messed on the carpet two or three times a week. This may have been the reason he was given up for adoption. In any event, Dad finally issued an ultimatum: "One more mess, and Topper will be put to sleep."

Sure enough, despite our best efforts to get Topper out more frequently, Topper soiled the new carpet again. I knew what that meant. I was old enough to cross the street, so I was headed for my grandparent's farm in Iowa, Topper under my arm.

I had taken the train by myself a number of times before, but with a ticket from Chicago purchased by my parents. I packed a suitcase with a couple changes and a small bag of dry dog food, then walked four blocks to the Burlington railroad station. The station was normally crowded early in the morning with men commuting to offices in downtown Chicago. It was completely empty by 9:30 when I arrived with Topper. All the money I possessed was in my pocket—eight dollars and fifty cents. I asked the stationmaster for a ticket to Gibson, Iowa. He knew immediately what my plan was, so he said it would take a couple of minutes to print a special ticket. While I was sitting on the waiting room bench, the ticket agent called the police, only two blocks away, directly across the tracks. In minutes a cop arrived and the jig was up.

Fortunately for Topper and me, there was hardly any punishment, and Topper was given a new lease on life. Over the next ten years his intestinal control improved greatly. It was helped by confining Topper in the kitchen, with tile floors, when everyone was away from the home and more frequent walks. Lots of praise for doing the "right thing" outside also helped Topper acquire good toilet habits.

Like Bill learned twenty years later, it takes serious planning to successfully run away from home.

Halloween

Americans spend hundreds of billions of dollars each year celebrating holidays, including Christmas, Valentine's Day, Easter, Mother's Day, Father's Day, and Halloween. Let's put this spending into perspective.

According to recent reports from the National Retail Federation, here's how the U.S. holidays rank in terms of spending habits. The figures are estimates for 2006–2007.
- Christmas (Hanukkah and Kwanzaa) $457 Billion / $800 per person
  - Valentine's Day $14 Billion / $116 per person
  - Mother's Day $13.8 Billion / $115 per person
  - Easter $12.6 Billion / $110 per person
  - Father's Day $9 Billion / $100 per person
  - Halloween $5 billion / $60 per person

Note: Thanksgiving spending is impossible to track separately as the weekend is included as the beginning of winter holiday spending.

Comparing to what Americans give to charities, American citizens donated $260 billion to charities of all kinds in 2005, the latest year for which figures are available. (Source: The Giving USA Foundation.)

The following was excerpted from CanWest Media Works Publications Inc.: "Halloween has evolved from an end-of-harvest holiday on the eve of All Saints Day to one of the top 10 spending sprees after Christmas, Valentine's Day, Easter, Mother's Day and Father's Day."

As I recall, my parents spent less than a dollar for giveaway candy and nothing for costumes when I was young. After he retired, Dad gave away shiny, new dimes.

Unlike the others, Halloween is not a gift-giving occasion, so the spending is purely for fun. According to a United States survey by the National Retail Federation, Halloween celebrants will spend an average of $65 U.S. per person this year, adding up to a total of $5.1 billion, including $1.8 billion on costumes and $1.5 billion on candy.

Some take umbrage at the commercialization of Halloween and lament the loss of its origins and ancient traditions."

"We'll be having none of that pumpkin or trick-or-treat rubbish," said Jack Ferguson, the man in charge of Halloween events at Scone Palace in Perthshire, Scotland, who derided the practice of going door-to-door for candy as representing "American big business and rampant consumerism."

Instead, children will be led around the grounds of the palace by someone dressed as the ghost of a Jacobite soldier, recalling the Jacobite Rebellions of 1715 and 1745 that failed to restore the House of Stuart to the thrones of Scotland and England.

What has that got to do with Halloween? Not nearly as much as the Celtic festival of Samhain (pronounced "sow-in"), marking the coming of the new year. As one year blurred into another, the Celts believed, the boundary between the living and the dead became less distinct, leading relatives long passed, and evil spirits, to return to the living.

The deceased relatives were carried back to their resting places in carved gourds, with candles lighting the way to ward off evil spirits. This tradition can be traced to an Irish myth about a man called Stingy Jack.

The Irish began to refer to the ghostly Stingy Jack as Jack of the Lantern, or Jack O'Lantern, and carved scary faces in turnips and potatoes to place in windows and near doors to frighten him away. Immigrants brought this custom to the New World and found that pumpkins, indigenous to North America, made excellent Jack O'Lanterns.

The reason we continue to carve pumpkins on Halloween then is not to invoke evil spirits, but rather to keep them away. This should put to rest the notion that Halloween is a demonic festival that celebrates witchcraft and the macabre.

While its association with horror and gore is a modern twist on Halloween, the ghoulish and gross now seem as integral a part of the holiday as apple bobbing, an age-old party favorite that has its roots in the Roman conquest of the Celts around 70 AD. The Romans incorporated into the Celtic tradition their own harvest festival, Pomona, named after the goddess of fruit, who is symbolized by an apple.

Now that Halloween has been demystified and undemonized, we can all enjoy the costumes and candy without fear. But beware of Stingy Jack.

The Veterinarian's Son   Halloween   67

Long before Halloween was an excuse to dress up the kids and go begging for treats, Halloween was celebrated as a time for teenagers—mainly boys—to play tricks on unsuspecting neighbors. As mentioned in a previous story, Uncle Wendell had the all-time trick by placing Grandpa's buggy on the church roof. We couldn't top that, but we had four great tricks—two common and two unusual.

Pin the Door Bell

This involved finding a house with the porch light off, but the inner house lights lit. Then, as now, people who are willing to pass out treats, left their porch light on. We were after the Scrooges. Nearly all doorbells were alike at that time—a two inch round metal plate with a push button in the middle. By inserting a bent straight pin in the side of the button—the doorbell would ring constantly until the pin was removed. After placing the pin, one runs across the street to survey the owner's frustration.

Set (Stick) a Horn

Most autos in the early '40s had round steering wheels with a central horn. Most autos were parked on the street or in the owner's driveway and were unlocked. The prank involved finding a two-foot-long flexible stick, bending it under both sides of the steering wheel, sliding it gently up and over the horn. The honking lasted until the stick was removed or the battery ran down. Here again, the fun was watching the owner realize it's his car making the ruckus and his frustration that followed.

The Invisible Rope Pulling, Tug of War Contest

Most of the time Phil and I went out with two or three other youngsters, ten to fourteen years old. This trick involved placing two or three teens on either side of a quiet but well lit street. As a car approached within two hundred feet all of the kids would shout in unison, "One, Two, Three—PULL!" Both groups would pretend to be engaged in a "Tug of War" contest. Each side pulling and straining backwards as if in a classic struggle, pulling the invisible rope as hard as we could. If we succeeded in stopping or markedly slowing the car, we figured it was a good trick.

Trap the Car Between the Leaves

This trick involves careful planning and execution. A long dimly light street is selected. Two large piles of leaves are placed on either side of the street at least 200 feet apart. Each pile is pushed toward the center of the street leaving a center gap of 10 to 12 feet to allow a car to enter the trap. The leaves are dosed with a small amount of gasoline. After the car passes the first opening, the far piles are pushed to the center and set on fire. Before the driver realizes what is happening, we close the second pile and set it on fire. Then run, run, run. Within a few minutes, the fires are out and the prisoner is released.

A conversation with my brother, Phil, reminded me of another diabolical Halloween escapade:

Flaming Paper Bag

This required identifying a villain—the neighborhood grouch. He never handed out treats. His porch light would be off, but he could be seen reading in his living room. We filled a paper bag full of dog poop—preferably moist, not dry—set the bag on fire, ring the doorbell or set it off with a pin and then run to the other side of the street. The unsuspecting victim opens the door and stomps on the fire. We thought it was hilarious at the time.

Sixty years ago, tricks were really tricks. Nothing really malicious was intended. I imagine we would be arrested and incarcerated for that foolishness today.

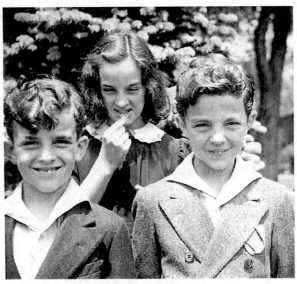

"Three little angels"
Phil, Marg, and John • 1940
Mari Yamamoto's book, 6-15-11

Why I Became a Vet

It never dawned on me as a young child that I would become anything other than a vet. Some of my earliest memories are of the living quarters attached to Dad's storefront animal hospital on Ogden Avenue in Brookfield, Illinois. From the age of five, I was intimately acquainted with veterinary medicine, either in the animal hospital or on my grandparents' farm in central Iowa.

When I enrolled in college in the fall of 1946, I was not yet 17. Most of my male classmates were veterans of WWII, five to ten years my elder. After cleaning kennels for the last few years, the last thing I desired was to continue in this messy profession. I was talented in math and enjoyed history and economics, so why not a degree in business? My first semester away from home was too much fun and not enough studying. I barley managed a C average. It was decided, mutually by Mom, Dad, and me, that I was not ready to strike out on my own. I enrolled in the local junior college whose semester started in 3 weeks. To pick up a little spending money, I took a job at Breen's, our local laundry and clients of Dad's.

Working in Breen's Laundry was a shock to my system—January cold outside, July heat and humidity inside—loading huge baskets of commercial/institutional laundry from washer to dryer to mangle to fold to packaging. Two ten-minute breaks and 30 minutes for lunch. Cleaning kennels and grooming dogs was a snap compared to this job. While the other, mostly white, employees were kind and considerate, they were next to illiterate and spoke a language I did not understand. What a difference from the clients in the animal hospital. Almost without exception, Dad's clients were well-spoken and engaging, and his patients were happy-go-lucky animals. The contrast was unavoidable. I gave my notice after two weeks.

Dad was not a great parent when it came to communication. We had very few "heart to heart" talks. I can only recall a couple of times playing catch or walks in a park. Working 60 to 70 hours a week left little time for bonding with his offspring. Only 3½ years separate my older sister, Margaret, and my younger brother, Phil. The early nexus we established was the glue that held us together for over 75 years.

Mom was the nurturer; Dad the disciplinarian. My brother and I were very happy when he switched from a straight razor to an electric—no more razor strop to the behind when we misbehaved. Kids today don't have any idea how lucky they are that straight razors have gone the way of buggy whips.

After dinner one evening, when I was complaining about the horrible working conditions in the laundry, Dad set me straight. He said, "Johnny, I want you to think seriously about veterinary medicine. Once you become a doctor, you will be one for life. People will show you respect, restaurants will find you a good table when they are overbooked and you will be given the benefit of the doubt until proven unworthy. You can't put a price on respect. After you get your degree, you can do anything you like—become a businessman, teacher, or banker—but you will always be 'Dr. Merrick.' " The light bulb went off in my head. I changed my course work to pre-vet and never looked back. It didn't hurt that Carol, my steady girl, agreed and encouraged my decision. Fortunately, my grades went from C's to mostly A's without the distractions of college life away from home.

> UNIVERSITY OF ILLINOIS
> COLLEGE OF VETERINARY MEDICINE
> URBANA, ILLINOIS
>
> August 13, 1949
>
> Mr. John Merrick
> 9115 Ogden Avenue
> Brookfield, Illinois
>
> Dear Mr. Merrick:
>
> This will confirm telephone call from your father advising of your interest in the student assistantship beginning September 1. I am passing this information on to Dr. J. O. Alberts of the Department of Veterinary Pathology and Hygiene, and unless you are informed to the contrary please report for work September 1.
>
> I am sure you appreciate that there is a probation period in connection with all assignments at the University.
>
> Very truly yours,
>
> Robert Graham
> Dean

By taking my elective pre-vet courses in economics, history and accounting, I was able to pursue those interests while building up the science credits to apply to vet school two years later. My grade point by that time was a respectable, but not great—4.4 where A = 5.0. I was not accepted into the first or second class at the University of Illinois vet school. The policy was only male veterans were given the few available slots—28 in the first two classes. Four of us young, non-veterans were given jobs in the vet school. We all had just missed the final cut. The story of finally achieving our goal will be told at another time. It involves a much earlier Illinois governor and the political dealing which goes around without end. My year in the autopsy lab was the best practical learning experience in vet school.

Quiz Kid? Margaret, Not Me!

It wasn't as bad as being identified as a Jew in Hitler's Germany, but the sign on our front door announced to the world "This Property is under Quarantine—Poliomyelitis" in large red letters. People using the sidewalk to go to town would cross the street to avoid coming close. My older sister Margaret Ann had been diagnosed with polio in the summer of 1941, soon after she had graduated from the eighth grade.

Until 1955, when the Salk vaccine was introduced, polio was considered the most frightening public health problem of the post-war United States

The field trial set up to test the Salk vaccine was, according to O'Neill, "the most elaborate program of its kind in history, involving 20,000 physicians and public health officers, 64,000 school personnel, and 220,000 volunteers." Over 1,800,000 school children took part in the trial. When news of the vaccine's success was made public on April 12, 1955, Salk was hailed as a "miracle worker," and the day "almost became a national holiday." His sole focus had been to develop a safe and effective vaccine as rapidly as possible, with no interest in personal profit. When he was asked in a televised interview who owned the patent to the vaccine, Salk replied, "There is no patent. Could you patent the sun?" In today's world, I wouldn't be surprised if someone tried.

Symptoms of polio may be major (paralytic) or minor. Most symptoms in younger children resemble an attack of the flu lasting a few days—fever, headache, vomiting and sore throat a few days after exposure. Major poliomyelitis usually strikes older children and adults. Symptoms may include aseptic meningitis (inflammation of the lining of the brain), deep muscle pain, hyperesthesia (abnormal sensitivity of the skin), paresthesia (abnormal skin sensations—burning or prickling), myelitis (inflammation of the muscle), urinary retention, and muscle spasms. This indeed was a dreaded disease.

Margaret woke up and fell on her face attempting to get out of bed. The active tomboy was suddenly transported into another world. Margaret was blamed for closing every public pool within 15 miles of our house. As kids, we loved to go swimming any day we could get away from household chores. In the two weeks prior to Margaret's illness, public nurses found out we had visited the three popular pools in surrounding towns. Word spread among our friends, it's all Margret's fault we can't go swimming this summer.

In her book detailing the amazing life of her mother, Dr. Marianna Scheffelin Yamamoto describes Margaret's remarkable recuperation and triumph as follows:

Margaret Merrick Scheffelin

Quiz Kid

In the summer of 1942, at the end of her freshman year in high school, and a year after she contracted polio, a new interest came to Margaret. A staff member of the *Quiz Kids* radio show called to ask if Margaret would apply to be a panelist on the program. The program was looking for girls, and one of the staffers involved in the "girlpower" search was Joan Brown. Joan had been a counselor at a camp that Margaret had attended, and remembered Margaret at nine as "The Demon Reader." Joan could only remember Margaret's first name, but through sleuthing found her. Margaret auditioned, and came on the program in July 1942 as the 111th Quiz Kid, making forty-five appearances until her 16th birthday (at which age Kids "graduated" from the program).

The *Quiz Kids* began in June 1940 as a half-hour radio program in which Quizmaster Joe Kelly asked five panelists, all under sixteen, to answer questions. Much of the show's interest and appeal was in the spontaneity with which the Kids answered these questions. The top three scorers were invited to come back the next week, and the contestants earned a $100 bond each time they appeared.

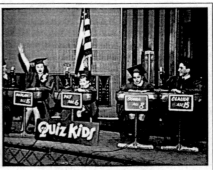

Margaret on the *Quiz Kids*

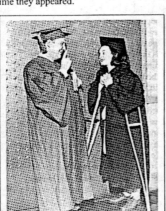

Quizmaster Joe Kelly & Margaret

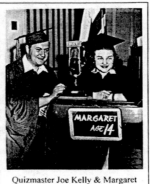

Quizmaster Joe Kelly & Margaret

Career counseling left a lot to be desired in the 1940s. Margaret was told, "Most women marry so it doesn't matter if they go to college or not. In your case, marriage is doubtful, so I don't know what you will do." Andy and Dorothy would not accept this pessimistic prediction and took Margaret to the Illinois Institute of Technology for vocational testing. This was a new field and used hundreds of interviews to analyze the likes and dislikes of people in 100 different occupations. One was given a score on the most likely and unlikely occupations of interest.

Many famous people were involved with the show, and the Kids were hosted by local and national leaders and personalities—Hollywood stars on the west coast, political leaders on the east coast, and industrial leaders between the two oceans. The show sometimes had Guest Quizmasters including entertainers such as Bing Crosby, Ed Sullivan, and Bob Hope. Guest Quizmaster Bob Hope had the distinction of "stumping" the Kids. He asked them who John Arthur Gordon was, and when no one knew, said, "You kids aren't so smart as I thought you were—he's my uncle who runs a hardware store in Pomona!"

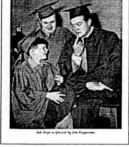

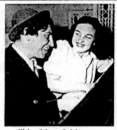

Chico Marx & Margaret playing duets

Chico Marx came on the show, and during the program talked about Margaret. Chico said, "Joe, there were a lot of things I thought I wanted to say tonight. But this afternoon I talked to some of the parents of these fine children and I'd like to tell just the story of one Quiz Kid." He talked about what an active life Margaret had led before being stricken with polio, playing all kinds of sports and winning medals. He said that the wonderful thing about Margaret was that she hadn't let polio get her down, but instead had turned to the things she *could* do—books and music and things like that, and built a new life for herself, and in fact had become one of the star Quiz Kid students. Chico said, "Joe, it's been an inspiration to meet a kid like that. And Margaret, you keep up that wonderful spirit of yours, and it won't be long before you're winning medals again!"

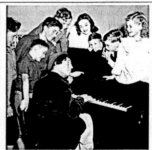

Chico Marx with Quiz Kids (Margaret is behind the piano.)

A number of Quiz Kids went on to make significant accomplishments. James Watson won the Nobel prize as one of the co-discoverers of the structure of DNA. Harve Bennett [Fischman] became a Hollywood producer, whose credits included several of the *Star Trek* movies, and TV shows such as *The Six Million Dollar Man, The Bionic Woman, The Fugitive*, and *The Mod Squad*. Richard Williams became a diplomat, opening the first American consulate in mainland China since the 1940s and serving as U.S. Ambassador to Mongolia. Vanessa Brown became a Hollywood star, as shown in a publicity shot for *Tarzan and the Slave Girl* (1950).

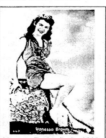

Vanessa Brown in the 1950 *Tarzan and the Slave Girl*

Margaret's report was entitled, "The Too Many Aptitude Woman." It was very appropriate. It also detailed her interest in science, engineering, and possibly architecture. After two years at Ohio State University in Columbus, Ohio, Margaret and fellow student Edward Scheffelin were married. Margaret's career was put on hold when she gave birth to the first of their eight children. Pretty good for a gal who was told she would likely never marry.

After marriage, Marg and Edward (Scheff) found it difficult to support a family and remain in college. Scheff reupped in the Air Force. There was no need for bombardiers, unfortunately, so he dropped from a 1st Lieutenant to a Staff Sergeant. Over the next 20 years Margaret managed to complete her Bachelors and Masters and receive a PhD in Special Education and Psychology on October 16, 1967, from the University of Illinois.

In 1968 Margaret started work as Assistant Professor in the Department of Special Education at California State University, Los Angeles. She was soon offered a position with the California State Department of Education. She developed the California Master Plan for Special Education, viewed as a model for the nation and the federal evaluation plan was later based on it. Over the next 25 years, Margaret served on peer review panels for the U.S. Department of Education's grant and contracts, and cooperative agreements.

In 1980, Margaret was awarded a Fulbright Scholarship, taking a six month leave of absence to conduct research on the employability of persons who are both deaf and blind at the University of Hamburg. Fortunately, Margaret's oldest daughter, Susan, had married a German National and both were teaching school in a suburb of Hamburg. For many years afterward, Margaret would attend the Annual Seminar of the Fulbright Commission, often giving lectures in German.

After some 30 years in the Air Force, Scheff retired soon after their move to California. This enabled him to become the role model for future "house husbands."

All eight of Marg's children are college graduates—many with advanced degrees—attesting to their parents' value of and commitment to education. Indeed, all of their fifteen grandchildren are on the same path.

Margaret passed to her eternal reward in July of 2009 after 62 years of "Wedded Bliss." At a family reunion in 2008, I told the assembled throng how much I and brother, Phil, enjoyed being with Margaret as she was recovering in the 1940s. Movies were the main attraction on Friday or Saturday nights, since there was no TV yet. There were frequently very long lines for the evening feature. Margaret and anyone helping her were always escorted to the head of the line. Margaret managed to limp a little more until we got into the darkened theatre.

After the Quiz Kids program closed, Professor Joe Kelly traded his cap and gown for a Coonskin Cap to host The Totem Club, an afternoon children's show on WTTW public TV in Chicago. Dad was featured weekly, bringing various animals to show and tell. My sister, Sue, was shown as his receptionist. I appeared frequently as his assistant in the mid fifties.

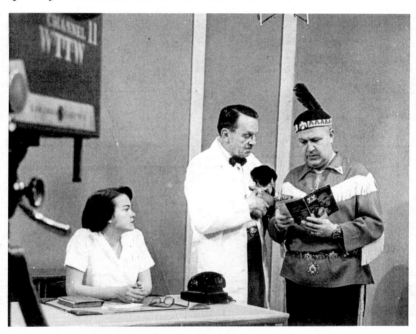

Susie Merrick, Andy Merrick, Jolly Joe Kelly
"Totem Club" • WTTW-TV • 1953

The "O House"

The smell from Mrs. Offenbacher's kitchen permeated the whole house. "She must fry everything in bacon fat," I thought. Both she and her husband looked as if their diet consisted of nothing but fried food. Samuel and Myrtle were in their 50s, unkempt and 40 pounds overweight. I doubt if they could support themselves if not for the student renters. The furniture was all "Goodwill." The bare floors were relatively clean. Two blocks from the east side of campus of the University of Illinois in Urbana, "O House" was typical of most students housing. Once a stately three story home of a well-to-do merchant, it had been remodeled into six study rooms on the first and second floors with an unheated, dormitory-style sleeping area on the third floor. The year was 1948. I had completed two years at Lyons Township Junior College and had just enrolled in the University of Illinois pre-vet program. The junior college did not offer many of the pre-vet required courses. Enrolling late—mid September for fall term, which began in the first week of October—meant campus housing was scarce. Colleges were overflowing with veterans of World War II, aided by the passage of the GI Bill. Mom drove down with me to assist in the search. The "O House" was the best we could find.

My roommate was a young Japanese/American (Nisei) from the south side of Chicago. Gene Shinosaki was to have a profound influence on my life. I would have never have passed physics without Gene's assistance. A second-year electrical engineering student, physics seemed easy for Gene, and he was able give me a rudimentary idea of the concepts. With his tutoring, I managed to get a C.

During the second week of the semester, I decided to write letters to Carol and my folks. I searched high and low but could not find any 3¢ stamps. I asked Gene if he had any. He replied, "Just a minute," and went out into the front hall. When he returned a short time later, Gene handed me ten stamps. I was shocked. I asked him, "Gene, where did you get these stamps?" He replied, "It was nothing." Then it hit me. Gene had walked two blocks to the corner drug store to purchase stamps. He wouldn't take any payment, saying, "You can do me a favor sometime." Sixty years later, I still am grateful to Gene for this lesson in unselfishness. To put the scene in context, America had just finished fighting a four-year war with Japan. Many of Gene's relatives had been interned in relocation centers (concentration camps) during the war. Other Nisei were members of the "Most Decorated Unit" in the U.S. Army during the war against Japan.

Previous renters had left many of their textbooks to be used by future students. Then it was not the now-common practice of ordering each new class to purchase ever more expensive textbooks. I remember using a book with the previous owners name inside, "Orange Apple." Les Bravermann, a junior, said, "I knew Orange. If you think that's funny, his two sisters were named May Apple and June Apple."

Growing up on my grandparent's farm in Iowa and the western suburbs of Chicago, my experience with Jews and "Orientals" (now called "Asians") was very limited. Les Bravermann was different from anyone I'd ever encountered. He was loud, self assured, articulate, and smart. Les was in business school and worked part time in the U. of I. athletic department. In those days, the athletic publicity department consisted of a director, a secretary, and Les, the part-time gofer. It was Les's job to hand out mimeographed press releases to visiting reporters, prepare halftime stats, and do any odd jobs required or requested.

Sixty years later, my granddaughter, Cc Robinson, had the same job with the athletic department of the University of Georgia. Working toward a Master's Degree in Journalism and Mass Communication, Cc was one of 60 people the UGA employed to send out information on the UGA "Dawgs" athletic teams. After graduating *cum laude* in May, 2011, Cc currently works for ESPN.

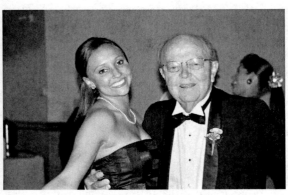

Cc Robinson and John Merrick • 2010

I was considering joining a fraternity. They had a winter dance scheduled for the week after Thanksgiving, and I was invited to bring a date. Carol, my steady date for the last two years, was a high school senior. She was my only choice for the prom, but there was a problem. Carol's parents would not allow her to travel the 120 miles to Champaign/Urbana on the train alone, but they would allow her to go if accompanied by a friend. Dee Hebert accepted Carol's offer, and it fell to me to find her a date. Les was a logical choice, and he was willing. He even arranged for Carol and Dee to spend the weekend at a girl's dorm. A very enjoyable time was had by everyone.

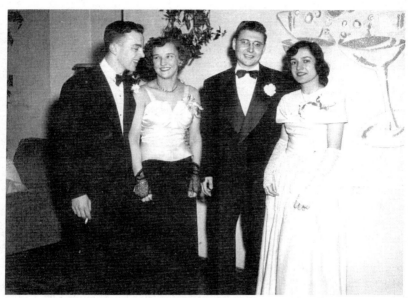

John Merrick, Carol Hough, Les Braverman, Delores Hebert
Christmas Formal • 1948

As I was preparing to go home to Western Springs for Christmas vacation, Les asked if Carol and I would like to go with him to Madison, Wisconsin during the school vacation time between Christmas and New Year. Illinois was playing Wisconsin in basketball and competing in gymnastics. Les and I would stay with friends at a men's dorm and Carol would stay at a nearby women's dorm. To my great surprise, Carol's parents agreed. The fact that Carol intended to major in physical education in college may have influenced their decision.

Carol and I met Les at the Northwestern train station in downtown Chicago for the four-hour ride to Madison. After checking into our rooms, we headed to dinner and the basketball game, to be followed by a dance at the women's dorm where Carol was staying. The basketball game was preceded by the gymnastics meet. They were both close and exciting, but I don't remember who won.

Arriving back at Carol's temporary residence, we entered a large foyer, typical of many of the fraternities and sororities. In the spacious living room were many couches and chairs. Each was occupied by a couple in various forms of embrace and love making. At the time, the rule at most college houses was "two feet on the floor." In other words, both individuals must have at least one foot on the floor at all times. This rule was enforced by an ever watchful housemother.

The "shock and awe" of the evening for Carol and myself was the presence of interracial coupling. At least 30 percent of the couples were of mixed race, with both sexes about equal—white guys with black girls and black guys with white girls. The only ones staring were Carol and I. Les said, "Remember, this is Madison, Wisconsin, the most liberal campus in the nation. Where else could an 18-year-old order a beer in the University Union?" I made a mental note: "Don't mention this to Carol's parents."

The Sunday morning train to Chicago was six hours late due to a huge winter storm in the northern Rockies. Instead of arriving at 6 PM, it was well after midnight when two exhausted teens walked the two blocks from the Northwestern to the Union Station.

Since Carol's dad had to work the next day, it was decided we could wait for the first commuter train to Western Springs leaving the downtown Chicago Union Station at 5 AM. Mom picked us up at the Western Springs' suburban station. We arrived home and collapsed.

Les got to ride back to Champaign with the team and missed all the excitement. When I spoke to Les about our trip, I asked him to prepare me for any other surprises in the future. He said something like, "It's time you and Carol learn how the rest of the world works."

I'm still learning.

Wedding Day

Weddings are supposed to be hectic; ours wasn't. Thanks to the planning of both parents, Carol and I enjoyed a relatively stress-free wedding day.

My mother had helped me buy a "going away suit." We journeyed to downtown Chicago's Hicky Freeman's—one of the better men's stores of the day—to select my outfit. Although perfectly tailored, it was, unfortunately, made of unlined wool—great for cold weather, but hot and itchy in summer. And August 26, 1950, turned out very hot.

Carol described her outfit in our wedding gift scrapbook: "My going away outfit was a checked suit with matching hat with brown accessories. It was a very dressy suit, so the accessories were plain. Mom gave me a new ?? set at Helen and Dee's shower for me. It was made of satin and lace with white satin house slippers. The lace and satin were the same material used in my wedding dress. My trousseau included numerous clothes and shoes, so it would be impossible to record them all. However, everything was beautiful and much appreciated." I'll leave it to the girls to imagine what Carol was writing about.

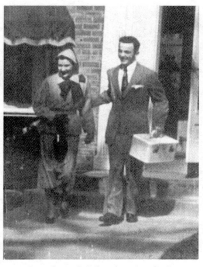

Carol and John begin their honeymoon • August 26, 1950

Carol's dad, Bill Hough, though disappointed in our decision to marry and thereby disrupt Carol's college plans, made the best he could of the situation. He began by offering Carol a wedding present of $2,000 if we would elope. That would be equal to $25,000 today. Carol refused on the spot. She didn't give it a moment's thought. I imagine most brides—even today—would make the same choice. So, the planning began soon after our engagement was announced at Christmas, 1949.

I remember the engagement well because it cost me my very first car. I was in school at the U. of I. part-time and working full-time at the vet school, waiting to be accepted the following year. My 1940 Chevy was my pride and joy. It carried me from Champaign, Illinois, 153 miles due east to Bloomington, Indiana, where Carol was attending Indiana University. When I asked Carol to marry me, I had no ring to seal the deal. In speaking to Carol's parents, they counseled us against an early marriage. We countered that if we didn't, they might be grandparents sooner rather than later. We had been "going steady" for over three years by then, and "The Pill" was still 15 years in the future. I promised Carol that I would deliver a ring as soon as I could sell my only source of cash—my car.

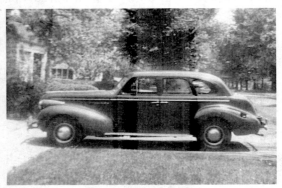

John's 1940 Chevy
Carol's Engagement and Wedding Rings

Soon after Carol transferred to the U. of I., we went to the best jewelry store in Champaign to pick out Carol's engagement and wedding rings. She also picked out mine. I had sold my Chevy for $225. Carol's rings cost $240. The jeweler remarked what a good investment I had made. I thought he meant Carol, but he probably meant the rings. Again quoting Carol from her account of the giving and getting of the engagement ring:

> The living room of the house at 3947 Clausen Avenue was lighted by the Christmas tree lights. The snow outside blanketed the ground in a beautiful white. The embers in the fireplace warmed the room. That was the setting where Carol Hough received her beautiful engagement ring from the most wonderful man in the world, Johnny Merrick, on Christmas Eve, 1949.
>
> Their first date was on April 27, 1946—the proposal on August 18, 1949. On their first date Carol was fourteen and Johnny was sixteen.

Immediately following the receiving of my ring, Johnny and I were congratulated by Mom and Dad Hough and my brother, Harry and his friend Ken Zagilski. Even though it was late at night, everyone in the Hough household was quite awake and really happy.

The next day was Christmas. Mom had the Merricks over for Christmas dinner. After dinner I heard a record playing, "I Love You Truly." Since we had no record player, I couldn't imagine where it was coming from. Mrs. Merrick, Doc, Phil, and Suzie had bought that record for me so we would never forget the night we got engaged.

Wedding days, then and now, are often preceeded by bachelor and bachelorette parties. Mine was held at my parents' home. I don't recall much except there was a present from my brother, Phil, of a large black bowling ball with a chain attached. He proceeded to affix the whole thing to my ankle. Dinner, drinking, and cards followed. I believe most of the group later went to Cicero to visit the strip shows, but I went to bed. I have no recollection about Carol's "bachelorette party," but I'm sure the girls were much better behaved.

Our wedding ceremony was held in St. Francis Catholic Church in the neighboring town of La Grange, Illinois. Both families were members of the parish. We had received premarital counseling from Father O'Hara, the assistant pastor. We felt that, being younger, he would be a better counselor than the Pastor, Father O'Connor. Over 250 attended the 10 AM ceremony in the cavernous building. I noticed that Father O'Hara said something to Carol before giving her communion. At the time I hardly paid any attention. Only 20 years later, at around the start of the women's lib movement, did Carol reveal his conversation. Father O'Hara said, "Carol, this is the one and only time in your life where you will be first. John is, and always be, 'the head of the house'." I really believe that started Carol on her quest to prove she was as good as any man and due the same respect. She was able to keep up with the men in tennis, golf, table tennis, and skiing. She was the only person in our family to letter in college, earning her "W" on the University of Wisconsin tennis team at the age of 41.

Following the wedding ceremony, the wedding party, relatives and out of town guests—approximately 120—were invited to a sit-down brunch at Frieden's, one of the nicer restaurants in the area. Their property included two acres of woods and flowers—perfect for wedding party pictures. We then had three hours to go home, relax, and change into our "going away" clothes before the reception at Carol's house. Bill Hough was a wonderful gardener, and Madeline was especially proud of her home, so the place sparkled with food, flowers, and champagne.

We posed for more photos with guests and family while awaiting the 5 o'clock hour, when we were allowed to leave for the drive to the Palmer House in downtown Chicago to spend our wedding night. The wedding party had decorated Mom's new Chevy Coupe with ribbons and tied tin cans to the rear bumper. We left the house in a shower of rice and, followed by half a dozen honking cars, sped away. Within a mile down Ogden Avenue, a police car stopped the procession. He pretended to give us a lecture about the perils of speeding, but he actually just advised us to slow down. He assured us that we need not be in a hurry, because he intended to lecture the group for the next five minutes, giving us plenty of time to make our escape.

We had previously packed the Chevy with all the luggage for our three-week honeymoon to Yellowstone, Salt Lake, and Pike's Peak. Carol advised me to have a small suitcase ready to bring into the hotel to avoid unpacking everything. Having never spent a night in a hotel, I was unsure of all protocol. I have never figured out why, but we had made dinner reservations in the Empire Room, the upscale dining and entertainment room ten floors below our twelfth floor room. We were the only patrons in the cavernous area at 6:00 PM. Neither of us were hungry, but we ordered something, ate half, and asked for the check. Neither of us had our mind on food at the time. The waiter asked, "Aren't you staying for the show?" I replied that we'd seen it last week with many in the wedding party. He gave me the look that said, "I wouldn't stay for the show either, if I had a chance to go to bed with that beautiful girl."

So finally, with all the formalities accomplished, we headed for our room, number 1214. Carol excused herself to the bathroom to change into the beautiful negligee she had purchased for the occasion. I opened my suitcase to find I had forgotten to pack any pajamas. So Carol was astonished to find me waiting in my skivvies. Since that experience, I've found sleeping in the nude was the way to go. If I woke up at an unusual hour and Carol was in the mood, there were less clothes to remove before she changed her mind.

In 1950 the rooms in the Palmer House were not air conditioned. To provide ventilation, windows could be opened. No screens were provided above the third floor. I opened the windows as soon as we entered. As luck would have it, the neighboring hotel directly across the street was the site of the National American Legion Convention. The noise from the parties carried through the night air. Fortunately, it didn't keep Carol and me from a good night's "sleep."

When I went to pay the bill the following morning, I discovered I had left my wallet at home when changing clothes. I had packed my checkbook, so I was able to settle our hotel bill. Now instead of heading for Yellowstone, Western Springs was our first stop. Since we would be stopping at my house for my wallet, Carol insisted we pay a courtesy call to her folks and thank them for their gracious hospitality. My mom thought the events of the wedding night were laughable. Carol's dad could hardly look us in the eye.

On the front seat of the car, Carol found an envelope with her name on it. Inside was this note from my mother:

> My Dear Daughter —
> I always think a girl should have some money of her own —
> Here's a start —
> Love —
> Mama Merrick

Inside the note Mom had tucked a $100 bill. I still treasure the note. It's pasted inside the "wedding gift" book that lists the 154 presents we received from friends and family.

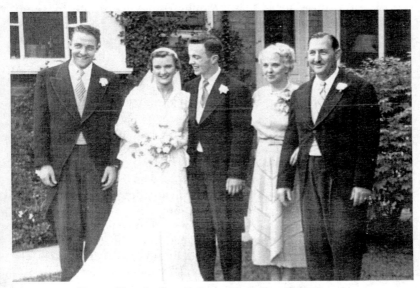

Harry Hough, Carol, John, Madeline, Bill Hough

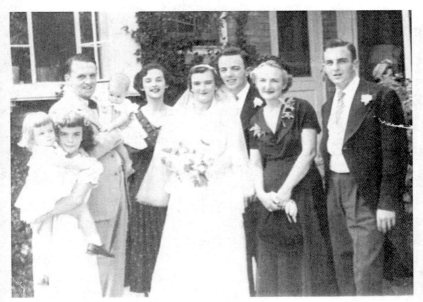

Sue Merrick holding Sue Scheffelin, Andy holding Katherine Scheffelin, Andrea Scheffelin, Carol, John, Dorothy, Phil

Peppermint Schnapps & Timing Gears

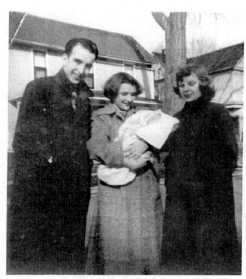

Ron Marshall, Carol, Dorothy, Carol Berge Marshall • Urbana, Ill. • Feb. 1952

Four friends in my '36 Chevy, homeward bound from Champaign, Illinois, to suburban Chicago for our 1950 Christmas break. Carol and I were in front; Ron Marshall and Carol Berge snuggled in back. Carol and I had been married four months. Ron and Carol were best friends with whom we frequently double-dated. They had been in our wedding party and were our respective college dorm roommates prior to our wedding. Their wedding was set for the summer of 1951.

The weather on this Saturday noon was clear but threatening to snow. Chicago had already experienced six inches in the last 24 hours. It was a straight shot up highway 45 thru Rantoul, Paxton, Kankakee, Frankfort, and finally Orland Park, to La Grange. It was a total of 130 miles—usually a two-hour drive. What could go wrong? We sang college songs all the way. At least, until the engine suddenly stopped. I knew we had gas, as I had purchased eight gallons for $2.00 this very morning. Ron said something like, "Don't worry, I'll handle this in a minute." Ron was a self-proclaimed mechanic. His only qualifications were his junior status in electrical engineering and a frequent visitor to junk yards for spare parts. Those prerequisites were not enough to help him solve our engine problem. Frequent attempts to start the engine were futile. Pushing the car and popping the clutch were unsuccessful. "We'll have to hitch to the next town for help," Ron said. I volunteered to go on ahead while Ron stayed in the car with the girls.

I had only walked 200 yards when a farmer with a pickup truck stopped and guessed our dilemma after seeing the car pulled over on the shoulder. He told me the next town was Lodi. I'd never heard of it. It turned out to be a "one-horse" town. Better yet, make that a two-tavern town. There was not a service station or garage in sight. I got off at the first tavern and inquired about a mechanic. The bartender replied, "Mike's Auto Repair is right

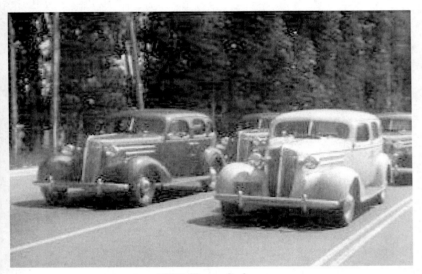

1936 Chevy Sedans

across the Illinois Central tracks." We were in luck, I hoped. Mike allowed he'd be happy to tow my car in and take a look. With that we were off in his truck down route 45—two miles in less than two minutes. In a flash, Mike had my Chevy hooked to the back of his truck and back to his shop—again at around 60 mph.

Mike said it would take awhile to diagnose the problem, so we walked back across the IC tracks to get something to eat at the Dew Drop Inn and Tavern. Unfortunately, George, the bartender, informed us the last restaurant closed about six months ago and he did not have a license to sell food. He did have peanuts and potato chips. We ordered both and decided to wash it down with peppermint schnapps and beer. Within thirty minutes, Mike showed up with good news and bad news. The good news was Mike found the problem and could easily repair the broken timing gear. The bad news: He doesn't have one in stock, and it can't be delivered from Kankakee until Monday morning. My car would be ready after 1:00 PM—almost 48 hours in the future. What to do?

My father was working until 6 PM, Carol's dad until 5. Bill Hough said he could take off a little early and pick us up about 6:00 PM. We settled in for a long wait. Two or three more schnapps and beers later, Bill Hough showed up in an angry mood. The fact that we were all half drunk added to his frustration. Ron, Carol Berge, and I piled into the back seat, leaving Carol to sit between her parents in the front. Two upset parents against one tipsy daughter—an unfair fight. The back seat riders missed all the dialogue as we were sound asleep in five minutes. Adding insult to injury, it snowed all the way to Carol Berge's house in Clarendon Hills, just 10 miles west of ours. As the car stopped and Carol Berge started to exit Ron loudly proclaimed, "Wait my princess, your Sir Walter Raleigh will place his cape over the snow to allow you safe passage." With that, Ron opened the rear door and slipped/fell into a three-foot snowdrift—the perfect ending to a very eventful day.

Associate Vets

Over the years, my dad, A.C. Merrick, DVM, hired many young associate veterinarians, including me, but never more than one at a time. The following stories illustrate the notion that one never fully knows the company one keeps, especially the extraordinary deeds and accomplishments to follow from those who have chosen the animal care profession as their own.

Les Fisher, DVM, later to become the famous television zoo vet, worked for my dad during the summer months before graduating from Iowa State University in 1943. During a stint in the Army from 1943 to 1945, Les's duties included care of General Patton's beloved horse, Willy, and the 2,000 pigeons assigned to Patton's Signal Corps's unit.

Les worked for a year in the Northwestern University Animal Research Center. In 1947, Dr. Fisher started his own practice, the Berwyn Animal Hospital, in Berwyn, Illinois, ten miles east of my dad's hospital. In the winter of 1946–47, Dad persuaded Les to provide transportation to a Christmas formal dance held at the Edgewater Beach Hotel on Lake Michigan, north of downtown Chicago, for me and my high school sweetheart and future wife, Carol. Dad was unsure of my driving ability in city traffic. My older sister, Margaret, home from her freshman year at Ohio State, was Les's date. The hotel was known for hosting big bands such as the bands of Benny Goodman.

Starting as a part-time zoo vet, Dr. Fisher later became the full-time director of the Lincoln Park Zoo in downtown Chicago. Under his tenure, from 1962 to 1992, the Lincoln Park Zoo was not only upgraded to a world-class zoo, but served as the home base for the award winning television show "Zoo Parade." Dr. Fisher's autobiography, *Life on the Ark,* describes his incredibly fascinating life in wonderful detail. The photo from Dr. Fisher's book shows his welcome at the zoo.

Years later, at my invitation, Les braved the worst snowstorm in Chicago's history to fulfill a speaking engagement for me in Kenosha, Wisconsin, about 60 miles north. Chicago's mayor, Mike Bilandic, was defeated that year by Jane Byrne, primarily because of the mayor's poor handling of the record 19-inch snowfall. I doubt that few of Les's world travels were more harrowing than that night's journey from Chicago to Kenosha and back.

My father developed cat scratch fever in 1949. These days, most people recognize that phrase as a rock and roll tune, but it was a very serious illness in the late '40s. Dad's treatment required lancing the pus pockets that developed on his hand, then letting them heal. As a result, he was unable to perform surgery for two months. During that time, routine spays and castrations for Dad's clients were taken to the Berwyn Animal hospital, where Dr. Fisher performed the surgery. Les never charged a penny for his professional services. Back then, veterinarians looked out for one another like farmers did. If a farmer's barn burned down, the neighbors all pulled together and built a new one. No one ever even thought of charging for their service, they did it to help a fellow community member. They did it because they knew it would be done for them if so needed. The veterinary community was much the same.

Berwyn Animal Hospital continues today as a success story in its own right. After Dr. Fisher became the director of Lincoln Park Zoo, the hospital was sold to Dr. Herb Lederer. Dr. Lederer expanded the hospital to its current 10,000 sq. ft. size, which now employs 16 veterinarians, including specialists who treat pets referred from area vets and around the country, and 60 support staff.

In 1943 Dad hired anyone he could find. Chuck Doyle had attended vet school in Ohio for two years. Today Chuck would be

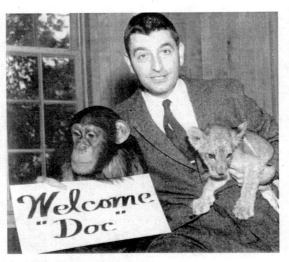

Welcome Doc!

The young chimp was growing increasingly restless sitting on my desk. He was grabbing at the "Welcome Doc" sign to my right and at the same time going for the pens in my pocket, as the flashbulbs threatened to blind both of us.

On my first day as Director of Chicago's Lincoln Park Zoo the media had been alerted to my arrival. The city's four major newspapers—*The Chicago American, Daily News, Sun-Times* and *Tribune*—all sent photographers who were crowded into my office

called a Physician's Assistant. Everyone, including Dad, called him Dr. Doyle. It's a wonder no one reported him to the authorities. "Dr. Doyle" mostly gave vaccinations and obtained histories for Dad. He was never allowed to do surgery. Secondary to his diabetes, Chuck suffered with a large open abscess on his shin, which never healed in the year he worked for Dad. Anxiety was a constant problem. He became very nervous during office hours. If more than two people were waiting, Chuck needed to go back to the kitchen and smoke a cigarette to calm down. Maybe his bouncing sugar levels affected his behavior. He had raised pit bulls—Staffordshire Terriers (the show dog type, not the fighters)—for years.

Dad had clients who fought dogs. I went with Dad to treat a wounded pit bull at Bill Cincinnati's house on the south side of Chicago. We arrived late Saturday afternoon, after office hours. After treating the wounded warrior, Mrs. C. insisted we stay for supper. The dinner plate must have been 26 inches diameter, heaped with spaghetti, and a red sauce on top. It was enough for two grown men—unless you're Italian. I finished about half. Mrs. C. pleaded, but I couldn't eat another bite. Dad finished some to lessen my embarrassment.

Ted Lafeber worked for my dad during summers before and after graduation from Iowa State in 1949. Ted was focused on vet practice. At this time my younger brother, Phil, and I were also employed by Dad. As brothers sometimes engage in horseplay, Ted would have none of it—no water fights with hoses for him. Clients loved Ted. They sensed immediately he not only loved their pet but his job as well. Try as he might, Dad could not convince Ted to permanently join his practice. Ted and I double dated prior to our marriages. Our first children were born the Christmas of 1951.

Within a year, Ted's father, an executive at DeVry University, built Ted a small animal hospital in Niles, Illinois, a Chicago suburb a few miles east of O'Hare airport.

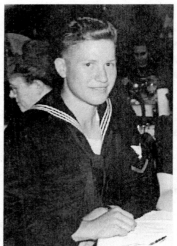

Pharmacist Mate 3rd Class
Ted Lafeber • 1944

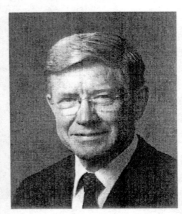

Ted Lafeber, DVM

Ted's most enduring quality was his enthusiasm. I know he must have had some bad days. In addition to losing his first wife, Molly, following a relatively minor surgical procedure, Ted had a young child drown in a backyard ditch. Despite these heartaches, Ted was unflappable. He would say, "I'm not about to let anything spoil my attitude. Clients and animals sense whether you are positive or not. I know I'm better when I project a positive attitude."

In 1956, soon after starting my practice in Kenosha, I called Ted about what he could tell me about training staff. I had just hired my first receptionist, Maureen Connolly, and I had no clue how to go about training her. Ted responded, "Send the young lady down here for a few days. I'll train her for life." She even stayed with Ted's family during the three-day visit. Maureen turned out to be one of the best receptionists I ever hired. Ted's lessons were simple and brief:

- Answer the phone within three rings.
- Smile when talking on the phone.
- The customer is right 99.9% of the time.
- Put the patient's interests above that of the practice.
- Always wear professional attire.
- Always use "professional language," such as:
  Butchers use "knives"; surgeons use "scalpels."
  Anyone can give "shots"; doctors give "injections" or "vaccinations."
  Any vet can do "spays"; small animal surgeons do "ovariohysterectomies."

Dr. Lafeber was also an early advocate for vets charging what they are worth. When I sent clients to Ted for an avian consult, I advised them to expect to pay for the best service they will ever receive.

Over the next 40 years, Ted became world famous. An early proponent of Avian Medicine specialty and Internal Medicine protocols in diagnosis, Ted published countless articles on Avian Medicine.

Ted was a much sought after speaker on the lecture circuit, expounding on veterinary management in addition to avian issues. Ted began Lafeber Bird Products in the early 1970s, building it into one of the premier companies in the pet food industry. Dr. Lafeber passed in 2001, but his family continues the business to this day.

A young English vet, Dr. Barrington R. Jones, was hired in 1950. Dad received a letter from the American Counsel in Wellington, New Zealand stating the process by which Barry could be hired. Barry updated Dad's knowledge concerning orthopedic surgery. Until Barry arrived, Dad had used only external fixation casts to repair broken limbs. Dr. Jones had spent the previous year at University of New Zealand Veterinary School, studying orthopedics. The new "Kirschner technique" involved placing stainless steel pins in the bones on either side of a fracture, then bolting them together externally.

Dad was surprised that this "tinker toy" assembly provided the excellent stabilization needed for healing. Meticulous care was given to sterilization. No more sloppy, possibly septic, surgery. Within a year, Dr. Jones headed to California and warmer climates. Pay has increased in the sixty years since Dr. Jones was hired for $300/month. Experienced vets now command $300/day or more.

Dad hired many other associate veterinarians over the years—most of them after I had struck out on my own. As a result, I did not have the opportunity to learn much about them, until he hired Eckart Reif.

Dad received a call from Bill Donavan, a client and VP of Swift Packing Company in Chicago—the same Swift Packing Company Dad had worked for as a meat inspector some 30 years previously. Mr. Donavan inquired if Dad needed any veterinary help. If so, he requested an interview for a young German vet, the son-in-law of Helmut Schnell, one of Swift's larger equipment suppliers. Dr. Eckart Reif had married Helmut Schnell's only daughter, Margaret. Mr. Schnell owned the largest sausage machine factory in the world.

As a wedding present, Herr Schnell had presented the newlyweds with "a year in America." He would pay all their expenses if young Dr. Reif could find a job. Fortunately for everyone, Dad was again in need of an assistant. It seemed that nearly every young vet Dad had employed, would leave in a year or two to start their practice. They evidently thought they had learned enough to test the waters themselves.

Schnell Sausage Machines were not the kind you might find in a butcher's shop. These were elephant-size models costing

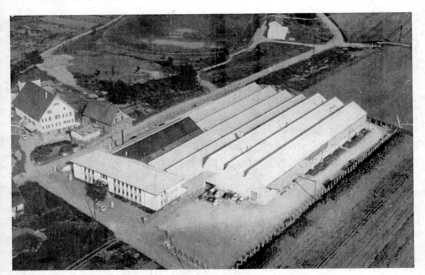

Schnell Factory • Winterbach, Germany • 1960

upwards of $100,000 in the days when that was a lot of money. Schnell products were sold worldwide—well, maybe not in China at that time. I imagine there are a number of them in major Chinese cities today.

Dr. and Mrs. Reif arrived in the summer of 1964. They moved in with Mom and Dad until they could find a furnished apartment. They ended up staying there the entire time they were in America. Eckart was a big man, 6' 2" and 200 lbs. He had a ruddy complexion, a contagious smile, and hearty laugh. Margaret was more subdued, but very self-assured. She was a beautiful woman who could have been a clothes model, except Margaret was "normal" size instead of gaunt-looking. Margaret had received a Master's Degree in Finance the previous year and was employed in her father's business.

Soon after the first snow, the Reifs decided they would like to going skiing in nearby Wilmot, Wisconsin, 12 miles west of Kenosha. Eckart allowed he could ski in his jeans. Margaret needed better. She borrowed one of Carol's ski outfits, and it fit to a tee. The Reifs spoke and wrote almost perfect English, having studied it for years in German schools. Eckart was readily accepted by Dad's clients and continued expanding Dad's knowledge of new techniques, especially in orthopedics. After eighteen months, Eckart informed Dad he would be leaving in the spring. He want-

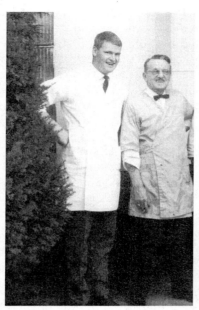 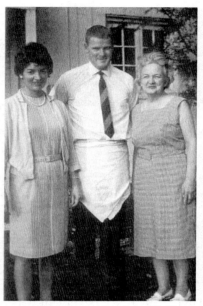

Dr. Eckart Reif, Dr. Andrew Merrick • Summer 1964

Margaret Reif, Eckart Reif, Dorothy Merrick

ed to give plenty of notice to allow Dad to hire another associate. Despite much pleading from both Andy and Dorothy, the Reifs had their mind made up. They were anxious to start a family and begin a practice of their own. To be 5,000 miles from home and relatives was unthinkable.

While waiting for his first "Klinik" to be built, Eckart became a worldwide salesman for the Schnell Company. During a trip to Chicago, Eckart persuaded Dad to accompany him to Buenos Aires for a week. Dad spoke no Spanish, but still had a great time on his first overseas trip selling sausage machines.

Eckart later wrote to my sister, Margaret, about an incident involving Dad. Dad had been in the hospital after a minor stroke. While helping him out of bed, a young nurse noticed there was a pig tattooed on Dad's right ankle. She said, "I've never seen a pig tattoo." Dad replied, "That's not a tattoo. It's a birthmark. My mother was deathly afraid of pigs." The nurse said, "I've got to bring in my mom to see this." Actually, Dad had the piglet tattoo done while he was in the Navy in 1918, but he thought the "birthmark" story was much more interesting. If he could keep from cracking up, most people believed him. My son, Bill, related that

Andy told him it was based on an old sailors' superstition that if one had a rooster or pig tattoo on their foot, they would not drown if the ship went down. When I asked him how such a silly tradition might have started, he explained that in olden times pigs and chickens were transported on ships in wooden crates. When a sailing craft sunk, these were often the few things that could float. When someone held on to such a piece of wreckage, they'd be more likely to survive.

Eckart established one of the larger small animal practices in southern Germany, specializing in orthopedics. His two sons also became vets. They were forced to attend vet school in Italy because German vet schools required one to perform military service prior to admission. The Reifs were pacifists. Because the boys had studied Italian in primary school, they were able to adjust to the lectures and text in a short time. Studying multiple languages is very common in European countries. It's one of the shortcomings of American education. It also helped that the Reifs owned a vacation condo in Naples.

Margaret opened an upscale women's clothing shoppe in their home town of Schwabish-Gmund. She told Carol on one of their many visits, "You must come to see my store. The shoes are fabulous. Many are priced under $200!" Carol told Margaret she would start saving money for our trip. Unfortunately, it wasn't until Eckart's 65th birthday celebration in 2003 that we were able to visit our long time friends.

In 1970 Eckart wrote to Dad and me for help. He wanted to be listed as "Dr. Reif" in Germany. Veterinarians, like most professionals, were not allowed to use the title "Doctor"— only MDs and PhDs had that honor. In America he had been called Dr. Reif, and he assumed the same would be done in Germany. Despite personal letters and articles we sent from the USA, his efforts were unsuccessful.

Eckart and Margaret's son, Dr. Ulle Reif, is now running the practice. After completing his veterinary studies in Italy, he spent two years in America becoming a board certified orthopedic surgeon at Michigan State Veterinary School, widely known for its veterinary orthopedic excellence.

Technical Knockout

Back in the good old days, a dependable kennel man was hard to find, and even harder to keep. They are still in short supply. Anybody who could keep hold of a 90-pound Mastiff or control an agitated 15-pound tomcat was special indeed. They had to be quick, good-natured animal lovers who didn't mind getting bitten or scratched once in a while. Needless to say, they had be willing to work for very little monetary reward.

Jesse Gulley was a first-rate kennel man and turned out to be a second-rate boxer. When he started working for Dad in the late '40s, his record in the ring was a mediocre two wins and three loses. A young, handsome black man (then Negro), probably 20 to 22, Jesse had worked for us six months when he informed us of his pugilistic pursuit. Moving to Chicago from Mississippi, Jesse was a welterweight class, 140–147 pounds, the same as future greats Ray Robinson and Sugar Ray Leonard.

Soon after telling us of his fighting endeavors, Jesse invited Dr. Andy (Dad) and me to witness his next fight. The small boxing arena in Cicero was typical of the era. Seating perhaps 300 people, the barn-like battleground had bleachers on all sides of a squared fighting area in the center. Boxing was the Friday night event, followed by Saturday night wrestling. The French Angel was often the "villain" on the wrestling card. Verne Gange was the wrestling champ—one of the few "real" wrestlers around at that time. Fighters were all up-and-coming young men looking to move up to the big time. The arena had a certain smell—stale tobacco smoke, sweat, liniment, cheap perfume—and an air of excitement. In the era before mass TV, the crowds were quite large on most weekends.

Jesse was to box in one of the "undercard" or preliminary bouts leading up to the main event. Each bout consisted of four action-filled, three-minute rounds. Winners received $20, or $25 if by knockout. Losers got $10. My guess is that at least half of the purse went to his trainer/manager/gym owner.

Jesse started well, landing more punches than his opponent, but ran out of gas by round three. The crowd had originally been cheering for Jesse, but they turned against him when he faltered.

Crowds are fickle like that. Jesse managed to survive a fourth round knockout only because of the fatigue of his opponent. On the ride home, Jesse informed us that he knew the reason for his defeat—he lacked a punching bag. He was only able to go to the gym three or four times a week, but if he had a bag at home, he could work out every day. In no time, he figured, he would build his stamina and skills enough to improve his record.

Weight bags sold for $50—well beyond Jesse's means—but he had a plan. In those days, veterinarians routinely groomed animals. I remember trimming as many as six or eight Cocker Spaniels in one day. Jesse would hold the animals when needed and give them baths. He informed me that he was going to save all that dog hair we threw in the garbage and make his own punching bag.

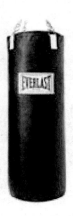

Over the next few weeks, Jesse meticulously swept all the loose hair and deposited it in a pillowcase to carry home. He gave glowing reports of his success in hanging the bag in his rented room and hiding it under his bed at night to keep his landlady, Ophelia, from discovering it. She was a very religious person who disapproved of liquor, gambling, and most of all, fighting. Jesse told us his jab was becoming quicker, his combination punches were having a more punishing effect, and his right cross was a sure knockout punch.

One Monday morning, however, Jesse informed us he was giving up his boxing career. His landlady had noticed bugs—fleas—in Jesse's room and found the weight bag stashed under his bed, along with hundreds of fleas. She promptly threw it and all of Jesse's possessions out on the front lawn. "I don't rent to @!*#%&*," she screamed. Supply your own expletives; Jesse never did tell us exactly what she said. It was probably the best thing that ever happened to a young man who badly needed a new hobby. As with many kennel workers, Jesse left after six months without explanation. I never saw his name in the sports pages.

Short Order Cooks & College Jobs

Earl was a good short-order cook. On second thought, Earl was a great short-order cook. He worked the morning weekend shift at the Downtown Grill. It was a typical greasy spoon place with six stools and five booths, located one block west of the train station in downtown Champaign, Illinois.

I had just been hired by the Champaign County surveyor, Ralph Vickers. After completing his regular duties during the week, Mr. Vickers was free to pick up surveying jobs on the weekends. I filled in when his regular assistants were not available. Mr. Vickers was an early bird, picking me up in his '36 Chevy pickup truck before dawn, then it was off to the Downtown Grill for a hearty breakfast, courtesy of Mr. Vickers.

The aroma of eggs, bacon, hot cakes, and coffee that hit the nostrils as you walked into the café almost made it worth getting up that early. Earl was at his usual place in front of the spotless grill. Gleaming pans hung from the ceiling. Some people whistle while they work. Earl hummed. "Nobody knows the trouble I've seen. Nobody knows but Jesus." "I've been working on the railroad, all my live long day." Earl was a small, wiry man. His face had as many lines as his forearms had tattoos. He had the look of a man who had spent many years in confinement as the result of a misguided youth. Misguided no more, Earl had found his calling.

Mr. Vickers suggested the pancakes. I'll always be in his debt for that. Earl produced the best pancakes I'd ever tasted, by far. Thick, golden brown and plate sized. You would have to be a bigger man than me to eat more than two.

After a month of devouring Earl's griddle delights—always followed by praise for his cooking expertise—I got enough courage to ask his secret formula. "Time to rest," he replied, "I make the batter the night before, let it sleep in the fridge overnight, then it's right and ready in the morning." My problem was remembering to make the batter the night before. When I did, I thanked Earl for his gift.

(A footnote from the present time: My local country club chef makes pancakes to rival Earl's. I asked him one day for his secret. He replied, "Aunt Jemima." When I asked about making them the night before to refrigerate, he replied, "Never." It seems the modern premixed pancake batter needs no overnight slumber.)

Surveyor's assistant was one of the best part-time jobs I had in college. Besides a hearty breakfast, we were in the outdoors, usually in rolling farmland, climbing fences, pounding stakes, and taking measurements—not unlike our first president 200 years before. The tools of the trade hadn't changed since George Washington's day. Mr. Vickers didn't work in the rain, so every day in the field was sunny and bright. Unfortunately, the job ended with the end of the spring semester when I went home to work in my dad's animal hospital. I needed more than part-time employment to support a growing family.

The fall semester found me again looking for part-time work. With two babies at home, Carol had her hands full keeping up with her household duties. I was not much, if any, help. Full time classes, studying, and a part-time job occupied all my waking hours. Carol decided to sell Christmas cards to friends and neighbors. This was in the day when most families sent and received dozens of cards during the holiday season. Contacting neighbors, fellow students and staff members, she netted around $200 for her efforts.

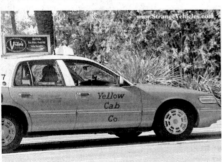

Answering an ad for a taxi driver in the Champaign Courier newspaper lead to my next employment. The hours were 5 PM to midnight, seven days a week. With that schedule, I had no doubt they had a hard time filling the position. I mentioned the job to my classmate and softball teammate, Jesse Payne. Jesse said that sounded like just the job for us together. Jesse said, "We could work from 5 to 9 and study from 9 to 12 every other day." And so we did. It worked out even better than Jesse had foreseen.

We could quit after 11 PM except on weekends. During slow times we would park by the train or bus stations, following the schedule of arrivals; books sat on the front seat ready for any breaks.

I learned every road and alley in the twin cities of Champaign and Urbana within the first couple of months. Even today, 60 years later, I still look for alleys to make my trips quicker.

Very early on I became acquainted with the Red Light District on the north side of Champaign. With the supply of university students and nearby Chanute Air Force Base, the "working girls" were never short of "johns." My most memorable delivery was in mid-May. Cabbies were often used for package delivery, especially from druggists or florists, so it was no surprise when I got a call to deliver a Mother's Day flower arrangement. The shock was when I realized it was to go to one of the "girls." I even got a surprisingly large tip. The madam always tipped cabbies well so we would bring customers to their house instead of the one down the street. "All in a day's work," Jesse remarked.

I started another job after reading an ad in the newspaper, "Delivery Man Wanted." I arrived at the used car lot to answer it. The owner said the job consisted of delivering sandwiches and drinks to campus dorms, fraternities and sororities. The hours were Monday through Thursday from 7 to 10 PM—a perfect fit for my schedule. The older model delivery van I was assigned at the used car establishment was drafty and cold due to a non-working heater. Around 6:45 PM I drove the van to Mrs. Childress's house on the north side of Champaign. She would have prepared dozens of preordered sandwiches (ham salad, egg salad, cheese, and peanut butter & jelly) and separated them as to which group went to which dorm. Drinks of orange juice, lemonade, or tea were also in separate groupings. My route sheet was typed up, so off I went. Most dorms had a designated pickup person to double check the order and pay my bill. Sandwiches cost fifty cents, drinks cost a quarter. Once in a while I'd get a small tip. The job ended at the Christmas break. When the new semester began, I searched for a warmer type of employment.

Take Two and Hit to Right

"Take two and hit to right." I'd played baseball all my life but I'd never heard that advice before. The words came from Jesse Payne, a classmate in school and second baseman on our interscholastic team, The Cremasters. In addition to being good baseball strategy, Jesse used it as a metaphor for life—like our current young, dynamic, thoughtful president. Think and explore the matter at hand before you act, then try to help advance your teammate instead of swinging for the fences and popping up.

I believe it was Jesse who thought "Cremasters" would be an appropriate name for a vet school team. We had just finished first year anatomy studies. The cremaster is the muscle which regulates the distance the scrotum is from the body. In the cold, the muscle contracts to keep the testicles warm, and the opposite in warm weather. We thought it was a wonderful joke. I imagine most of our opponents thought it referred to cream rising to the top.

In the early days of veterinary medicine at the University of Illinois in Champaign-Urbana, the environment was very loose. I was a member of the third class, accepted in the fall of 1950, and the first class to admit four of us who were not veterans of WWII. As a consequence, many of my classmates were older than our instructors. Some had been ranked officers; one, a full colonel. The academic classes were held in a converted sorority house. Clinics were held in a converted horse barn across the street from the architecture building and adjacent to the marching band's practice field. As a result, there was a camaraderie between faculty and students unlike anything on the rest of the campus. Between classes and on breaks, everyone retired to the band field in good weather. Footballs and baseballs were flying all around.

Someone suggested forming a team to compete in intramural athletics—softball, flag football, basketball, and table tennis. Jesse and I entered in the table tennis competition. We won a few matches but were eliminated in the quarterfinals. The Cremasters had a similar experience in basketball. Stan Spesard, Walt Nehrkorn and Tom Folkerts were great all-around basketball players. Unfortunately three good players do not make a team.

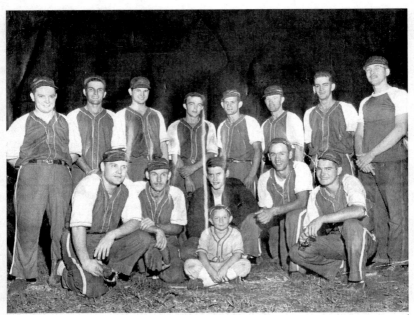

This rates as a big and busy week in the season of Hart Oil's softball team, which last Saturday captured the St. Joseph district championship. Monday night the Oilers whipped Swift & Co., 11-1, to clinch second-round honors in the Champaign Industrial league. Wednesday some of them may be in an exhibition game with the Champaign Moose at Switzer Field at 7:45 p.m. Thursday they're scheduled to make their sectional tournament bid against Tolono in the meet at Pesotum. And Saturday night they're slated to clash with Clifford-Jacobs, first - round Industrial champs, to settle that loop's 1951 title. Front row, left to right — Tom Folkerts, Jesse Payne, Dale Sollars, Capt. Walt Nehrkorn, W a ' Fehrenbacher. Back row— an Lykins, Ray Taft, Walt at cher, John Merrick, Earl Kingry, Harold Heffernan, J o h n Elder, Manager Morris Cover. Batboy—Shelby Williams.

We had many classmates who had been varsity athletes in high school, and a couple in college, but we did not have a softball pitcher. Without a great pitcher, the best team is only average. Enter Dale Sollars, a friend of one of our players and a business major. We quickly made him an honorary vet student. Dale had all the tools—blazing fast ball, deceptive change-up, both a riser and sinker pitch—the complete package. We breezed through the intramural league, easily winning the first-place trophy. I made the student paper as "Maverick." Leading off in the seventh inning of a scoreless game, I singled to center, reached second on a passed ball, third when the catcher overthrew the second baseman and scored on a fly ball to right. Game over!! The real hero was of course our brilliant pitcher, Dale. His ERA approached zero. Most of our wins were by shutouts or scores of 10 to 1.

Many of my classmates, including myself, were married. Some even had a couple of kids in school. As a consequence, few left campus to go home for the summer. A number of us took construction jobs at nearby Chanute Air Field in Rantoul, Illinois. The government was building housing for the anticipated airport expansion. With most of our players available, we searched for a sponsor to allow us to play in the city summer softball league. Sponsors supplied entry fees and uniforms, and sometimes a pre- and postseason party. One of our younger instructors, Dr. Maurice Cover, had become our manager/coach/faculty advisor. He convinced his neighbor, the owner of Hart Oil Company, to become our sponsor. Our Cremasters intramural win was the persuading factor.

Hart Oil won our league, but it was much harder this time. Unfortunately, we lost 1 to 0 in the sectional finals against a pitcher equal to Dale. Most other teams had pitchers almost as good as Dale. Fortunately, we had very good hitters. Our shortstop, Walt Nehrkorn, had played minor league baseball. Tom Folkerts played on the Navy team. Our left Fielder, Walt Thatcher, who was getting his PhD in advanced chemistry, had been a triple letter winner in high school. Walt Fehrenbacher scooped every ball hit toward left. Jesse Payne was a magician of the double play at second. Raoul (Ray) Taft, Johnny Lykins, John Elder, Harold Heffernan, and I alternated in center and right field. I often relieved Earl (Buck) Kingry as catcher. Most are now playing in that heavenly ball field in the sky, where a game is never called by rain.

The Men's Old Gym

When I enrolled in the University of Illinois Pre-Veterinary School in the fall of 1948, the university required every student to take one semester of physical education. I had participated in tennis, golf, cross country, and lettered in wrestling in high school. I decided to try something different—gymnastics. Lyons High School had not offered this sport in the '40s. As it turned out, this was an unwise decision. Wrestling and gymnastics were conducted in the Men's Old Gym.

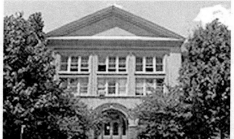

The H. E. Kenney Gym was built in 1902, in the Renaissance Revival style. The building was originally named the "Men's New Gymnasium" until Huff Hall opened in 1925, at which time its name was changed to the "Men's Old Gym." In 1974, the Board of Trustees named it after Harold Eugene "Hek" Kenney (1903–72), who wrestled for the Illini from 1923 to 1926. Located two blocks north of the Union building, next to the engineering campus, the Men's Old Gym was the site of my first tragedy at the U. of I.

Playing with Carol and the kids in her neighborhood, I had attempted to do a cartwheel the previous summer. I suffered a mild ankle sprain for my effort. Carol and the youngsters were all able to cartwheel and walk on their hands like circus acrobats. I should have learned my lesson.

The session involved running to a partner on the floor and being catapulted over him, like a somersault. I landed awkwardly. I fell and fractured my forearm, both radius and ulna, midway between the wrist and elbow. For the life of me, I can't remember which arm; I believe it was my right. After a short trip to nearby Burnham Hospital, radiographs revealed the extent of the injury. By this time my arm had swollen to twice its normal size, indicating a torn blood vessel. Treatment required a four-day stay in the hospital with my arm in a temporary sling to allow the swelling to subside. I was in an eight-bed ward similar to the scene in *One Flew Over The Cuckoo Nest*. My next-door neighbor was in the third week of treatment for a fractured back. His therapy was "lying as quietly as possible" and being rotated twice a day to avoid bedsores. I felt fortunate by comparison.

Out of disaster came a little good luck. The day after my accident, my first physics test was scheduled. I was sure I'd flunk. Gene Shinosaki came to my rescue again. He spent a couple of hours going over the concepts with me. After leaving the hospital, I managed to get a C on the test.

In the fall of 1950, my brother, Phil, rented a room in the house on Elm where Carol and I were living. Phil remarked that he was having a hard time fitting a P.E. class into his schedule. He mentioned that he was told he could skip the mandatory class if he could prove proficiency in a sport. He proposed I take his place and save him the trouble of enrolling in something we both considered a waste of time. Since Carol had been my only wrestling opponent for the last two years, I thought a real opponent would be a nice change.

With Phil's student ID in hand, I entered the Men's Old Gym where wrestling practice was held. I was assigned an opponent of my weight class and we proceeded to wrestle like a real match, under the watchful eye of one of the coaches. Instead of three 3-minute rounds, we did three 1-minute workouts.

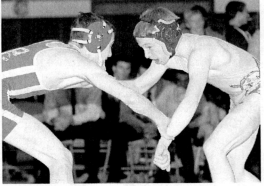

First from a standing position, then alternating crouching to begin, I held my own—but I suspect my opponent allowed me to score some points. After the session, it was handshakes all around. The coach followed me into the locker room and asked me to report for wrestling practice the next day to try and qualify for the varsity. It was a nice boost to my ego, but "Phil" was going to have to decline. I've forgotten the excuse I gave the coach.

I'll admit I missed the action of combat, but wrestling with Carol was a lot more rewarding

Large Animal Practice

Many of my classmates were "farm boys"—guys who had been raised on a farm and knew all about the trials and tribulations of the life of a country vet. My farm experience was limited to three years from the age of four through seven, and summers as a teenager on my maternal grandparents' farm in Iowa. I didn't think seriously about large animal practice, but I wanted to give it a try. The summer of 1953, after my junior year, I had the opportunity to see what would determine which path I would follow.

Dr. Lynn Freeman had a mixed animal practice in the neighboring town of Rantoul, Illinois, some 15 miles north of the university. Carol was pregnant with our second child, Bill. By staying in Champaign, Carol could keep her same doctor, Gernon Hesselschwerdt, and deliver in the same Burnham City Hospital as she did 18 months earlier.

I began my clinical education in large animal medicine in late May. I accompanied Dr. Freeman on all his farm calls. We vaccinated cattle, castrated and vaccinated pigs, dehorned cattle, and treated a variety of illness in cows, pigs, chickens, and an occasional horse. Since I had done literally hundreds of spays and castrations while working at Dad's practice, I was probably more experienced at that than Dr. Freeman. After I mentioned this to Dr. Freeman, he was glad to let me do most of the small animal surgeries. The practice of veterinary medicine was much less restrictive in the '40s and '50s. The country had gone through an extended period with a severe shortage of qualified professionals. Something like this would be unheard of today. I only revealed my secret to my surgical team during our junior year.

Junior surgery was divided among teams of three students. My group included Walt Nehrkorn, a farm boy from northwestern Illinois, and Don Strombeck, raised on a small farm near Zion, Illinois. Neither had any surgical experience. Walt had managed his mother's dairy farm after his dad died. After graduation, Walt had such a successful practice that he ended up owning two farms, two KFCs, one bank, and a car dealership. Don was a brilliant student who later became head of small animal clinics at the vet school in Davis, California. Some of us were envious of

Don's ability to study so little and get all A's. We assumed Don must have a photographic memory.

I explained to them—but not the professors—that I had been doing surgery since I was 16. At first, it was just closing the skin after Dad had performed the surgery, then I progressed to minor wound repair or removing skin tumors. This gradually led to castrations and finally ovariohysterectomies (spays). I kept an accurate count for the first three years. After I had done 500 surgeries, I quit counting. I'm sure I had done more routine surgery than some of our young professors.

Most veterinary schools and medical schools now teach students on simulators. As of September of 2010, fewer than 10 of the 28 veterinary schools in the United States still include terminal procedures in their core surgical training. The following describes training at Michigan State.

Virtual Surgery in Veterinary Medicine
by Dhruti Thanki, M.A.
Media Interface and Design Lab
Department of Telecommunication
Michigan State University
East Lansing, Michigan

The veterinary students prepare for surgery class. But they are not washing their hands or sterilizing their instruments. Is this characteristic of one of the best veterinary programs in the country? Actually, yes.

Michigan State University is establishing a curriculum for its School of Veterinary Medicine that will transform surgical instruction. The technology behind the new teaching methods is virtual reality. Virtual reality is a fairly new science, involving the creation of a three-dimensional, interactive, computerized environment. Among its hundreds of applications, medical procedures have been among the first to be developed.

Virtual Reality

In order to create a virtual environment, one must have two basic elements. The first is the hardware, such as head-mounted devices and tactile instruments. The head-mounted devices (HMD) are worn by the user, and are used to view the three-dimensional virtual environment. HMD come in several forms, such as helmets and special goggles. Tactile instruments give the user the illusion of touch. For example, a wand can be used as a scalpel; the user cuts into the virtual patient's muscle and can feel when the scalpel "hits" bone.

The second component is software, which is used to create the environment. Today, several graphics packages offer the detail and three-dimensional quality that can be used to reproduce everyday objects.

In July, 2011, the Physicians' Committee for Responsible Medicine asked District Attorney Bill Cox in Chattanooga, Tennessee in a letter to investigate and stop violations of Tennessee's animal cruelty statute. The Washington, D.C.–based physicians' group promotes alternatives to animal research.

"Of the 177 accredited medical schools in the United States and Canada, only three use live animals to train students in surgery clerkships," according to the letter signed by Dr. John J. Pippin, the committee's director of academic affairs, and two Tennessee physicians, Dr. Robert Burns of Memphis and Dr. Jennifer Ellis of Clarksville.

The letter contends that using pigs in the training violates Tennessee's animal cruelty law but Cox said the state statute excludes livestock.

"We received the letter and we reviewed the statute and the Legislature has deemed swine to be classified as livestock rather than domesticated animals," Cox said.

Officials at Johns Hopkins have responded to a similar complaint in the past, and the Uniformed Services University in an e-mail statement said they use a "limited number of animals in our research and education programs; however, whenever it is deemed appropriate we use simulation and computer models."

The statement said the program strictly follows animal welfare guidelines. "We take very seriously the care and use of animals here at the university and limit their use as much as reasonably possible," the statement said.

My personal opinion is the use of live animals is much more realistic then operating on models. When the patients are treated humanely and later sacrificed, I fail to see the "animal cruelty" argument.

I was even left to "run the practice" by myself when Dr. Freeman and family left for a long weekend. Fortunately, no great problems were presented. The day Dr. Freeman arrived home was hot for late June, 90° by noon. Dr. Freeman had been called to see a sick cow. As he was about to leave, a client called with a dystocia (difficult birth) case in a cow. Dr. Freeman told me to attend to the dystocia, and he would drop by after his call was finished.

The cow turned out to be a "first calf" Angus heifer accidentally bred in her first heat to a large Angus bull. Delivering this calf was going to be like threading a rope through the eye of a sewing needle. She had been in labor for six hours when I arrived. Stripping to the waist, I slipped into the protective rubber sleeve which extended up my right arm over my shoulder. Thankfully, the farmer had moved the heifer into the barn, where she was tied in a stall. Delivering young heifers bred to large bulls is difficult in the barn lot or pasture.

Palpation revealed a live calf in a Torticollis position where the fetus's head is twisted back upon the neck. Treatment involves pushing the head back and straightening it into the normal nose-first position. Cattle have long front legs, so they are usually presented first with the fetus assuming a "diving" presentation. After straightening the head, the forelegs need to be coaxed into position.

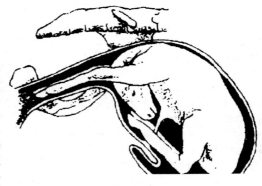

I struggled for over two hours, finally repelling the head and getting one leg thru the cervix with the aid of a chain attached to the leg and assistance of a "calf puller." By this time the calf showed little signs of life. Dr. Freeman finally arrived, analyzed the situation, spoke to the farmer, and asked for a sledge hammer. One swift blow to the heifer's skull ended her misery. The farmer was instructed to call for her immediate delivery to the packing plant so he could salvage something. If I had any pleasant dreams before about life on the farm, this cured me of them.

Carol soon delivered our first son, William Andrew, named after both granddads. Within two weeks, Dad called to see if I could come home to help him for the next two months. With Dr.

Freeman's okay, we headed for Brookfield—myself, Carol, Dorothy, and newborn Bill.

After two months of farm practice, I decided to limit myself to treating small animal pets in the future. My motto was, "If you can bring it in the door, I'll treat it."

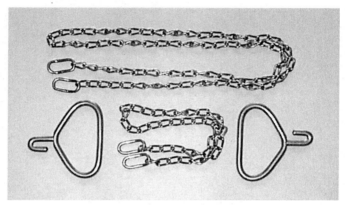

A "calf puller" for difficult births.

Explosions in Vet Med

"Hot pepper," Phil said, as he tossed the sack of margarine my way. The time was the fall of 1950. The place was the apartment of my new bride, Carol, and me in Urbana, Illinois. I had just started vet school at the University of Illinois. My brother, Phil, had rented a second floor room from Mrs. Darrow in the same old house four blocks from campus. We walked up an outside staircase to the kitchen entrance to our second/third floor rental. Phil often took meals with Carol and me. On this occasion we were sitting in the kitchen as Carol prepared supper. "Here, make yourself useful," Carol said, as she tossed a small plastic bag full of white margarine to Phil. She expected him to pop the small orange color bubble inside the sack and mix the contents with the bland fat until the entire mass obtained the color of freshly churned butter. It was illegal at the time to sell colored margarine in most of the United States, Illinois included.

After the war, the margarine lobby gained power and, little by little, state by state, the main margarine restrictions were lifted, most recently in Wisconsin. One reason for allowing color additives to margarine was the fact that the same color was added to butter during the winter months. Cows need green hay to produce the milk that could be processed into yellow butter. The dried hay fed in the winter produces white butter. Feed additives can now be used in order to compensate for variance in color due to beta carotene (provitamin A) content.

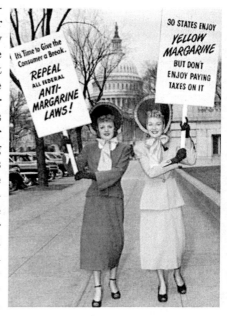

However, some vestiges of the legal restrictions remain in the United States. For example, the Food, Drug, and Cosmetic Act still prohibits the retail sale of margarine in packages larger than one pound, and the sale of yellow margarine remains illegal in Missouri.

I caught the missle from Phil and returned it in the same motion, continuing the task to mix the margarine. Brothers being brothers, the game rapidly increased in speed and intensity as the sack flew back and forth between us. As I recall, Phil missed my toss. When he tells the story, it's my error, not his. Either way, the sack hit the kitchen wall with such force that the contents splattered all over the wall and floor below. Phil and I spent the next hour cleaning up the mess and the following hour walking to the A & P grocery store for more margarine. Carol forgave, but she never forgot.

Nearly 50 years later, in 1998, Phil was visiting in Kenosha. Among other things, Kenosha and nearby Racine are famous for Danish Kringle.

Wikipedia defines Kringle as "a pastry in Scandinavia, a Nordic variety of pretzel, which came to these countries with the Catholic monks in the 13th century, and especially in Denmark, developed further into several kinds of different sweet, salty, or filled pastries. The word origins from *kringla,* meaning ring or circle. In fact, the pastry is usually baked in a circle or oval shape."

On November 22, 1998, the Kenosha News carried the following story under the headline, "Post Office Cautious With Kringle." The reporter, Debbie Metro, was a friend and client.

The second shipment arrived in good shape, without any warnings. Phil reported they tasted great. For the uninitiated, Google "Kringle" on the Web. Your taste buds will thank you.

Post office cautious with kringle

I can see the bumper sticker now...

"Kenosha, Home of the Explosive Kringle."

At least that's the message Kenosha veterinarian Dr. John Merrick received when he tried to send some of the pastry to his brother in Virginia.

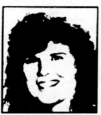

From the Metro Desk

Debbie Luebke Metro

Usually Dr. Merrick sends his brother, Phil Merrick, a retired military officer from Williamsburg, Va., home with some kringle. But during a recent visit, he forgot to get some, so he called Polentini's Bakery and ordered a few to mail to Phil.

A few days later, a member of the Polentini family called him.

"She said the package had been returned to the bakery marked 'Do Not Open — Explosives,' or something like that," Dr. Merrick explained, laughing. "She said that's never happened to them and she'd try to send him a couple more."

Wives' Revenge

All jobs require "down time" activities. Veterinary school is no exception. Junior and senior year, in addition to regular classes, demand a great number of hours be spent in the clinic. Those hours can fly by when patients are lined up for treatment, or drag when business is slow. This is especially true in the evening and night time. As a diversion, it became accepted practice for students to play cards. Euchre was the common game, and stakes were minimal—nickels, dimes, and quarters.

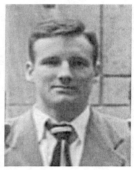

Stan Spessard
Sept. 1950

Classmate Stan Spesard and his wife, Mavis, suggested this story and sent me the following letter—handwritten, as Stan refuses to join the 21st century and buy a computer. His kids bought him one a few years ago. It sat and gathered dust until one of them took it back.

The Great Stolen Car Caper

In our junior year in veterinary school, several classmates made a date to play euchre at the apartment of classmate Tom Gunhouse. Merrick and Elder came in Spesard's car, enjoyed an evening of low stakes cards, then exited Tom's to go home. My car was missing. We all walked a few blocks to the Urbana Police Station to report the car stolen.

We then left the station to proceed to our respective apartments. Spesard arrived at his apartment to discover his car parked on the street out front of his residence. The police manhunt was called off and the story of the missing car unfolded.

All of the card-playing classmates had married in the past year or two.

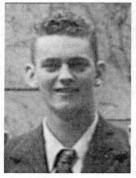

John Elder
Sept. 1950

Leaving spouses at home alone to go enjoy a few games of cards was apparently a "No-No." Spesard and Elder's spouses, Mavis and Marge, called Carol Merrick to find out the card game location. She knew and revealed the Gunhouse apartment location. Mavis and Marge then walked several blocks to the Gunhouse apartment. Mavis had a spare set of keys. Having no driver's license didn't deter her mission of mischief and revenge. After driving a short distance, the girls parked the car and watched as we left the apartment, discovered the car missing, and began walking to the police station.

Mavis and Marge drove home to await the return of the victims of the stolen car caper. I can't recall another night out for cards, ever.

I don't recall this great adventure, but I'm sure it happened. What fun the girls must have had watching the boys walk to the police station, then all the way home. Having to call the police and report their wives had "appropriated" the car must have been equally embarrassing. In the future, most of the card playing was done in the break room at school.

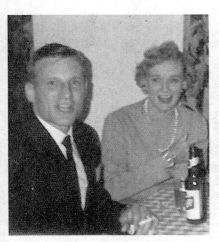
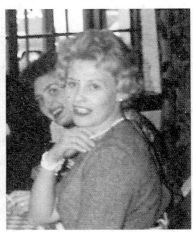

Stan Spessard, Carol Merrick • Marge Elder, Mavis Spessard
Phren's on Oregon • Vet school reunion • 1965

Senior Trips

"The City of the Big Shoulders" was what Carl Sandburg called Chicago. Most people have forgotten his classic poem's first line, "Hog Butcher to the World." One half of a section—320 acres—put together by a consortium of nine railroads in the 1860s, the Chicago Stockyards would decline after the completion of the interstate highway system. In 1954 the Chicago Stockyards was still a must-see for any farm visitor to Chicago.

Two senior trips were the highlights of our vet school senior year in 1954. One was to Indianapolis, with a visit to the sprawling Pitman-Moore drug company. At the time Pitman-Moore was one of the largest drug companies in the world and a leader in producing drugs for veterinary use. I imagine PM thought they would influence our use of their brand over competitors like Jen Sal, Fort Dodge, or Upjohn. There was the usual product sales pitch, a look at the spotless, sterile production line, good food, pleasant lodgings—nothing out of the ordinary. PM had already hired one of our classmates to be the "student host." He later took a job with PM.

Swift and Company in Chicago was a different matter. After an early-morning, two-hour bus ride from Champaign, we checked into the Stockyards Inn in the heart of the Chicago Stockyards. Entering the inn was like entering a European castle. Ornate carvings and massive framed paintings hung amid tapestries on wooden walls. Nearing the noon hour, we were directed to the inn's dining room for our midday repast.

Lunch was in the same elegant spirit. Everything first class—tuxedoed waiters, sterling silver service set on linen table clothes, crystal goblets filled with sparkling water—just what one would expect in the Ritz, but not in the heart of the Chicago Stockyards! The best was yet to come.

Our meal consisted of a marvelous tossed salad followed by pepper steak—pieces of choice sirloin simmered in a delightful mixture of onions, green peppers, and tomatoes—with rice or potatoes swimming in a sauce of beef broth, soy sauce, and garlic. By far, this was the best luncheon meal I had ever eaten. The aroma was exceeded only by the gustatory effects on my taste buds. For one who had grown up on eating leathery steak cooked on

Grandma's wood-fired stove, the contrast could not have been more profound. I recall the farm boys in my class had seconds and thirds.

Our afternoon tour began on the top of the slaughter house. Pigs were driven up the inclines to the killing area. Chains were looped around one hind leg and slowly pulled up to the ceiling. The pig is pulled along the conveyor, its throat slit, blood drained, then into a boiling water bath to remove the hair, followed by many knives rendering the carcass into meat.

Cattle meet death in small enclosures. One blow between the horns with a sledge hammer and the steer crumples to the floor. Within a minute they are hoisted up on the trolley like the pigs. The steers destined for Jewish tables are treated differently. Kosher slaughter, or shechita, is performed by a person known as a shochet, who has received special education and instruction in the requirements of shechita. Shechita is the ritual slaughter of mammals and birds according to Jewish dietary laws. The act is performed by severing the trachea, esophagus, carotid arteries, and juguar veins using an extremely sharp blade (chalef), and the blood is allowed to drain out. The animal must be killed with respect and compassion.

The shochet kills the animal with a quick, deep stroke across the throat with a sharp knife. When performed properly, shechita appears all but painless and quickly renders the animal unconscious. This brought to mind what our anatomy professor told us years before. Dr. Sinclair said, "If you're ever in a mind to commit suicide, never cut your wrists—slit your throat. There are almost no sensory nerves in the area of the jugular vein. It's relatively painless." As we watched, rabbis performed the Jewish rituals to ensure the meat was kosher. A couple of us snuck back to observe them sitting and smoking—no kosher ceremony when visitors were absent.

Wikipedia tells the following amazing story:

In the latter part of the twentieth century, the layout and design of most U.S. slaughterhouses has been significantly influenced by the work of Dr. Temple Grandin.

While Grandin's primary objective was to help slaughterhouse operators improve efficiency and profit, she suggested that reducing the stress and suffering of animals being led to slaughter may help achieve this aim. In particular she applied an intuitive understanding of animal psychology.

Grandin now claims to have designed over 54% of the slaughterhouses in the United States as well as many other slaughterhouses around the world.
Grandin's design reduced the stress on the animals and workers alike.

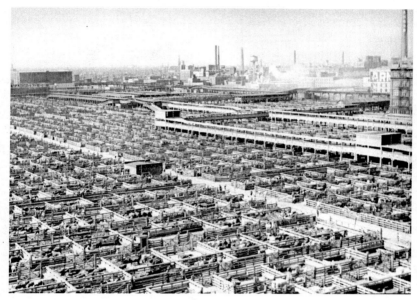

Chicago Stockyards • 1947

We watched federal meat inspectors perform both ante-mortem and postmortem exams on the cattle and hogs. Altogether, it was a noisy, messy, smelly job. I decided that this is not why I spent six years in college. Little did I know that this on-the-job education would come in handy 20 years later when I was asked to fill in for the local meat inspector in Kenosha when he became ill. With the help of his assistant, I was an adequate "pinch hitter." One man's meat is another man's poison. If meat inspection was not my calling, Jesse Payne followed his schooling by taking a job with the Federal Government as a Meat Inspector for 35 years, eventually becoming president of the Federal Veterinary Association.

After another wonderful meal, our group tried to decide how to spend our evening. Someone remarked, "Merrick's from Chicago. Ask Johnny where to go." With a group of 32 young guys away from wives and girlfriends, there was only one choice—the strip clubs in Cicero. Off we went, with the bus driver along for the show.

If you've been to one strip show, you've seen them all—a loud MC/comedian, a three-piece band, scantily clad girls of various ages and beauty, and lots of smoke. Midway through the show, Johnny Elder remarked, "I forgot to call Marge. It's her birthday today. I wonder where there's a pay phone." John, a farm boy from southern Illinois, was recently married to Marge, a very Italian city girl from Rockford. Marge's first words were, "John, what's all the noise? Where are you calling from?" John yelled to me, "Where are we?" I responded, "At a restaurant in Cicero." Marge screamed something in Italian followed by, "I know damn well where you are—at one of those damn strip joints. Just wait 'til you get home!"

Poor John! He was teased all the way to Champaign. As I recall, John slept on the couch for the next week. At least he didn't starve. Marge was an excellent cook and continued to fatten up her farm boy.

State Boards

Taking and passing the State Boards is a necessary "rite of passage" for graduating veterinary students. I took and passed the exams in three states—Illinois, necessary to practice with Dad in suburban Chicago; Minnesota, after two good friends had recently moved to St. Paul; and Wisconsin, after purchasing a practice. The exams in the '50s covered everything one had learned—memorized—in the previous four years, from the anatomy of the horse and chicken to biochemistry and parasitology, from clinical diagnosis to antidotes for poisons. Somehow, most of us passed.

The current practice of taking national veterinary exams after two years of covering the non-clinical material is a much more common-sense approach to testing a student's grasp of the subject. The exam covering the final two years of clinical medicine and surgery is given by each individual state and covers the nuts and bolts of everyday practice. Many states will give reciprocity to veterinarians who have passed the boards in other states. This is generally true for states looking for vets, which does not include states like California and Florida.

Dr. F. was a classmate of Dad's at Ohio State in the '20s. His friends and colleagues considered Dr. F. a very successful veterinarian. Two years after setting up a large animal practice 30 miles west of Chicago, Dr. F. married the banker's daughter. Dr. F's new job was to become a gentleman farmer and money manager. He was very attentive to his new duties.

Soon after his election as Illinois governor in 1950, William Stratton called his next-door neighbor to request a favor—would Dr. F. accept the governor's appointment to the Illinois state veterinary examining board? This presented Dr. F. with a dilemma. Turning down a newly elected governor's appointment would seem very rude, but accepting the appointment would expose Dr. F. to the world as a know-nothing vet. A quarter century had slipped away since those merry days in vet school. What to do?

Dr. F's solution was to call his old friend, Andy Merrick. Dad readily accepted the task of preparing questions for Dr. F. to submit to the veterinary licensing board. Dad already knew the governor very well. They had worked together for many years, starting the veterinary school at the University of Illinois. Dr F. obtained copies of previous exams, which he forwarded to Dad. Using the past tests as a guide, Dad wrote up the dozens of questions to be given to the anxious applicants. Dr. F. picked up the completed exams, signed his name and sent them on their way.

After two years, Dr. F. felt he had done his duty and resigned his position on the Illinois Veterinary Examining Board and recommended Dad as his replacement. The governor appointed Dad to the examining board in 1953, where he served until the governor left office.

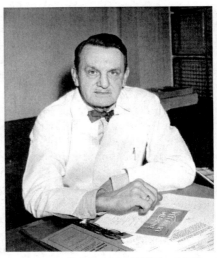

Andrew C. Merrick, DVM • 1953

Even though Dad was on the examining board when I took the test for my Illinois vet license, he never gave me a hint as to what the questions contained. I really didn't need any help; at that age, I thought I knew everything there was to know. As most professionals learn, it takes four or five years of practice to become comfortable in your field. By that time you've learned what you don't know and where to go for answers.

I had been in small animal practice in Kenosha, Wisconsin for ten years when I received a call from Bill Sinclair, a client who had moved from Kenosha to 100 miles north of Madison. He wanted my opinion of the care his two year old Dachshund mix was receiving from his local vet. The dog had fallen and injured his front leg two weeks prior. He had been treated by Dr. H. at the time but was not bearing any weight on the leg, which was cast in what sounded like a modified Thomas splint.

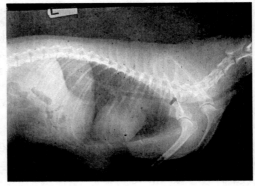

I asked Bill what the x-rays showed. He replied, "There weren't any x-rays." I said, "You must be mistaken. I'll call Dr. H. and call you back." Imagine my surprise when my telephone inquiry to Dr. H. produced a barrage of expletives!!! "What the @#$ was I doing meddling in his case?" "How in the @#$ did I dare to question his treatment?"

This went on for a couple of minutes until I finally got the doctor to admit that no x-rays were ever taken. He had diagnosed a proximal ulnar fracture and applied the Thomas splint.

I was brief and to the point in my follow up to my ex-client:
1. Under no circumstance ever take this or any pet to Dr. H.
2. Seek another local vet. (I suggested two or three in the area.)
3. Make sure x-rays are taken prior to any fracture reduction.
4. Call me with your new vet's diagnosis and treatment advice.

Bill reported that the radiographs revealed a non-healing fracture of the distal humerus. A modified Thomas splint would almost guarantee that healing would be next to impossible. This splint would actually make the fracture worse, and the animal would be in constant pain.

The kicker to this tale is that Dr. H. was not only a member of the Wisconsin Veterinary Examining Board for eight years, he was its current chairman. I'm sure there's a moral here, but I'm afraid to look.

Uncle Russ, Chicago Bears, and Golf

My uncle Russ was a great teacher, a stern taskmaster, and wonderful role model. He had the makings of a "Renaissance Man." My dad's older brother, unlike my father, was an active sportsman. Golf was one of his passions; football was another.

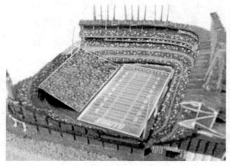

Russ had season tickets to the Bears—four seats, about ten rows up, behind the Cubs dugout, on the west side of Wrigley Field. Once a year he would take Phil and me to a game. Wrigley Field has not changed much in the last 70 years. For football, the field was striped to run north to south along the left field foul line. Temporary bleachers were installed along the east sideline. There were no corporate sky boxes; everyone sat in the weather—rain, sun or snow.

An old program lists the average lineman weighing 220 pounds—almost 100 less than today's "Refrigerator Perry." Sid Luckman was the star quarterback. Ken Kavanaugh played both offense and defense on the end of the line. He was the last player in the NFL to play without a helmet. He and a number of Bears were clients of Russ.

One early Sunday morning in the fall of 1944 Uncle Russ, Aunt Ann, Phil, and I boarded a Northwestern RR "Bears' Train" in downtown Chicago to travel to Green Bay to watch the Bears play the Packers. The Packers compiled a record of 88-41-7 (.673) at City Stadium, including NFL world championship seasons in 1929, 1930, 1931, 1936, 1939, and 1944. Notice the "high school" stands, leather helmets, and lack of shoulder pads. These guys looked like us.

The Old City Stadium was a horseshoe-shaped structure made of wood and originally did not have any toilet facilities. It stood

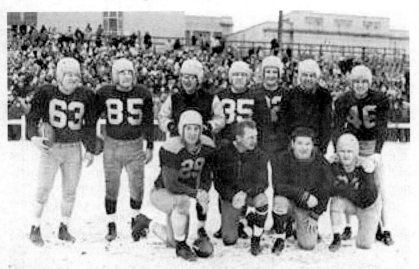

behind Green Bay East High School and next to the East River. The Packers used the school for locker room facilities. Visiting teams often dressed at their hotel before the game rather than use the lockers at East High. The stadium originally seated 6,000. Its capacity would be gradually expanded to 25,000.

Following Don Hudson's retirement in 1945, Green Bay's fortunes took a turn downward. While its playing surface was consistently praised, by the 1950s City Stadium was seen as too small and inadequate, even after expansion. The leaders of the NFL, including George Halas, informed the Green Bay club owners that they needed to improve their stadium facilities, or else the Packers would be moved to Milwaukee or elsewhere, permanently.

The residents of Green Bay responded by voting in 1956 to build a new City Stadium, which opened the following year, as "old" City Stadium became a high school field. The new stadium would be renamed Lambeau Field in 1965, after the death of team founder Curly Lambeau, and has become one of the most revered venues in all of American sports.

The Packers have won 13 league championships, more than any other American professional football team. They have also won four Super Bowls. Their arch-rivals, the Chicago Bears, are second, with nine NFL championships (including one Super Bowl). The historical rivalry with Chicago extends to the Hall of Fame—the Packers have the second most Hall of Famers (21, behind the Bears' 26). The Packers are also the only team to win three straight NFL titles, which they did twice (1929–31 and 1965–67). Most NFL teams play in cities with population in the millions. Green Bay, population 102,000, is by far the smallest city to support a major sports team. When I moved to Kenosha in 1956, the waiting list for tickets was around 30,000. I figured why bother to get on the list. It's now 86,000.

In early December, 2011, the Packers launched their fifth stock sale, seeking 62.5 million dollars. The first shares were sold in 1923, when 1,000 people bought $5 shares. Green Bay Packers, Inc., has been a publicly owned, nonprofit corporation since Aug. 18, 1923, when original articles of incorporation were filed with Wisconsin's secretary of state. A total of 4,750,937 shares is owned by 112,158 stockholders, none of whom receives any dividend on the initial investment. No one will be allowed to purchase more than 200 shares, including ownership from previous sales.

The team initially offered 250,000 shares for sale starting December 6, 2011. The money will be used to expand and update Lambeau Field and the Packers Hall of Fame. But the allotment is nearly gone, even though the shares cost $250 each and have virtually no resale value. I bought three shares—one for myself and two for my boys. We plan to attend the Board of Directors meeting next July in Green Bay at the start of preseason training camp. Sales of Green Bay Packers stock have been so brisk since an initial offering that the team is making another 30,000 shares available.

One of the more remarkable business stories in American history, the team is kept viable by its shareholders—its unselfish fans. Even more incredible, the Packers have survived during the current era, permeated by free agency and the NFL salary cap. And, thanks in large part to Brown County's passage of the 2000 Lambeau Field referendum, the club will remain solvent and highly competitive well into the future due to its redeveloped stadium. Fans have come to the team's financial rescue on several occasions, including four previous stock sales: 1923, 1935, 1950, and 1997.

The "Bears Football" special train was a raucous ride. Anticipation, fueled by plenty of alcohol, was sky high. The game figured to be close, with the Bears a slight favorite. Arriving in Green Bay by noon, then a waiting bus to the stadium. The game turned out to be a disappointment—Green Bay Packers 42, Chicago Bears 28. The train ride back to Chicago was more somber.

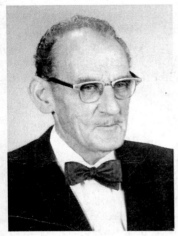

My brother Phil reminded me, "We were driving to the Bears game on Sunday, December 7, 1941, when news came on the radio about the attack on Pearl Harbor. We were playing the Chicago Cardinals at Comiskey Park. The Bears won that game, 34 to 24, and the league championship."

Uncle Russ had hard and firm rules when it came to golf: The only opponents are the course and yourself. He insisted on counting every stroke; you only cheat yourself if you don't. Play the ball where it lies, unless the local club rules allows lift, clean and place. Never use a cart; golf is meant to be walked, carrying your clubs. Maybe a pull cart if old and infirm. Russ remarked, "Every time you put your bag down and lift it up, it squeezes your liver and adds days to your life." Plan ahead; try to place shots that will avoid future trouble. Aim for the center of the green; don't take too many chances.

Russ believed seven clubs were all anyone needed: driver, spoon, cleet (2), midiron (5), mashie (7), niblick (9), and putter. The entire group, including cloth bag, weighted no more than ten pounds. Russ's wife, Ann, was a good golfer in her own right, also. She was never far from 95–100 strokes for 18 holes. Every shot was 100 to 125 yards, straight down the middle. She played bogey golf—something we aspired to.

Great Books discussion groups were another passion. Russ founded a Great Books Club both in Cicero, Illinois, and after semi-retirement, to the Marblehead Peninsula on Lake

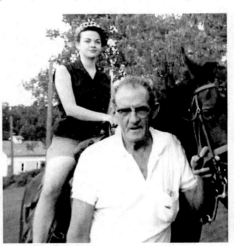

Sue Merrick Creamer and Russ
Marblehead, Ohio • Circa 1962

Erie, Ohio. Russ was a member of Kiwanis, Civic Theatre, and president of the County Board for Retarded Children. He was also a member of the Marblehead Metaphysics Club and many other civic groups.

Russ was a true wordsmith. He believed in learning one new word every day, then practice using it in conversation until it became habit. He was also an accomplished poet, submitting many works for publication. One of his poems appears below.

Russ suffered a fatal heart attack on January 14, 1967, one week prior to his 75th birthday.

> Friends, Acquaintances, Callers
> Our House is interesting
> If only for one pleasant thing
> We have visitors galore at our house on the hill
> And our jolly coffee pot is never still.
> Some of the callers we knew long ago
> Others recently we came to know.
> We love this mélange, Bess and I
> For their well of stories never run dry.
> Some of them come who have travelled far
> Some who never got past their favorite bar.
> Some come who are happy and full of fun
> Some with tales of woe to be spun.
> With my relatives and those of Bess,
> They number into the hundreds I guess.
> When relatives sit around playing that old family game
> Like, I wonder what Nephew Jim sees in That Dame.
> Or some past event which with sorrow our hearts filled
> At which we now laugh, bitterness long distilled.
> Some of our visitors are humble, poor as can be
> Some distinguished and of nobility.
> Others appear prosperous, smack of success
> Aye, in our guest book we boast a princess
> We have entertained teachers, actors, writers galore,
> Some scientists and painters have entered our door
> Some made us laugh, some made us cry
> But we loved entertaining them, Bess and I.
>
> JRM — 1-11-58

And Baby Makes 3, 4, 5, 6, 7, 8, 9, and 10

Linda and Charles Cunningham were the ideal clients. Their recently acquired black Lab was definitely their "baby"—a member of the family in every sense of the word. While many dogs were kept in outdoor kennels, Precious—yes, a hunting dog named "Precious"—had the run of the house and slept next to her "mom and dad" in their bedroom. Like all new parents, Linda and Charles were eager to learn everything I knew about feeding, behavior, toilet training, and vaccinations—the best way to bring up a perfect "child."

Precious lived up to her name. Smart, alert, obedient, and affectionate, with just enough mischief to remind us she was really a puppy. Her first year was uneventful. It included the routine vaccinations, worming, grooming, and obedience training. Charles had wanted to include field training for hunting ducks, but Linda vetoed that idea. She didn't want her baby exposed to firearms. "After all," she said, "accidents do happen."

Precious's mom had been a champion show dog. She was also an excellent mother to Precious and her ten siblings. I explained to the Cunningham's that the disposition of the mother is much more predictive of the offspring's behavior than the father. As a result, Precious should make a wonderful Mom.

Fortunately, the owners of Precious's mom had an unrelated Labrador who could serve as a stud. The usual routine involves taking the bitch to the stud dog's residence about the seventh day after she shows vaginal bleeding. Breeding is attempted daily until the two are successfully "tied," then every other day for two more matings. Precious refused Duke's attentions for two days— growling, nipping and sitting down. She allowed Duke to mount and penetrate on the third day, then again on day five. The Cunningham's were exhausted by this time and concluded that twice would have to do.

When Linda brought Precious into the office for her four-week checkup, I could palpate eight or ten embryos. She was beginning to show signs of motherhood, weight gain and breast enlargement. I counseled Linda on what to do in preparation for the delivery:

1. Delegate Charles to construct a plywood whelping box about 6 inches longer and wider than Precious. Since Precious measures 24 inches at the shoulders and 30 inches from nose to anus, the box should be 30" × 36" with 6- to 8-inch sides. This does two things: It makes a small area so Mom can easily reach any pups that stray, and it contains the pups until they are 3 to 4 weeks old. Precious will make a nest out the copious amount of torn up newspapers you place in the box.
2. Dogs usually deliver in 60 to 65 days after breeding; that is, approximately nine weeks or two months.
3. Allow Precious to use the box at least one week prior to whelping.
4. Have a clothes basket with a covered heating pad ready for the first pups to be born.
5. Quiet is a good rule in the delivery room. Children should be encouraged to watch but talk and ask questions in a low voice.
6. Allow Precious to clean her newborns and eat the afterbirth (placenta). The placenta is chock full of hormones which stimulate uterine contractions and milk production.
7. As a rule, the umbilical cord does not need to be tied. The grinding action of Mom's teeth will stanch the hemorrhage.
8. Pups can be delivered within 5 to 10 minutes of each other or as long as two or three hours between births.
9. Mom will usually get up, drink a little, and urinate after the last pup is delivered.
10. Help each pup find a nipple. The first few hours are critical.
11. Some mothers refuse to nurse or care for a runt. This is nature's way of eliminating deformed or very weak individuals. These pups can sometimes be saved by good nursing. Some Moms may again then assume her duties. Unfortunately, many of the rejected babies die in the first 48 hours. It's wise to prepare young children for this possibility.

I promised to be available for the big day. Linda assured me she would call at the first signs of labor. Moms usually quit eating and begin to make a nest 24 to 48 hours prior to delivery. Precious quietly delivered her first girl while the Cunningham's were eating dinner and listening to the radio. By the time I arrived at the home at 7 PM, two more babies had entered the world with no help asked for or given. Over the next three hours Precious delivered ten pups—five girls and five boys. The Cunningham's were ecstatic.

Precious proved to be an excellent mother. Linda an equally proud "grandmother." Little did she know the problems that lay ahead.

The unwritten rule of dog breeding is: The stud's owner gets the "pick of the litter" (POL) or a cash price equal to what a good quality pup would sell for on the open market. Among friends it's usually the POL. This pup is usually delivered to the stud's owner at around 6 to 8 weeks of age. Linda was reluctant, but she resigned herself to seeing one of her boys leave. The Cunningham's placed ads with an asking price of $100—a little high, I thought. After no sales for two weeks, five were sold for between $50 and $75. That left four fast-growing pups almost four months old. They had long outgrown their whelping box and now had full run of the spare bedroom. Linda decided—after an ultimatum from Charles—that she needed to be much less picky about which families were "good enough" for her pups. By the time the two remaining pups were five months old they had destroyed the window sill and desecrated the floor in the bedroom. Charles made the window into a dog door and finished fencing the back yard. The pups and Precious now had free access to the outside, making everyone's job a lot easier. The floor would be refinished at a later date.

Precious was spayed (ovariohysterectomy) before her next heat. The Cunningham's decided raising two legged children would be easier, and maybe even cheaper.

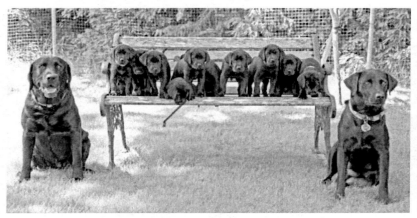

Proud mom, attentive dad, and their canine Brady Bunch.

Dog Whisperer

I never knew Mr. Crawford's first name for sure. He was always just "Mr. Crawford." A small, spry, dapper, black man—Negro in those days—he was the best "dog trainer" I ever knew. Meticulous in manner and dress, he always wore a suit, tie, and hat. He spoke in a deliberate manner. His accent was impossible to identify. A hint of British, Jamaican, and Louisiana Cajun, a result of either moving around the country or practiced eloquence. Much like Barak Obama, you could almost see his mind shifting gears before putting his mouth in motion. He claimed to have been a horse trainer, but I never was able to verify it. British television made dog trainer Barbara Woodhouse famous in the 1980s, when she was in her 70s. Twenty years later, Cesar Millan would fascinate American TV audiences with his ability to treat problem dogs. Mr. Crawford was 40 years ahead of his time.

Mr. Crawford believed you train an animal by love, repetition, and reward. His voice was stern, not loud, and commanded respect. He would take two or three patients, usually dogs, back to his house on Chicago's Southside for days or weeks. He imposed no time limit; the training took as long as it took. When he was finished, one could be sure the bad habits were extinguished and replaced with good behavior. He charged by the job, not an hourly rate, with results guaranteed—no questions asked. If he could not produce the results as promised, there was no charge.

Mr. Crawford was a rare breed—a black Republican. In fact, he was the Republican precinct captain in his district. As precinct captain, he would be expected to canvass the precinct for votes—difficult at best on the south side—and work with the Democratic precinct captain to solve neighborhood issues, etc. He also was employed by the local Democratic captain as a Cook County Deputy Surveyor. He told me his job required him to drive to a certain spot in the Cook county forest preserve and move a series of stakes exactly 3 feet 6 inches. Then next month he would move them back to their original spot. For this "work" he received $20.50 per week. He called this his "job," but he knew better. That's the way it was in Cook County and probably all over America. I doubt if it's changed much over the last 50 years.

"A young vet with two small children should have a dog," Carol said soon after I started working for Dad. I agreed. In due time we found a cute, 8-week-old, female, Field Springer Spaniel—not the large show type. She had a short-haired liver-and-white coat.

Duchess was a delight, a typical puppy with typical puppy problems chewing everything in sight, jumping in the tub to bathe with the kids, coming only when she deemed it necessary, etc. On one of his visits, I related to Mr. Crawford how difficult Duchess was to train. He asked if I would like him to train Duchess. He said he would take her home for as long as it took to make her into as dog we would really enjoy. After discussion with Carol and the kids, we decided to opt for training.

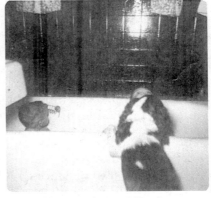

Bill, Dorothy, and Duchess

Three weeks later Mr. Crawford delivered a "new" Duchess. She was much calmer, sat on command, obeyed "come," "sit," etc. Mr. Crawford saved his best trick for last. Taking Duchess outside, he walked with her at heel to the edge of our side street. "Duchess," he commanded, "go sit on the curb across the street." In a flash, Duchess obeyed the order. We were impressed. Duchess continued to behave perfectly for the next few months. She would be a "horse" pulling a wagon one minute, and a pillow to nap on the next. Duchess was indeed, the perfect pet—quiet, well behaved, obedient, and loving.

One fall morning, Duchess and the kids were playing in the front yard when our four-year-old daughter, Dorothy, came crying inside. "Somebody took Duchess!" Carol ran outside and searched the area. No Duchess. A neighbor down the street reported she had observed a strange

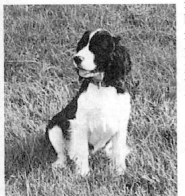

Duchess at 14 weeks old

car stop near our house, observe the play in the yard, and simply called "come." Duchess instantly ran and jumped into their car, and they drove away with our baby, never to be seen again. Buckets of tears followed.

Lesson learned. Sometimes you can train too well.

Private Zoo Vet

My dad, A. C. Merrick, DVM, opened his first small animal hospital in Brookfield, Illinois, 15 miles southwest of Chicago, in 1935. Our family occupied the back apartment of the typical brick business building located on a busy suburban highway.

Dad had no connection to the world-famous Brookfield Zoo, but my brother and I loved to walk the mile or so to the zoo and spend a summer day with the animals. In 1937, the Chicago Herald Examiner was doing a feature article on the zoo. We were approached by a zoo attendant asking if we would like to participate in a "walrus race." I was eight and my brother, Phil, was six. We made the front page of the newspaper that day with a photo of us riding two walruses—very large and, thankfully, very tame—in a staged race. (The full story appears on pp. 31–32.)

One of Chicago's biggest family attractions of the 1950s was Hawthorn Melody Farms, located in northeast Illinois about 30 miles north of Chicago, in the outskirts of Libertyville. Adlai Stevenson, former presidential candidate and U.N. Ambassador, was a close neighbor. Hawthorn Melody was not only a successful dairy farm, but also a mini theme park, incorporating a petting zoo, steam train, wagon rides, sports stars, cowboy heroes, and western town. It provided visitors with a glimpse into farm life.

John Cuneo Sr. was a wealthy man who made his money in the printing business in Chicago. He purchased the Samuel Insull mansion and estates near Libertyville, Illinois, in 1937. Part of the estate had been used for farming, so Cuneo decided to make farming his hobby. He became a "gentleman farmer." Dairy farms were not an uncommon sight in Lake County at this time and, just like neighboring Wisconsin, known for their dairy production even today. Cuneo wanted to do something in the dairy industry with his farm that would make it stand out from the rest. He determined that not only was he going to have the best cows in the dairy, but he planned to build the most modern facility as well. He was very proud of his modern milking parlor and decided to put in a large glass window in the milking barn so the public could observe the process. He encouraged people from all around the area to come visit the farm, and take a tour to see how

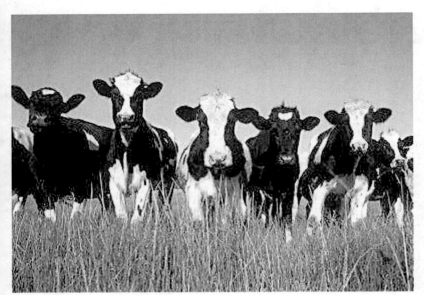

the milk was produced. People who visited could see the new machines at work. He hoped they would be impressed enough to purchase Hawthorn Melody milk.

In 1948 Cuneo began his "A Day at the Farm" program and invited "disadvantaged children from the city out to the farm for educational purposes, as well as for them to have fun." Many people that lived in the city never really ventured out to the countryside and knew very little about agriculture and the dairy industry. Hawthorn Melody Farm was their opportunity to see a farm up close and experience country life. There were tours of poultry, hog, and horse barns—which ended with milk and ice cream treats—a miniature railroad, and hay rides. In 1951 Cuneo added a children's zoo, and in 1955 he added a Wild West town. All of this just coincidentally happened to serve as great advertising for Hawthorne Melody Milk products.

Mr. Cuneo (affectionately referred to as "Mr. C.") understood opportunity when he saw it and took advantage of it. He had created a small-scale theme park, before Disney, to give families in the growing city of Chicago a chance to familiarize themselves with country life while having fun together. This experience educated children and adults alike about the dairy business and promoted the Hawthorn Melody brand. Cuneo put his money where his mouth was, so to speak, spending extensive capital to mod-

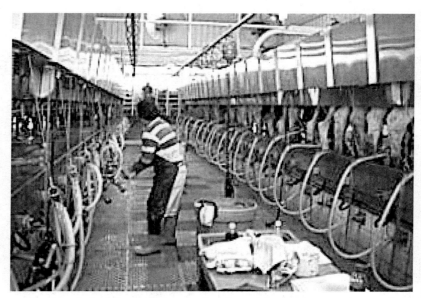

ernize his dairy, demanding technology advancements to produce a better, safer, higher quality product, and to make it more efficiently. His innovations in the dairy business became the industry standard in milk and dairy production. Hawthorn Melody Farm is remembered fondly by a generation of city kids who experienced country life and a realistic agricultural production within its boundaries.

Chief among the many exhibits was the "Boxing Kangaroo." This particular marsupial had been trained to entertain visitors by wearing children's boxing gloves and pretending to fight a small trainer. As soon as the 'roo landed anything that resembled a punch, the trainer dropped like a rock and was counted out to the cheers of the crowd—like cheering for the "good guy" at a pro wrestling match. The current problem was the animal's refusal to assume the typical boxing stance, sitting back on his tail and pawing at the trainer in front of him. The show began with the animal chasing the trainer around the ring, then stopping for a treat after one or two circles. This part of the act presented no problem. However, when the 'roo stopped and assumed a fighting position, he showed evidence of pain.

Dad routinely treated Mr. C's pets and Fox Hounds, but he was not the "zoo vet." Even so, when the "Boxing Kangaroo" developed problems, Dad was called in for advice. I was the junior member of the practice, having started immediately after graduation from the University of Illinois in 1954. Dad said something to the effect of, "you must know more than I do about kangaroos, so go up to Libertyville and get the 'roo back on his feet and into the ring."

The boxing kangaroo is a national symbol of Australia, frequently seen in popular culture. The symbol is often displayed prominently by Australian spectators at sporting events, such as cricket, tennis, and football matches, and at the Commonwealth and Olympic Games. The flag is also highly associated with its namesake national rugby league team, the Kangaroos.

A distinctive flag featuring the symbol has since been considered "Australia's sporting flag." The idea of a boxing kangaroo originates from the animal's defensive behavior, in which it will use its smaller forelegs (its "arms") to hold an attacker 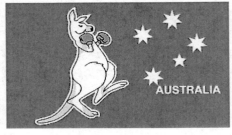 in place while using the claws on its larger hind legs to try to kick, slash or disembowel them. This stance gives the impression that the kangaroo appears to be "boxing" with its attacker.

Examination of the kangaroo revealed nothing special except acute pain upon palpation of the lower spine. No other symptoms were presented. Portable x-ray equipment was not available, so radiographs were not taken. The animal was eight years old, middle age for the species. I surmised "Roo" had arthritis or intervertiberal disc problems. With a serious diagnosis in hand, a fitting treatment plan was suggested: Declare Roo retired as the "Undisputed Kangaroo Boxing Champion," train a new young protégé to take his place, and carry on with the show.

Hawthorne Farms ran stories in the local press announcing Roo's retirement and his immediate replacement. The new 'roo was a crowd pleaser for the next decade.

The Hawthorn Melody Farm attraction was closed in 1970, after just two years of new management. "Decreased attendance, competition from newer facilities in the city, difficulty in maintaining good help, liability factors, and aging animals" were all causes of the downfall cited in the local press. Dairy production moved to Wisconsin, and the barns and attractions in Libertyville were torn down. The farm lives on as an exhibit at the Cuneo Museum and Gardens, once the home of Mr. Cuneo and his family.

Carol Hough Merrick

Bill Hough stopped his car to pick me up hitchhiking two miles from Lyons Township High School in La Grange to my home in Western Springs. I thought I recognized the pretty girl as I slid into the front seat beside her. I remembered Carol as the annoying little sister who wanted to play football or baseball with us boys. Carol's older brother, Harry, had been in my class since sixth grade. Carol had the good looks of her mother, but was an athlete at heart, just like her dad. I thought, "Wow! How girls change in a couple of years!" She smelled great and looked even better. After wrestling practice, I probably smelled like liniment and a locker room towel. Mr. Hough asked if I was one of the Merrick boys, and I responded affirmatively. He introduced Carol. We sat in silence until we got to their corner where he dropped me off. I tried to remember Harry's little sister, but I could not get the image of the changed young woman out of my head. This was not the first time I'd met Carol, of course, but it was the first time I noticed her.

Carol's parents, like mine, were an unchurched family. Madeline Hough was a nominal Roman Catholic; Bill Hough, a nominal Baptist. My father, Andy, had been raised Catholic, Dorothy was raised in the Quaker faith. At that time, the 1920s and '30s, it was common for the Catholic church to demand the children of such unions be raised Catholic.

Carol and I first met in St. Francis Catholic Church in LaGrange, Illinois. The family dog, Spotty, was a patient of my father's. Dad would drop us three kids off at church on his way to his animal hospital for Sunday office hours. We were expected to walk the two miles home. On occasion, Mr. Hough would give us a ride home from church.

It was the spring of 1946. I was a senior; Carol was a sophomore. I needed a date for the high school senior prom, but I had a problem: skipping two early grades left me the youngest and one of the smallest kids in my class. I had wrestled 105 pound class as a sophomore and had now worked up to the 115 pound class, but I had not built up enough inner strength to invite a girl on a date. When I told my brother, Phil, about meeting Carol and how she

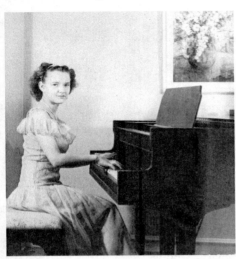

Carol Hough, Age 14 • Spring, 1946

had changed, he said, "Why don't you invite her out?" After much deliberation, I took the chance. Carol answered the phone and reported she would have to ask her parents' permission. A minute later, she agreed. So began a courtship, friendship, partnership, and marriage that would last over 60 years.

Years later Carol informed me she had told her Dad that it was Phil, not John, Merrick on the phone. Carol was not allowed to date seniors and since Phil was a sophomore, it would be okay. She says it was just a slip of the tongue, but I guess we'll never know for sure.

Since the prom was six weeks away, I asked Carol to go with me to the Saturday night dance at The Corral, the student run youth center in La Grange. I agreed to pick Carol up at 7:30, but I didn't arrive until almost 8:00. Carol's Dad greeted me with, "You're late, Merrick." I apologized and explained that I had gone to confession and there was a long line in the church. Madeline Hough beamed and remarked, "What a nice young man." Bill Hough had the look that said, "What a great story. I don't believe a word of it."

Two years later we were still dating when Carol graduated from high school and headed to Indiana University to major in physical education. I was in pre-vet school at the University of Illinois in Champaign, exactly 153 miles west of Bloomington, Indiana. Fearful of losing Carol to some Hoosier, I made the three-hour drive between our universities at least twice a month. These were the days prior to birth control pills. Our relationship was getting serious. I decided to sell my beautiful 1940 Chevy and buy an engagement ring. We asked her parents' permission to marry, explaining that it was a either a proper wedding, a possible elopement, or a shotgun wedding in the near future. Madeline and Bill Hough reluctantly agreed to a summer wedding and Carol got her ring. She also transferred to the U. of I. for her second semester of college, but it would be 20 years until she could begin to complete her higher education. Starting after the last of our six children, Peggy, entered second grade, Carol enrolled in the University of Wisconsin, Parkside in 1968. She was so unsure of her ability to compete against the younger generation, she only took one class the first semester, music appreciation. Carol had studied piano for eight years, giving her own recital at the age of 14, so music appreciation was a class right in her "sweet spot." She aced the class, found out that she could compete, and she was off and running.

Six years later Carol had received a Bachelor of Science in

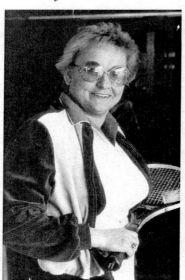

Carol's Letter Jacket • 1977

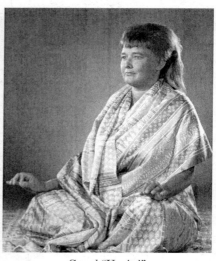

Carol "Yogini"
Shivananda Ashram
Val Morin, Canada • 1973

Liberal Arts, a Master's Coaching Certificate, and a Master's in Guidance and Counseling. Carol earned her varsity tennis letter at the age of 39. She also managed to spend one summer at a yoga ashram outside Montreal, getting her Yoga Teacher's Certificate. This enabled Carol to teach yoga at the University of Wisconsin for ten years. Many of her classes drew 70 to 80 students—by far the most of any P.E. class at the university.

After working for the state as a job counselor, Carol was employed as a "head hunter" in Chicago before starting Merrick Temporary Services. Her company had as many as 500 employees working as "temps" in businesses in and around Kenosha. Carol was also a cofounder of the first shelter for battered women in Wisconsin.

Carol injured her back playing golf; after hitting what she described as, "the best drive I've hit in ten years. Surgery to remove a prolapsed spinal disk ended up giving her an "in-house staph infection" that almost cost Carol her life. After six months of agonizing therapy, Carol was able to walk around the house, but she used a wheelchair outside. This unfortunate illness ended Carol's sport and Yoga career. Even in retirement, Carol remained active in promoting programs which helped women and the poor around the world.

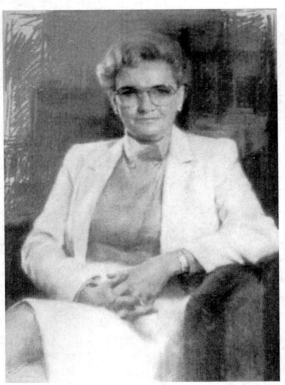

Carol passed in July, 2006, suffering a fatal heart attack in the hospital while recovering from a severe bout of the flu. We had been married 56 years and together for over 60.

The family and friends gathered at a local hotel one month after Carol died to "celebrate" her life. Friends and family gave moving descriptions of Carol and her effect on them and their community.

One of the more hilarious moments was a granddaughter's description of the scene in Carol's bedroom the previous day when all the "girls" went shopping in Carol's closet. Fortunately, most were close enough to Carol's size that minor alterations would suffice. Ohhs and Ahhs could be heard in the next county. Carol would be soooo happy.

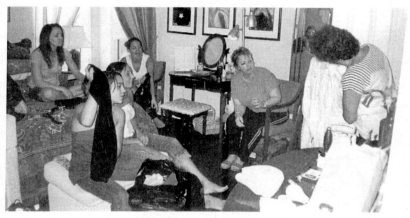

Daughters and Granddaughters
Carol's bedroom • August 2006

Community activist passes away

Carol Merrick led efforts for women

BY EMILY AYSHFORD
eayshford@kenoshanews.com

Whether advocating for women, counseling residents or serving on committees in the community, Carol Merrick was "the one who did whatever needed doing."

Carol Merrick

"She was very good at that," said former County Board supervisor and community activist Eunice Boyer. "We'll miss her in the community."

Longtime local businesswoman and women's advocate Merrick died Monday in Georgia. She was 75.

Merrick, who grew up in Illinois and came to Kenosha with her husband Dr. John Merrick, became known throughout the community as a good-hearted, optimistic person who cared about her family, business and community, said local real estate agent Colleen Deininger.

After working in her husband's veterinary practice, Merrick raised six children, went back to school to complete her bachelor's degree, received two master's degrees, and became a counselor and business owner.

"She was quite an active person," said longtime County Board member Anne Bergo. "She was always thinking ahead."

Merrick's forward thinking led her to help create the Kenosha Women's Network in 1980. In a 2000 interview with the Kenosha News, Merrick said she was moved to build a women's network after hearing a speech by Gene Boyer, a co-founder of the National Organization for Women in Wisconsin.

"They challenged us to start our own groups, and I love a challenge," Merrick said in the interview. "This was before women were allowed into Kiwanis or Rotary. It took us a year to start up the club, to get our ducks in order. It was an exciting experience. It still is, every time I go to a meeting."

Merrick also founded Displaced Homemakers, an organization that helped former homemakers find new careers in the early 1980s.

"There weren't nearly as many working women then," Deininger said. "She helped a lot of these women get training to get back into the work force. She did a lot with the women in the community."

In a 1991 article about problems facing Kenosha women, Merrick said, "If we are going to make any headway in helping women become economically strong — and that is what this is really all about — we must have people in key positions who are sympathetic to our cause."

In addition to helping women, Merrick also taught yoga at the University of Wisconsin-Parkside and served on the Gateway Technical College Board in the 1990s. She also served on a Kenosha County Growth Management Task Force and on numerous other committees and councils.

"She got more done in a day then maybe a lot of people get done in a week," Deininger said. "She was just a very active person."

Kenosha News
July 19, 2006

City Girl

Kenosha, just over the Illinois border into Wisconsin, 50 miles north of Chicago, was a contrast in lifestyles. In 1956, the city of 60,000 had a number of unionized manufacturing plants—American Motors (Nash), American Brass, Snap-On Tools, Simmons, Jockey, and more. The county, with a population of 40,000, was rural, with a few small communities, lakes, and dairy farms. Just as today, the Democratic labor unions (United Auto Workers, etc.), dominated the City Council and the Republicans offset their power with firm control of the County Board.

It took me a year or two before I could identify a native Kenoshan coming into my new practice in Kenosha. In the mid '50s, the majority of native Kenoshans seem to think their glass—whether one half full or half empty—had a hole in the bottom. No matter what they did, they just knew the water (good times) would soon be gone. Eventually, I learned to tell a native Kenoshan, both city and rural, by their pessimistic attitude. If times were good, "Just you watch, it will get worse." Conversely, if times were bad, "See, I told you it would get worse." New clients, especially from the Chicago area, were just the opposite. Almost all had a positive outlook on life. They hadn't lived through the last 30 years of the ups and downs of the auto industry. American Motors Corporation (AMC) had recently been formed by a merger of Nash/Kelvinator and Hudson Motors. Production of their very successful automobile, Rambler, was begun in 1956 under AMC president George Romney. Better times were on the horizon.

Carol learned her lesson less than a week after we moved to town. Ruthie Trowbridge, whose husband owned a local lumber yard, was a new neighbor across the street from our rental house, one-half mile south of my animal hospital, on the outskirts of Kenosha. Ruthie came over one morning and asked if Carol would watch her two preschoolers while she went downtown. Carol said she'd be happy to, and she organized something for Ruth's two and our three youngsters to occupy them while she did the laundry and breakfast dishes. Within an hour Ruth was back in the front door with a couple of shopping bags under her arms to show off her loot. Carol remarked, "How could you possibly be back from downtown Chicago in one hour?" Ruthie laughed, "Not Chicago, silly, downtown Kenosha." It never dawned on Carol that there was any other downtown than Chicago.

In the late '50s and early '60s, most women were "homemakers"—still working inside the home. They would often enjoy a midday coffee klatch. Soon after moving into our three bedroom prefab in Kenosha, Carol met daily with the neighborhood "girls." After the usual gossip about kids, husbands, and celebrities, Helen Estill said, "So tell us, Carol, how does it feel to be married to a doctor?" Carol's immediate response was, "Doctor? Ha! I knew Johnny before he was old enough to shave."

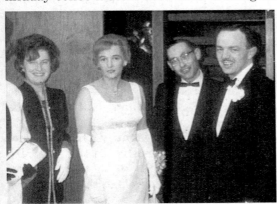

Nadine Herz, Carol, Dr. Richard Herz, and John Headed to the Symphony Ball • 1965

A war bride from India was new to the neighborhood. Jyota spoke excellent English but was quiet and reserved during the free-for-all conversation. Verna Jacobs questioned Jyota, "How do you like living in America with all our modern conveniences?" "It's quite different," responded Jyota, "In my home in India, I was 14 years old before I had to comb my own hair. We had servants to perform most of the household tasks. So yes, it has taken me a while to get used to the change."

Less than a month later, Carol decided she needed a new housedress. Stopping in at one of the small family owned dress shops in midtown Kenosha, Carol inquired about house dresses. The owner showed Carol a number of typical, practical, $5.00 models. Carol then spotted some new styles on a neighboring rack, and asked, "What about those?" The clerk responded, "Those are new this week, but they are $7.50." Carol declared immediately, "I'll take two." To Carol's chagrin and later delight, the clerk replied sarcastically, "You must be a city girl!"

Ever since that day, when a new client ends her office visit with a remark like, "Is that all?" or "I expected you'd charge more than that," I know I have another "city girl" for a client—one who will not only expect, but demand the best of my abilities, and be willing and able to pay a premium for the service. It reminds me of the professional business counselor's advice, "Don't worry about keeping all your C and D clients coming back. As a rule, it's next to impossible make a good living catering to C's and D's. Concentrate on the A and B clients. Charge a premium fee and offer first-class service. That way you'll be able to attract and keep excellent employees, afford to purchase the best equipment, take a needed vacation more than once a lifetime, and save for your kids' college and your retirement."

I believe the number of "city girls" has increased exponentially since women have become emancipated in the last 30 years. Women also seem to have a much more emotional attachment to their pets. Women tend to think of pets as family members. Many men still tend to put their pocketbook ahead of their heart. They think of pets as expendable, like another tool or possession. As part of its ongoing "FemiNation" dialogue into the lifestyles and attitudes of contemporary women, Lifetime Networks recently announced a survey on the relationship between women 18–49 and their pets. The poll found that 89% of women indicate they will spend the same amount or more on their pets in the next 12 months, while 24% plan on spending more money.

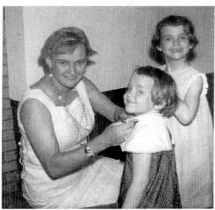
Carol prepping two future "City Girls" • Peggy, 3, Ginger, 5

"This poll shows that pets are no longer viewed as mere companions, but as integral parts of their families," said Mike Greco, Executive Vice President of Research. "Underlining this powerful emotional bond, 87% of women consider pets members of their family, with 59% willing to risk their lives to save their pet." The survey also reveals that just under one third (28%) of women put the needs of their pet ahead of their own. Given a choice between human or animal companionship on a deserted island, 13% opted for their pet—perhaps because 30% say their pet is the best listener! Findings of the survey include:

1. **Reigning Dogs and Cats**
   - Roughly seven out of ten women (69%) between the ages of 18 and 49 own a pet.
   - One-half (51%) of women 18–49 own at least one dog, and one-third (33%) own at least one cat.
2. **Pets Are People Too**
   - Most women pet owners 18–49 (87%) consider their pets to be members of their family.
   - More than half of women pet owners 18–49 (59%) would risk their lives for their pet.
   - One-in-ten women pet owners 18–49 (12%) have sacrificed a relationship for their pet.
   - More than one in four women pet owners 18–49 (28%) put the needs of their pet ahead of their own.
3. **Pampered Pets = Purchasing Power**
   - The majority of women pet owners 18–49 (58%) claim that they "always pamper their pets with the best products."
   - In the past year, 81% of women pet owners 18–49 have purchased their pets toys (66%), professional grooming (26%), organic food (22%), outfits (16%) and/or some type of spa service (4%).
   - Among women pet owners 18–49, more than two-thirds (68%) buy their pets holiday or birthday presents, one-third (36%) takes their pets on vacation, and 20% dress their pets up.
   - On average, women pet owners 18–49 report having spent $160 on a gift for their pet (37% admit to having spent more than $100).
4. **Woman's Best Friend**
   - More than one-in-ten women pet owners 18–49 (13%) would choose to have the companionship of their favorite pet over another human being if they were stranded on a deserted island.
   - A third of women pet owners 18–49 (30%) say that their favorite pet is the "best listener."
   - Half of women pet owners 18–49 (49%) let their pet sleep in their bed.

As with most all professions, veterinary medicine is becoming "feminized." In the summer of 2009, over half of the veterinarians were female. Seventy five percent of all veterinary students are female. I have seen the future of vet med, and it's wearing a pantsuit or a dress!

Dyna Mite, Canine Variety

The girls in Lehman Lodge, Carol's dorm at the University of Illinois, found a small, white Fox Terrier wandering on a sidewalk near campus ten days before Christmas break in 1949. Inquires at houses in the neighborhood failed to find its owner. Probably no more than six weeks old, she stayed in Carol's bedroom for two days until the housemother found out. "Johnny's in pre-vet," she said, "He'll know what to do." Rules were more relaxed in the men's dorm, Four Columns, where I lived across the street from Lehman House. It was not exactly "Animal House," but we could have kept a pet pig with no trouble from the landlady, Mrs. Coleman. Christmas break was upon us before she discovered the new boarder. The tiny precocious pup was soon the delight of the dorm. She wolfed down canned puppy food and entertained the boys until exhaustion took over. Unlike the dormitory sleeping area on the third floor in the "O House," Four Columns had bunk beds in the student rooms. She slept in a shoebox at the foot of my bed.

Carol's parents, Madeline and Bill Hough, had lost their 14-year-old Beagle mix, Spotty, to cancer the summer before. Dad performed the euthanasia. Spotty was buried in their back yard behind the garage. It didn't take too much persuasion to convince them this pup would be a perfect replacement for Spotty. They agreed to take the new puppy when we came home for the Christmas vacation.

Dyna got her name within the first hour of her arrival in her new home. She tore around the house as if she had been born there—up and down the stairs, on and off all the furniture—such energy. She had slept the two-hour drive from Champaign to suburban Chicago. Carol's dad, Bill, remarked, "This pup is really dynamite." The name stuck.

Over the years, Dyna—short for Dynamite—grew into a 15-pound Fox Terrier who was a lively attention-getter at our wedding the following summer. Dyna enjoyed her "only child" status. She asked for and received coffee with cream and sugar after her morning treats, took regular walks—on demand—often four or five times a day. She served as the fill-in grandchild when the real thing wasn't available. Tragically, 12 years later, Carol's dad,

Grandpa Hough, fell from a ladder while cleaning his gutters. He'd suffered a stroke, and while recovering in the hospital, passed away from a heart attack. At first Dyna was a comfort to Grandma Madeline Hough. As the months passed, it became evident Madeline could not care for herself adequately, let alone a pet. We decided to bring Dyna home to Kenosha to live with our growing family.

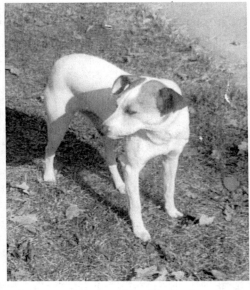

After 13 years, Dyna was back with her original owners. It took a few weeks before Dyna became accustomed to and was accepted by our resident dog, Pixie, and cat, Sooty. Both were young enough to allow Dyna to assume the role of matriarch. Our family didn't drink much coffee in the morning. That soon changed. Dyna would not be denied her morning caffeine fix. Perhaps I can blame Dyna for the caffeine I learned to enjoy. Instead of daily walks on a leash, Dyna also relished the freedom of five acres of woods. We had recently moved into our new house built behind my animal hospital. She could put her terrier skills to use chasing squirrels, annoying birds, and digging for grinnys (ground squirrels).

Her favorite time was 3 PM, awaiting the school kids trekking home through the woods after school. She would meet and greet neighbor children as eagerly as our own.

As with many terriers, Dyna lived a long, healthy life. At the age of 18 she developed an acute illness. Age had taken its toll on her heart and kidneys, with both systems showing signs of the wear and tear of the aging process. As luck would have it, Carol and I were on one of our infrequent ski trips to Aspen, Colorado. Our baby sitter, after consulting with us by phone, called my friend and colleague, Dr. Jim Nordstrom. He made a house call that evening. Jim phoned us at our lodge with a very grim prognosis: Dyna's kidneys had shut down. She was suffering from uremic poisoning. After explaining to the family that Dyna had no chance to regain her happy life, the decision was made not to prolong Dyna's suffering. Her life ended as it had begun, in the arms of her loving family. The fuse, lit so many years ago, was extinguished.

Mrs. Doherty—Compliments

I had skipped two grades in grade school, so I was always the youngest and smallest in my class. Our family was split up during the height of the depression in 1934. Margaret, age six, went to live with Aunt Jo and Uncle Byron in Berlin Heights, Ohio. I was sent to live with my grandparents on the family farm in Gibson, Iowa. I was 4½ that summer. Phil, age three, ended up with Aunt Manon and Uncle Gerard in Forreston, Illinois.

For reasons unknown, Grandpa Santee enrolled me in the local one room schoolhouse a quarter mile down the road. There were 23 students in eight grades. I had two other children in my first grade class. I have no idea why I was placed in school before the age of five, but I suspect the motive was not only to start me on the path to higher knowledge, but also to provide babysitting relief for Grandma Santee.

By the summer of 1935, my father had opened his first animal hospital in Brookfield, Illinois, enabling the family to be reunited. Enrolling in St. Barbara's Catholic grade school at the age of 5½, the nuns assigned me to first grade. "But he finished first grade in Iowa last year," my mother explained. "In that case," Sister Mary Joseph said, "John can start in second grade. If he can keep up with the other pupils, he can stay."

This acceleration of my education had a profound effect on me—not so much in the early years as in middle school and high school. When my peers were experiencing growth spurts and teenage angst, I was still in prepuberty. As a result I was somewhat shy, but not introverted. Wrestling, organized by weight, was the only sport where I could have a chance at a varsity letter. Wrestling in the 115-pound class and winning an "L" in my senior year was the fulfillment of my goal.

In my senior year—I was not yet 16—I took Mrs. Doherty's class in English literature. Unlike some kids who jumped up with all the answers, I was not one to speak up in class. Mrs. Doherty's practice was to have students read out loud, a page or two of Beowulf or whatever work we were studying. When my turn came, I stood up and somehow got through my performance without too many mistakes. Mrs. Doherty remarked, "Mr. Merrick, you have a wonderful speaking voice. I want you to practice reading aloud at home every day."

Those words—that compliment—literally changed my life by changing my perception of myself. Indeed, my voice had changed in the last couple of months, thanks to the testosterone now flowing in my veins. I can still picture Mrs. Doherty and the moment in my mind. Indeed, I did as suggested, reading aloud daily for the next few weeks. I auditioned for parts in school plays and joined the Western Springs Little Theatre. Like most endeavors, practice makes perfect. Mom even insisted I take singing lessons. Since that day I've had countless people remark about my voice. "You should be an announcer," etc. Most business or government leaders have a baritone or bass voice. I think we are programmed to respect the alpha male voice. I can't think of any world leader with a squeaky, nasal voice. The lion's roar shows whose in command.

After writing the story of Mrs. Doherty's effect on my life, I tried to find out if she was still alive. Doubtful, as she would be at least in her nineties by now. I often thought through the years, "Why don't I call the Lyons Township High School to inquire about her whereabouts." Sadly, procrastination won the battle.

Ms. Sally Kapso emails from LTHS, "Yes, her name was Grace Doherty. She died in 1980 in Western Springs, according to the Social Security Death Index. Born in 1888, according to the yearbooks, they say her name was Grace W. Doherty. She had two degrees, from A.B. Eastham College and A.M. University of Chicago. It looks like she started at LT in 1926 and taught through 1954. I don't find her in any of the yearbooks after that."

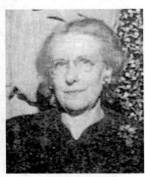

Grace W. Doherty
1888–1980

Even though she will never hear my praise, I'm sure her spirit lives on through the thousands of students she influenced.

What gives compliments their power?

Webster defines compliment as, "An expression of praise, admiration or congratulations; a formal act of civility, courtesy or respect." Some people exude compliments.

Howard Brown, the publisher of our local paper, the *Kenosha News,* could not meet anyone on the street or in his office without expressing two compliments—three if it was a woman. Meeting Carol and me, Howard would invariably say, "Dr. Merrick, how are you and your lovely young bride today? What a beautiful dress you're wearing, Carol." Carol would say something like, "Howard, you're so sweet to notice." Howard would reply, "And your hair... is that a new style? It's very becoming of you." Carol knew full well Howard was always full of compliments, but she relished the praise.

I never left a meeting in Howard's newspaper office without a small gift. Sometimes it was a bag of jelly beans, once a delightful book written by the "Obit" editor of the *New York Times,*

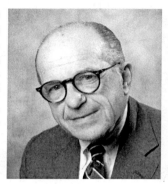

Howard Brown
1923–2011

often a memento for Carol. I once teased his charming wife, Betsy, "Don't you get upset with Howard's flirting with all the girls?" "O, my goodness, no. He's not flirting. That's just Howard being Howard," she responded with a laugh. Howard passed away in April, 2011, after a long battle with stomach cancer. Hundreds of condolences were received and published in the *Kenosha News.* Most all described "Uncle Howard" as: Humorous. Attentive. Charming. Compassionate. Intelligent. Honorable. This is how they remembered their beloved "Mr. Brown."

There's a lesson there: When in doubt, compliment.

Marty Bach would now be called a school guidance counselor. In 1962 Marty was the truant officer for Kenosha High School. Marty was a friend, neighbor and member of our nickel-and-dime poker group. Marty told us of a problem he had that day with one of his "clients."

"I try to start off talking to these kids with a compliment. It throws them off because they assume I'm going to yell, lecture, and threaten. Today, this young punk had me stumped. He was ugly, dirty, overweight, had a scraggly beard, and smelled. I was at a loss for a compliment, so I blurted out, "So what's your reason for skipping school?" He answered, "I got my girlfriend pregnant and I needed to find a job if I'm going to get married." "I almost fell off my chair," Marty said.

He continued, "If this sorry excuse for a human being can find someone to love and care for, there's hope for the human race after all. It really made my day."

I've found clients invariably smile when I compliment them or their pet as they enter the exam room. I have no scientific evidence, but I'd wager clients are less likely to dispute a fee when the visit is begun with a sincere compliment. Look at it this way: You've given them a gift. Only the person on the receiving end can judge its value.

Why is it that many of us find it hard to praise, admire, or congratulate? Do we worry we won't be believed? Is it poor parenting? Are we just plain lazy? No, I think it's a lack of effort and practice. Anyone can learn to show the respect that a compliment imparts. As that New York Cabbie replied when asked how to get to Carnegie Hall, "Practice, Practice, Practice."

The Music Box Vet

Doc Byron Merrick's babies came in all shapes and sizes. Unlike most vets who have puppies, kittens, calves, and foals, Dr. Byron (Buzz) Merrick's family was made up of music boxes—well over 300, but who's counting? Inspired by playing with a neighbor's music box as a young boy in Columbus, Ohio, his collection was the fulfillment of a childhood dream, to own a music box.

After serving as a first sergeant in the Balloon Corps in WWI, Dr. Merrick graduated from Ohio State University School of Veterinary Medicine in June, 1923. He married Josephine Brown on that same day and began a mixed animal practice shortly thereafter in Berlin Heights, Ohio, near Lake Erie, halfway between Toledo and Cleveland.

Mrs. William Olds called Dr. Merrick to the Olds's farm to treat a sick cow in 1929, paying for the successful treatment with a music box from her antique shop. This was the impetus for his hobby/quest/obsession.

Not being blessed with children, Dr. Merrick and his wife Josephine started their worldwide scavenger hunt in the '40s with a few routine musical boxes. By the time of his retirement, they had established the largest private collection in the United States. One five-month tour involved driving 8,000 miles around Europe in 1962, included stops in every European country, and ending in Lisbon. From Lisbon they flew to Cairo, Jerusalem, and Beirut. Flying home in time for Christmas in Ohio, they met their car at the airport, which had been shipped ahead.

The remarkable collection spans the entire development of mechanical music players from early Swiss musical watches to juke boxes. Some of Edison's early works are included. Dr. Merrick had a special "museum room" added to their house to accommodate the 300-piece collection. Dr. Merrick helped found and was the first president of the International Society of Music Box Collectors. The first meeting of the society was held in 1956, in his newly remodeled addition. Looking as if it had been transported from a chalet in Switzerland, the room held the doctor's incredible menagerie of musical boxes, ballerinas, singing birds, dancing clowns, watches, and Burmese glass. Dr. Merrick loved to give guided tours to clients and visitors.

The collection was arranged in chronological order, starting with musical watches, the first musical instruments, dating back to about 1770. Advances in technique were shown in a rare music box made in Switzerland in 1840 by A. Malignon. When the first tune was completed, the cylinder automatically shifted to line up a new set of pins to play a second tune. By 1850, Geneva and St. Croix were the music box centers of the world. Craftsmen began making larger cabinets. Ratchets were used to wind up springs instead of keys. He had one of the first "orchestra" music boxes. Made by Paillard in Switzerland in 1873, it combined an organ, drum, seven bells, and a castanet. One piece, presented to Theodore Roosevelt when he was Police Commissioner of New York by the Swiss government, played 12 tunes including the "Star Spangled Banner." The bells were struck by golden eagles.

The auction of Dr. Merrick's collection, held after the death of Josephine in 1993, set a new record for music box sales. Over 500 people came to Wolf's Fine Arts Auctioneers in Cleveland from all over the world—Japan, Belgium, England, France, and Monaco. The record-setting item was a rare Pierodienique telescoping interchangeable cylinder musical box. Swiss manufactured, circa 1880, it sold to international interests for $66,000. Over $1.6 million dollars was raised for the Merrick estate.

My niece, Margaret's daughter, Ms. Mari Scheffelin Yamamoto, is writing a book detailing the extraordinary life of her mother. As Margaret was very close to Byron and Jo throughout their entire life, she received a number of mementos following their death. Mari sent me the following communication:

> An unusual way of contributing to national defense came after the death of Margaret's dear Aunt Jo. Byron Merrick's world war uniforms were found in a box in the attic where they had lain for nearly eighty years. The uniforms and other World War I items included a rare panoramic photo of the 29th Balloon Company during World War I at Fort Monroe. Margaret donated all of the items to the U.S. Army Center of Military History (CMH), which was particularly happy to have the collection, saying they have very little about the balloonists in World War I. CMH transferred the items to the U.S. Army Aviation Museum at Fort Tucker, where the donation would be known as the "Merrick Collection."

Dr. Byron Merrick was honored as Veterinarian of the Year by Ohio State University in 1958 and received the prestigious OSU College of Medicine Distinguished Alumni Award in 1964.

Over 50 years have passed since the day in 1956 when I purchased the animal hospital in Kenosha, Wisconsin, enabled by a $4,000 down payment loan from my uncle, Dr. Byron P. Merrick. The terms were fair—8% interest, $48.50 a month, for ten years. I never missed a payment and retired the debt five years early. Being both generous and entrepreneurial, I'm sure Uncle Buzz brought music into the lives of many young vets like myself.

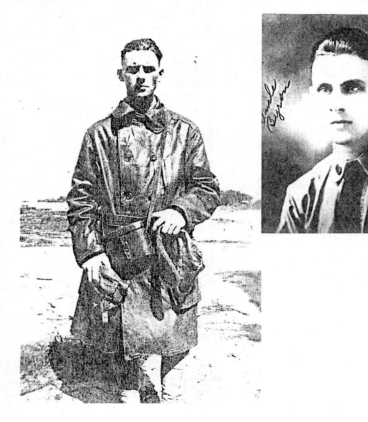

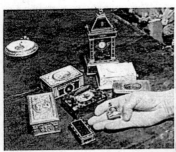

Ornate snuff boxes double as music boxes. Music also emanates from the private letter seal shown in Dr. Merrick's hand.

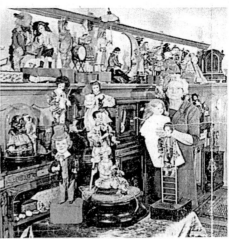

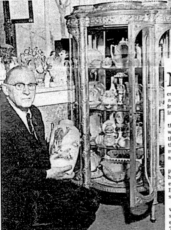

Burmese glass, made for only six years, is another Merrick hobby. Unusual color is result of gold and uranium added to the mix. They have over 109 of the expensive pieces.

A House

By ETHELBERTA HARTMAN

MUSICAL BOXES, Burmese glass, Staffordshire cottage figures, lithophanes—any one of these could make a lifelong hobby but Dr. and Mrs. B. P. Merrick of Berlin Heights, in Erie County, have notable collections in each of these fields.

Doc and Joe, as they are called by their fellow townsmen, live in a modest white house. Several years ago, when their musical boxes threatened to put them out on the street, they added a room in Swiss chalet style almost as big as the original house.

Its large log-burning fireplace, exposed rafters, casement windows and hanging lamps are reminiscent of Switzerland, home of the musical boxes. Especially built cabinets with sliding shelves hold many of the larger boxes.

The Merricks (he is a widely known veterinarian) have musical pieces as small as a thimble, and one that is large enough to be a handsomely carved desk. There are watches, fobs, snuff boxes and lockets that were made to be used as gifts.

Pressure on a small gold locket causes a wee bird with iridescent feathers to pop out. It opens its bill, vibrating as it sings.

A rare sedan chair watch belonged to King George III. It has a carved filigree band edged with pearls and amethysts. Five bells strike a tune on the hour.

Many years after these small pieces someone hit on the idea of a cylinder with projecting pins. These cylinders were built into all sorts of cabinets. Bells, organ effects, castanets and drums were added. One of Dr. Merrick's boxes sounds like a whole orchestra.

One piece, presented to Theodore Roosevelt by the Swiss government when he was police commissioner of New York, plays 12 tunes, including the Star Spangled Banner. Golden eagles strike the bells.

Musical pieces include a large number of automatons, or animated toys. These were created for adults in great variety. One fellow raises and lowers

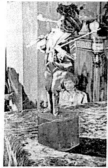
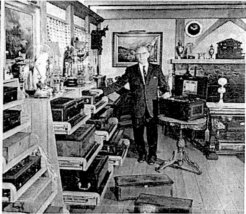

Unique velvet-clad doll smokes cigarette, inhales and blows the smoke.

Specially designed cabinets with sliding drawers cover the length of the recently added chalet room which houses part of Dr. Merrick's music box collection.

THE PLAIN DEALER SUNDAY MAGAZINE SUNDAY, JULY 5, 1964   Photos by DWIGHT BOYER

Full of Collections

his arm to puff on a cigarette, with actual smoke. Two gray kittens, wearing glasses, play and sing.

Musical boxes were the first Merrick addiction—about 35 years ago—but they have become so scarce and so expensive that he has added little to that collection recently. During his most recent trip to Europe, he drove 8,000 miles and spent six months on the trail of objects to be collected.

MRS. Merrick's favorites are the Jumeaux dolls, created by a famous doll maker of that name from 1860 to 1880. They were noted for their natural-looking eyes. One has her ears pierced for earrings. Another plays with her fan and smells her flowers. Edison's talking doll (no Jumeaux) with the cylinder inside, sings a lullaby.

The tops of the cabinets hold dozens of Staffordshire cottage figures. These were turned out in quantity in the area of this English county. They depict the acters of the 19th century.

Burmese glass was only made for six years after it was patented in 1885. The Merricks have over 100 pieces of this glass which is found in all shades of salmon pink blending to lemon yellow. It owes its unusual coloring to gold and uranium in the mix, and was called Burmese because it was supposed to resemble a Burma sunrise. It was made only in New Bedford, Mass. and—at the request of Queen Victoria—in London.

The Merrick collection includes numbers of bud and rose bowls, a lamp base, candlesticks, fairy lamps, an ornate epergne and two unusually large vases. They are decorated with birds and flowers.

Although many thousands of lithophanes were manufactured in Germany and France between 1835 and 1890, few of them remain today. They were panels made of porcelain and were used styles and customs and historical char- in lamp shades or simply hung in a window as decoration. Light shining through revealed beautiful pictures in gradations of gray, controlled by the thickness of the porcelain.

The first of the lithophanes were carved directly on the porcelain. Soon, however, a method was developed whereby one design carving could be duplicated.

THE Merricks have about 70 of these. The designs include copies of famous paintings, children at play and many scenes of rural America.

Dr. Merrick was instrumental in organizing the International Musical Box Club and was its president two years. In the summer of 1961 the Merricks entertained 76 members at the annual meeting.

While the Merricks were in Europe last fall they visited two Swiss in San Croix who had repaired many of their boxes.

The Merricks happily share their treasures with anyone who is interested. They ask only that arrangements be made by mail ahead of time.

PROFFER OF GIFT AGREEMENT
For use of this form, see AR870-20

| November 30, 1995 | REGISTRATION NUMBER: CMH 1995.068 | Page No. 2 |

DESCRIPTION OF PROPERTY:

1. COAT WOOL OD KHAKI WOOL USA 1917 Complete Good
2. BREECHES OD KHAKI WOOL USA 1917 Complete Good
3. COAT KHAKI KHAKI WOOL USA 1917 Complete Good
4. BREECHES KHAKI KHAKI WOOL USA 1917 Complete Good
5. BREECHES KHAKI KHAKI WOOL USA 1918 Complete Good
6. COLLAR KHAKI WOOL USA 1918 Complete Good
7. CAP AMERICAN LEGION KHAKI WOOL USA 1920 Complete Good
8. PHOTOGRAPH 29TH BALLOON CO KHAKI WOOL 29TH BALLOON COMPANY, FT MONROE, VA PAPER USA 1918 Complete Good

Donor Signature: *Margaret Scheffelin, Ph.D.*   Date: *Dec 11, 1995*

Museum Representative: *Judson E. Bennett, Jr.*

UNITED STATES ARMY AVIATION MUSEUM
UNITED STATES ARMY AVIATION WARFIGHTING CENTER
P.O. BOX 620610, FORT RUCKER ALABAMA 36362-0610
(205) 255-2893/3036   FAX (205) 255-3054   LIBRARY (205) 255-3169

May 31, 1996

U.S. Army Aviation Museum

Margaret Scheffelin, Ph.D.
Visual Tutor Company
3015 Root Avenue
Carmichael, California 95608

Dear Dr. Scheffelin:

Thank you for your concern and interest in the Army Aviation Museum. The donation of your uncle's World War I uniforms and memorabilia has greatly enhanced our collection and our ability to tell the story of Army Aviation.

Enclosed are two copies of the Proffer of Gift Agreement. Please sign one copy and return it to the museum for our records. The second copy is for your records.

A list of cataloged items are listed on the gift agreement form. The 29th Balloon Company picture has been placed in our archives. The uniforms and memorabilia will be known as the "Merrick Collection."

Again, thank you for your interest in preserving Army Aviation history.

Sincerely,

R. S. Maxham
Director
U.S. Army Aviation Museum

Enclosure

Dinner Guests and Visitors

It was the custom in the '50s and '60s for husbands to "work" and wives to "keep house." I don't recall that there was ever any intention to deny that women "worked." Maybe we unconsciously thought so, but I know I never thought women were slacking in their efforts to manage the lives of their families. I'm sure farm families never wondered about which gender worked more than the other. There was always more than enough work to go around. Kids were welcome and needed to do the myriad chores.

Six kids in ten years kept my wife, Carol, busy in the home. She still found time to be an occasional emergency surgical assistant, receptionist, bookkeeper, etc. in my practice. Being home full time, Carol enjoyed cooking for the family, breakfast, noon, and night. She encouraged my proclivity to invite clients, salespeople, and others to a "home cooked" meal at our house—down the 500-foot path behind the animal hospital, through five acres of oak woods to our Frank Lloyd Wright–style house, built in 1963. The approaching west side was almost completely open to view the woodland by sliding glass doors on the first and second floors. Meals were taken in the "family kitchen" facing the woods.

In the early days of practice, salespeople were often considered friends, bringing in news of new products and techniques and gossip about colleagues and medicine in general. People like Jim Duffy, detailing for Chicago Vet Supply, later Holmes Serum and beyond, were frequently over to our house for lunch. I imagine some of the guys found it convenient to make their stop at my practice late in the morning.

I also made it a practice to invite strangers who came to our house from religious organizations to family meals. I thought exposing the children to various points of view would encourage critical thinking and discussion and result in open minds. One evening two representatives of Latter Day Saints came by and were invited in to give their pitch during our evening meal. As luck would have it, the older "talker" sat by me and conversed during the entire meal. The younger "listener" sat next to Carol and farted continuously. "Those will be the last Mormons we serve in my house," Carol announced after they left.

In the spring of 1973, I received a letter from a young Australian vet, explaining his plan to drive across the county from Seattle to Maryland, where he had the prospect of a job. He was looking for places to visit and stay along the route to meet people, explore the country and cut down on expenses. I wrote him back to come ahead—we would look forward to seeing him and putting him up for a couple of nights.

Months went by and I had completely forgotten his letter or my promise. Our 13-year-old daughter, Ginger, was having a sleepover with 12 girls in attendance when the young lad from down under, rucksack in hand, ambled through the woods and appeared at the sliding glass doors to the living room where the young ladies were in various stages of preparing for bed. Needless to say, pandemonium erupted.

Years later Ginger told me the rest of the story. Sometime after midnight, when the household was fast asleep, the girls crept out of the house on a TP mission. TP, for the uninitiated, is the act of throwing rolls of toilet paper around, over, and through the trees of the homes of two girls who were unable to attend the sleepover, three boys they liked, and two boys they "hated." Their biggest fear was waking the grownups or our two huge Lab-Shepherd dogs. Fortunately, the adults and dogs were blissfully unaware of the midnight marauders. Before he left, the young traveler presented us with a boomerang as a thank-you present.

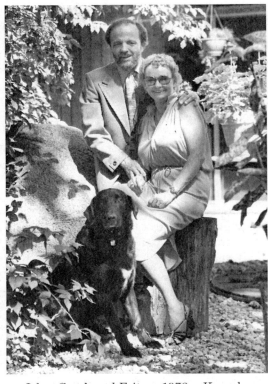

John, Carol, and Fritz • 1978 • Kenosha

Scenes like that are difficult to imagine today. While sleepovers remain popular, home-cooked meals are a rarity today. TV ads show families around the dinner table. TV ads pitch the idea that "Mom can prepare supper in only ten minutes" with the company's products.

Today the majority of women are employed outside the home and have very little time to entertain. Both sexes are expected to—and usually do—share the parenting and housekeeping duties. Women's liberation and Title IX has changed the entire landscape. Those of us who lived through that time period can reflect and enjoy the memories of a slower-paced time.

The Art of Bartering

Pablo needed a new suit. In fact, Pablo needed his first suit. He had a big date in Paris and he was desperate to find a tailor. The date was April 4, 1901, the Pablo was Picasso, and the occasion was the future modern art icon's first Paris showing of his paintings. He had been painting near Barcelona in southern Spain, but the art Mecca was Paris.

When Picasso explained to the local tailor his need for clothes without any ready cash, the tailor replied, "Let me see your work." He agreed to make Picasso a suit and received two paintings in return. Over the years, he traded for Picasso's work whenever Pablo need a wardrobe addition.

Even though Picasso's prices were far beyond the cost of a tailored suit, Pablo repaid the tailor's original generosity by continuing a one-for-one trade. Needless to say, the tailor became both "rich and famous."

The preceding story was told in *Time Magazine* in the mid-60's. Upon reading it, bells and whistles went off in my head. My wife, Carol, and I had recently joined the Kenosha Art Association and were taking weekly painting classes. Many of the local artists were clients. Some were very accomplished craftsmen. Maybe I could trade vet services for art, one pro with another. Most of the art clients I approached readily agreed and a tradition was born. The walls of my animal hospital and residence were eventually covered with the proceeds of ovariohysterectomies, fracture repairs, vaccinations, and the like.

Trading vet services for farm produce has long been a tradition, especially when times were tough and cash was in short supply. My uncle, Byron Merrick in Berlin Heights, Ohio, got his first of over 300 music boxes in a trade for saving a sick cow. A story in the Des Moines Register about my dad's "Expensive Animal Hospital" in suburban Chicago, costing $50,000 in 1935, compared that price to his getting paid for vet services in walnuts and potatoes a few years earlier in Oskaloosa, Iowa.

I'm sure most veterinarians swap services with a few tradespeople—plumbers, garage mechanics, and the like. In those cases we already know the individual's skill and price of the service to be exchanged. It's a very personal exchange—a barter based on agreement between two professionals who respect one another's work. In the case of artistic work, I always wanted to make sure Carol or I appreciate the artist's work before entering into any trade. I had a number of favorites who would keep a running tab until I had enough credit to trade for an especially wonderful piece of blown glass, sculpture, weavings or paintings.

I regret that downsizing in retirement cost me the wall space required to keep all the wonderful art. Children, friends, relatives and charities benefited from our move from Wisconsin to Georgia.

I traded with the very talented Allen Schabel for the tryptic which adorned the reception area of my animal hospital for many years.

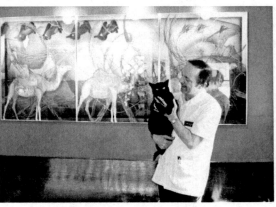

Tryptic "Camels, Sheep & Nudes"
Allen Schabel • Kenosha, Wisc. • 1978

Carol made the newspaper with her acquisition of John Farnham's work "God in the Box." The artists' conception of how many people seem to be following God's word on Sunday, but put him in a box for the rest of the week. John and his talented wife, Ruth, have made California their home for many years.

The art of bartering is something I will always have with me.

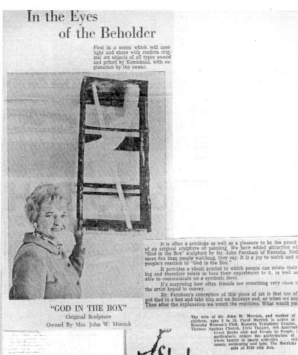

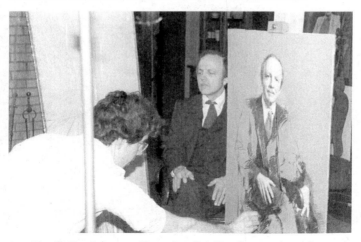

Jim Pollard from a Kenosha family of portrait artists
(He must have taken 100 photos!) • Kenosha, Wisc. • 1990

Sweet Georgia Brown

"Sweet Georgia Brown." Hum, whistle, or sing the tune, and it's a good bet most people imagine seeing basketballs flying around the court, propelled by the Harlem Globetrotters. The troupe, now 85 years young, was in town to perform their magical routines and rout the hapless Washington Capitals again. This was not a team of basketball clowns. The Globetrotters beat the premier professional team, the Minneapolis Lakers.

The year was 1958. Our newly formed service club, Western Kenosha Kiwanis, was searching for a fund-raiser to add to our annual peanut sale at the Labor Day parade. Peanuts brought in about $500 profit. Not bad for a one-day, three-hour event, involving most of our 25 members.

Jerry Pfarr, the sports editor of the Kenosha News and a frequent golfing companion, called me with a fund-raising idea for my Kiwanis Club. He showed me the promotional material he had received from the Harlem Globetrotters. In those days the 'Trotters played anywhere they could get an audience. Big time sports arenas were ten years in the future. I called the 'Trotter's office and spoke to the owner, Abe Saperstein. Yes, they could work Kenosha into their schedule. He recalled the Globetrotters playing in Kenosha 15 to 20 years ago. "A return visit," he said, "was long overdue." After meeting with the Kiwanis Board of Directors, we set a mid-February date, five months in the future. The contract we signed called for a 50/50 cash split of the gross receipts. We would need to cover the expenses from our half. As often happens, the guy who suggests a project gets put in charge, so I was off and running.

A new Catholic high school had opened in the fall. I figured their gym would be a good place to hold our first major fund-raiser. Father Olley, assistant principle and sports director, agreed and gave us a discounted rental price of $100. Abe advised me the "small town" going rate was $3.00 for adults and $1.00 for kids under ten. Thanks to great publicity from the *Kenosha News* sports department and the members of our Kiwanis Club, we had a standing-room-only crowd of 1,100.

Sam, a large, black man who could pass for a middle linebacker today, stood with me while we collected the walk-in ticket money. I had already turned any checks into cash and divided the first two thousand into stacks of one hundred. Sam must have been a distant cousin of Ronald Reagan—trust but verify. He counted every pile, banded them just like a bank, then put them into small envelopes. We both signed and dated the receipts. I imagine the players were paid in cash; Sam intimated as much. I didn't ask about withholding or other things that I considered none of my business. By 10:30 PM the players were on their bus and headed to Oshkosh, 120 miles north. What a happy bunch!

Quoting Wikipedia:

> Among the players who have been Globetrotters are NBA greats Wilt "The Stilt" Chamberlain, Connie "The Hawk" Hawkins, Nat "Sweetwater" Clifton, as well as Marques Haynes, George "Meadowlark" Lemon, Jerome James, Reece "Goose" Tatum, and Hubert "Geese" Ausbie. Another popular team member in the 1970s and 1980s was Fred "Curly" Neal, who was the best dribbler of that era of the team's history and was immediately recognizable due to his shaven head. Baseball Hall of Famers Bob Gibson and Ferguson Jenkins also played for the team at one time or another. In 1985, the Globetrotters signed their first female player, Olympic gold medalist Lynette Woodard, and their second, Joyce Walker, just three weeks later.

The evening was a total success. The 'Trotters pulled all their usual gags, trick dribbles, and shots—the dribbling wizard, the hidden ball in the sweatshirt, the bucket of water (confetti) into the stands, etc. In those days there was even an exhibition of two-handed set shooting from around mid-court. The Washington Capitals played valiantly, but lost again.

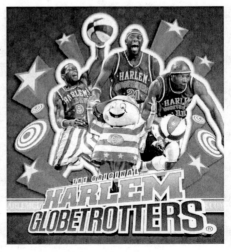

Western Kiwanis made just over $1,150 net profit. The club was overjoyed.

I became its third president the following fall.

Sweet Georgia Brown

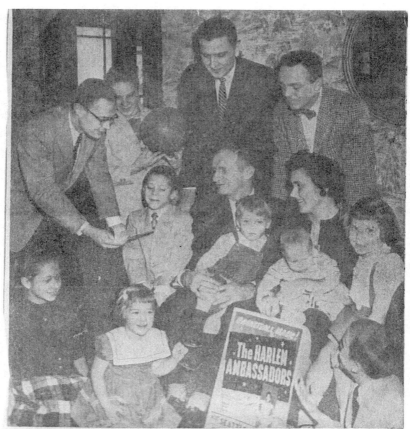

— Evening News Photo

MAYOR'S FAMILY BUYS TICKETS FOR HARLEM AMBASSADORS GAME — The Kiwanis Club of Western Kenosha filled several seats for Saturday night's Harlem Ambassadors basketball attraction during the weekend when they sold tickets to Mayor Eugene R. Hammond and his family. Seated on the floor are Mary, Carol and Louis Hammond (holding poster). Kiwanian Bill Kamler (left) shows tickets to George, the mayor (holding Ralph), Mrs. Hammond (holding Gary) and Ruth, who prefers to look at the photographer. Standing in the back are Eugene Jr. (holding basketball), and Kiwanis Club members Gregg Vigansky and Dr. John Mernick. The Harlem Ambassadors, formerly Harlem Globetrotters, will play the Seattle Stars in the feature game Saturday night at St. Joseph's gym. Sixth graders from Grant and Jefferson schools will perform in a preliminary game. Halftime entertainment also is planned.

Barry Z—Hidden Talents

I'd been practicing in Kenosha five years when I was elected president of the Kiwanis Club of Western Kenosha. The newsletter announcing my election is reprinted below.

KIWANIS CLUB of WESTERN KENOSHA

JOHN MERRICK
PRESIDENT
AUGUST SCHEPKER
VICE-PRESIDENT
HELMUTH SCHAEFER
TREASURER
VERN PEDERSEN
SECRETARY

2224 Roosevelt Road

Kenosha, Wisconsin

OFFICE OF THE SECRETARY
Telephone OLympic 7-6077

DIRECTORS
RICHARD BUNDIES
ROBERT CRAWFORD
ARTHUR HEINZE
RONALD JENSEN
WILLIS LEITCH
RALPH RUFFOLO
GREGG VIGANSKY

January 23, 1961

Dear Kiwanian:

LAST WEEK - Two momentous events took place last week-- first, John Merrick was installed as President of our club by Lt. Gov. Helm and second, but of equal importance, John Kennedy was installed as President of the United States by Chief Justice Warren. Truly a week that will go down in history. Lt. Gov. Helm "briefly" inspired us with a four point program and John Kennedy inspired us with a "get the point" program. Was an inspiring week too! ?

In the shadow of these great events Dr. George Koster managed to chew away at the door prize donated by Dr. Bob Crawford.

THIS WEEK - A representative from the Kenosha Insurance Agents Assn. will discuss the advantages and disadvantages of the "Package" Insurance Policy.

With this program Ron Jensen retires as Program Chairman and he sure did a good job, so, if I may borrow a few words from Winston Churchill, may I say to you Ron -- "By Jove, Good Show."

Remember March 1, is LADIES NIGHT -- find those ladies now!

--Wife: "I'm sorry to phone you at the office, but you have a special delivery letter which just arrived marked Private and Personal,"
  Husband: "Okay. What does it say?"

--Salesman: "Sir, this used television set is like new -- It was owned by a little old lady with weak eyes."

See you Thursday,

Dick

DOOR PRIZE DONORS

This week -- Andy Fennema
Next Week -- James Gourley

As a recently founded service organization, we were always looking for civic projects, so when Sister Mary Francis called from St. Joseph's High School with a request, I was anxious to hear her story.

Sister Mary Francis was the head of the art and music department of the new Catholic high school in Kenosha. She explained that one of her students, Barry Zoromsky, was a very talented musician but could not afford the tuition to attend the Chicago Music Conservatory and study under the famous Dr. Rudolph Ganz. Sister had been able to find about half of the $5,000 needed for the Barry to attend and receive lessons for one year.

I arranged for Barry to perform at my house one Saturday afternoon. In attendance were representatives of the four other service clubs in Kenosha: Lions, Rotary, Downtown Kiwanis, and Optimists. After hearing Barry perform, we decided to make Barry a joint club project. We managed to get approval of three of the four clubs to give $2,500 total. Western Kiwanis gave $800.

The first year was very successful. Barry preformed at one of our luncheon meetings prior to getting a renewal of his scholarship for his senior year in high school. We received glowing progress reports from Sister Mary Francis. There was talk of a future concert tour.

Then three years passed with no word about Barry. Rumor had it he had dropped out of college.

I received a call from a newspaper reporter—a client—that I should check out the new act at The Roadside, a gay bar on the north side of Kenosha. I was intrigued. I'd never been to a gay bar. Remember, this was 1964. There was not even the hint of acceptance of gays or lesbians in society, let alone in a union town like Kenosha. Carol and I couldn't resist. With two other couples for support—for what, I don't know—we arrived at The Roadside after a Friday night fish fry at our favorite restaurant, The Bartley House.

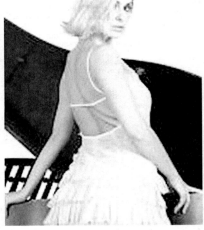

The featured performer was a female impersonator/piano playing–stripper, none other than our Barry—now called

"Bubbles Zee"—complete with silicone implants that would rival Dolly Parton's. Barry (Bubbles) was an outstanding performer. His act would almost rival Liberace's. We sat entranced through one set. The regular patrons loudly voiced their approval. We were surprised at the large crowd in attendance. I tried not to notice if any of my friends or clients were there.

I've often wondered what happened to Barry over the next many years. Did he succumb to the AIDS epidemic? Did he go back to music school? Did he end up in Vegas doing a Liberace-type act? Google was unable to provide the answer.

The Corral Story

"I've been ordered to cease and desist," Father Olley said when he called to inform me of the cancellation of our meeting. We had great plans for a youth center in Kenosha, but now, it seemed, all our work was for naught.

I thought of that quote from Plato, "What is happening to our young people? They disrespect their elders, they disobey their parents. They ignore the law. They riot in the streets, inflamed with wild notions. Their morals are decaying." Indeed, things haven't changed a lot in the last two thousand years.

The time was 1960. I had started my year as president-elect of our Kiwanis Club. We were in need of a new project. The Globetrotter basketball fund raiser was successful, but only a one-time event. The club was searching for a project that would fulfill our mission of service to community and children. That's when Carol mentioned that the kids had that classic complaint, "There's nowhere to go and nothing to do. It's a shame Kenosha doesn't have a youth center like La Grange has, the Corral." The only thing resembling a youth center was the Protestant Youth Center (PYC), a building converted from the German-American Center after WWI and used for sports and crafts, not socializing. It got its name from the funding source, the local Protestant Churches, and I'm not sure if Catholics or Jews were welcome.

In 1944, when Carol and I were attending Lyons Township High School (LTHS) in La Grange, Illinois, there was a similar outcry from the teenagers, "There's nowhere to go and nothing to do." Much to everyone's surprise and delight, these teens did something about it. Encouraged by Chuck Cassell of the La Grange Recreation Commission and other public-spirited adults, the LTHS students put their enthusiasm to work, calling a student mass meeting. Quoting from a press release, "In a surprisingly short time, they formed the Lyons Township Youth Organization, Inc., elected officers, appointed a board of adult supervisors, organized a drive for funds, and searched for a location for the youth center. They raised $7,000 ($70,000 in 2010 dollars) by calling on their parents and neighbors, and rented, remodeled, and equipped a vacant garage building in La Grange, which was their home until 1957. The interior was transformed into a knotty-pine, ranch-type lodge with a raised dance and recreation area in the center, surrounded by a huge log rail which gave the building its name, the "Corral." The Corral's board was made up of officers and directors elected by members from the four high school classes. All authority, final decisions, and action rested with the student Board of Directors; the Adult Advisory Board had power to listen and advise (when asked).

Three years later, when their lease was about to expire, the Corral faced a crisis. The owner refused to renew the lease because demand for real estate had increased. Finding another location in a few months seemed impossible. The Corral's Board decided to exercise a clause in the lease option—buy the building.

The "Save the Corral" campaign of 1947 raised $27,465 (over $250,000 in 2010 dollars) in three months—more than was needed to purchase the building for $25,000. That would be the last time the students had to appeal for contributions.

I presented the "Corral Story" to my Kiwanis Club and received their endorsement to proceed. Carol and I met with the student councils and faculty advisors of both local high schools. Mary D. Bradford was the public school, and St. Joseph's was the newly opened Catholic high school. Both groups gave their immediate, enthusiastic blessing to further explore the project for Kenosha youth.

Kiwanis supplied funds to hire a bus to transport 16 students from each school, plus four parent couples, including myself and Carol, as chaperones. We had a very productive meeting in La Grange with four members of the Corral Student Board and two parent advisors. We met in the "New Corral," a stand-alone building on the recently erected south campus of LTHS.

Our group was very impressed by the Corral Board, the building, and their policies. We could not image the students owned their building. After a member of our group lit a cigarette, one of the students from LTHS politely informed him there was a no smoking policy in the Corral. I couldn't believe my ears. The Corral I remembered was usually filled with smoke. The students explained that last fall their insurance was going to be raised $550 a year because of a minor fire caused by careless disposal of cigarettes butts. The student Corral Board figured they could put the money to better use. A vote by the board was upheld by the student members. I'm sure if the recommendation had come from an adult board, there would have been a mild riot.

We returned to Kenosha with great anticipation. A meeting was planned for the following week. Then I received that fateful call from Father Olley. I asked, "Are you kidding?" "No," he replied, "I'm relating to you just what Bishop Cousins told me." "Did he give a reason?" I asked. "Yes, he said it would promote intermarriage and was against Catholic policy." I could not believe my ears.

That effectively ended our dream of a youth center for Kenosha. The Bradford HS student group, parents and the Kiwanis members determined without the cooperation of one half of the youth in Kenosha, there is no possible way for the Corral idea to flower.

Within five years a new Pope, John 23rd, convened The Second Vatican Council, which declared ecumenism to be the new watchword for Catholics. The Council sought to restore unity among all Christians. We were a little ahead of our time.

Today, in the spring of 2011, the LTHS home page reports:

> The peak years of the Corral were from the '60s to the mid-'70s. During this time, the Corral boasted over 3,000 paid members per year and was open over 130 nights. On any given weekend night, 300—1,000 students could be present. Such musical talents as Styx, Muddy Waters, Chicago, and other local groups entertained the students. The facility was student-owned and -run, with 26 elected officers. A community board served in an advisory capacity, and the student board hired a director of the facility from the high school staff, Mr. Burt Kraus. The annual budget was met through Corral Pass fees, large dances, events, and an annual Corral Show. Several alumni of the Corral have gone on to careers based on their involvement in the Corral, the most notable being David Hasselhoff, of *Baywatch* and *Night Rider* fame.
>
> The late '70s saw the retirement of Mr. Bert Kraus as the director. When his strong relationship with the Corral stopped, student interests changed, and the membership numbers dropped significantly. With the decline in student involvement came the decline in activities offered. Finally, the demise occurred when the Lyons Township Youth Organization sold the facility, which needed several costly maintenance repairs, to the high school.
>
> The Corral is still a student activities center for all LTHS students, located right next to the south campus.

Students can find all sorts of stuff in the Corral, like video games, pool tables, ping pong, foosball, air hockey, cable TV, outdoor basketball, concessions, and much more. The Corral hosts all sorts of events, including dances, tournaments and even private parties. The Corral is open every day after school from 3:15 to 5:00 PM and on Friday nights from 7 to 10 PM."

The following article appeared in *The Kenosha News* describing in glowing detail the trip to the Corral.

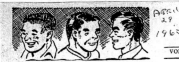

April 29, 1960

'Corral' for Teens A Possibility Here?

Overhearing talk about a "corral" has baffled some students at Mary D. Bradford and St. Joseph's high schools the past few weeks. However, this "corral" has nothing to do with rangelands and cattle.

The "corral" in discussion is a youth center in LaGrange, Ill., run by a successful non-profit corporation. All the officers, directors and members of the corporation are teenagers.

A movement spearheaded by Dr. John W. Merrick, who as a teenager belonged to the Corral, has been started by the Kiwanis Klub of Western Kenosha for consideration of possible establishment of a similar center here.

Dr. Merrick recently talked to sessions of student councils at both high schools and organized a trip to visit the LaGrange building. In addition to students, Mayor Eugene R. Hammond and several civic leaders visited the Corral.

Maureen Connolly, MBHS senior and member of Interclub President's Council who made the trip, described some of the center's activities. While Maureen was there, a rehearsal was going on for the annual variety show presented by Coral members. In past years, much of the operating capital has come from the variety shows.

They have made as much as $5,700 from performances.

After seeing the center and hearing an explanation of its workings, Maureen commented that "the parents and other adults in the community seem to be 100 per cent behind the kids in their project." Maureen was also impressed by the immaculate appearance of the building and the grounds, located next to LaGrange Township high school.

She liked the idea of the "Corral Pledge," stating general rules for conduct which is carried by all members. Admission without membership is not allowed, and guests are permitted only with the permission of the Corral Director.

The Corral Pledge states:

"As a member of the 'Corral,' I will:
1. Help to uphold the reputation of the Corral to the best of my ability.
2. Abstain from the use of alcohol before and during my presence at the Corral.
3. Refrain from loitering outside or in the vicinity of the Corral.
4. Cooperate with the officers and chaperons in maintaining proper order at all times.

Failure to follow the above rules will subject me to suspension from the Corral and its privileges."

Mitzi Cox, a member of the SJHS student council that visited the Corral, was impressed by the tremendous spirit of cooperation between the teenagers and the adults involved with the Corral. An Adult Advisory Board of 16 members assists the teenage members of the Corral Board. The adults are invited to serve and do so in an advisory capacity. Four chaperons are present on the Friday and Saturday evenings that the corral is open during the school term.

Mitzi stated that all the teenagers at the center seemed clean-cut. She felt that the town itself, because of its fairly small size, had a minimal problem with "rowdy" teens.

The fact that the high school and the center cooperate together extensively was commented on by Mitzi. Since the high school does not have a great deal of extra-curricular activities, the Corral organizes many outside projects that are normally undertaken by schools.

As a group, the SJHS students were more skeptical about the chances of an organization such as the Corral succeeding in Kenosha. Robert Heller, SJHS senior class president, felt that too many problems were involved in getting a similar project started in Kenosha.

"Buzzy" also felt it was to the advantage of the youth center that the high school did not have many outside activities.

An elaborate hi-fi system provides music for dancing during open hours of the center. For special events, name bands or local combos are scheduled. Permanent features of the Corral are non-profit canteen service, television donated by the LaGrange Lions Club, and table tennis in club rooms.

In addition to the student written, directed, and produced variety show, the center stages special parties and dances throughout the year.

Ken Turk, MBHS student council president and member of InterClub President's Council, said the operation of the present Corral is a "tremendously big project." When the Corral movement started in 1944, LaGrange teenagers raised $7000 and transformed a vacant garage into a knotty-pine recreation building. Four years ago the need arose for a larger center. Engaging the help of the community, $96,000 was donated to build the present modern headquarters.

Ken feels that a project on the level of the first Corral building would be feasible in Kenosha with the help of a large number of students working on it.

Ken was particularly interested in the way in which a part of the funds were raised. In a community bond drive, the students sold certificates, mostly in $10 and $25 denominations, redeemable in 10 years. They planned, at the end of 10 years, to be self-sufficient and to be able to pay back the borrowed money.

When letters were sent informing investors that bonds could be redeemed, the majority of the purchasers donated the money to the project, not wishing to ask for it back.

The present Corral has a membership of about 2600 students from LaGrange and surrounding towns, and operates on an annual budget of $17,000 raised entirely by students from dues, dances and parties, and variety show profits.

The Night Before Christmas

In the days before pet cemeteries were common, dogs and cats were buried at home or disposed of by vets at local rendering plants, just like farm animals. In the wild, scavengers, microbes and time eventually complete the "dust to dust" cycle, but in civilized society, rendering plants perform this needed function. Rendering is the process of cooking raw animal material to remove the moisture and fat. The yellow fat, or tallow, is skimmed. The cooked meat and bone are sent to a hammer mill press to remove remaining water and pulverize the remains into a gritty powder. The remaining yellow grease, meal, and bone meal are a good source of protein and other nutrients in the diets of poultry, swine, and pet foods. It was then, and is still the usual method of disposing of dead farm animals.

During the warm months, whenever I had a euthanasia or dead animal dropped off after being hit by a car, it required me to take a trip to Koos's Rendering Plant in Kenosha, Wisconsin. During the winter months animals could easily be kept for weeks until I had a trunk-full to deliver. If a client asked what would happen to their pet at burial, I usually said, "They will end up being disposed of on a local farm. Dust to dust—that kind of thing..." It was the truth, more or less. If someone insisted on knowing exactly what would happen, I told them. The fact was, most people really didn't want to know.

It is now common for pet owners to bury their companions in pet cemeteries not unlike those for humans. It is also permissible in most communities to bury your pet in the backyard, but you cannot declare that the site is now "sacred ground." Caskets are produced in all sizes for pet burial. Many grave sites are marked with expensive gravestones and statues.

On the Fridays before Christmas in the early '60s, I usually closed the hospital around 7 PM. One particular winter, Kenosha experienced an early arctic blast of cold—below-zero temperatures in the middle of December. Bodies of deceased pets were stacked like cord wood behind my animal hospital's back door, under a blanket, to await delivery to their final resting place. After tallying the day's receipts for my routine bank night deposit, I loaded the trunk of my '54 Chevy sedan with the stiff, lifeless bodies of six dogs and cats. As usual, I planned on making my night deposit before dropping the animals off at Koos's Rendering Plant.

Downtown Kenosha was brightly lit with Christmas decorations, and festive music filled the air. The Kenosha National Bank was a few feet off the main street. "Branch banks" did not exist in that era. After slipping the envelope into the night deposit slot, I noticed, to my surprise, that one of my rear tires was flat. I had not noticed any steering problem. The piles of snow on the pavement may have masked the developing flat tire. Without thinking, I started to open the trunk just as a group of shoppers were walking by. One of them inquired, "Hi, Doc, do you need any help?" The last thing I needed at that moment was help from a well-meaning client! Not wanting them to see what was in the trunk, I quickly closed it and politely turned down their offer. This was decades before cell phones, and since we only had one car anyway, my wife would be of no assistance.

I was puzzled as to how I could get to the spare tire without anyone seeing carcasses in my vehicle. After sitting in the car for a few minutes I decided on a plan. Across the street from where I was stranded was the a little bar called the "Corner Tap," which despite its name, was located in the middle of the block. As luck would have it, the owner was a long-time client. Wisconsin had, and still has, a law allowing cities to grant one liquor license for every 500 residents. At that time there were 120 bars and restaurants in Kenosha serving drinks. With that many bars available, I wouldn't have had to walk far to find one. Just for fun, I also counted the churches in town—64.

After using the bar owner's phone to ascertain that my garage/service station was closed, I settled back and ordered a peppermint schnapps with a beer chaser. One hour and one refill later, the street had cleared, as it was approaching closing time for the shops—9 PM. The company at the bar, the music, and the alcohol buoyed my spirits. In those days, I, like many of my generation, imbibed, though only on evenings and weekends. My wife had once read that if you have two or more drinks a day, you might have an alcohol problem. We solved that dilemma by buying bigger glasses! Some ten years later after Carol had started teaching Yoga at the University of Wisconsin, we gave up alcohol altogether.

Using an old blanket to provide cover, I smuggled the spare out from between the cadavers and managed to change the tire.

Thankfully, the spare was full of air. The street remained deserted, and no one came by or offered to help this time. The ride to Koos's Rendering was uneventful except for my concern about being stopped by the police—now for DUI. Arriving home, I felt as if I'd been on a farm call and delivered a calf in the barnyard. A long soak in a hot tub provided needed relief.

Carroll Rikli and Immanuel Magomolla

Carroll Rikli, director of the Christian Youth Center (CYC), called to set up our occasional table tennis match. Located in the old German American Sports Center on 52nd avenue, the building was renamed during WWI and purchased by a group of Protestant churches. Sometime in the early '60s the Protestant Youth Center (PYC) became the CYC. This may have been a funding issue, as Kenosha was about one half Catholic at the time. I imagine Jews and Muslims were allowed in if they kept their identity quiet.

Carroll had a Master's Degree in Physical Education. As a youth, he, his Dad, and his three cousins traveled the Midwest as

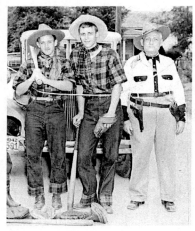

a four-man softball team, The Oklahoma Cowboys, challenging local hotshots to a contest. The events were usually charity fund-raisers with the Riklis winning over 90% of their matches. As is still the case today, the outcome of most softball games is determined by who has the best pitcher. Carroll was among the best. His dad, Col. Oscar Rikli, was the manager and trick shot expert who added to the entertainment. Carroll was asked why did they need four players? He replied, "If our first three players get on base, someone has to be able to drive them in."

Carroll had owned a 1965 Mustang—his pride and joy. By 1970 it was showing its age, as rust ruined the car's flashy appearance. The brakes needed relining, the clutch slipped a bit, and the transmission was in need of repair. Reluctantly, Carroll traded it for a new model Rambler, made in Kenosha, of course. Six months later, while driving by the dealeship, Carroll spotted a shiney 1965 red Mustang. His heart raced with excitement. He had to turn around and take another look. Sitting in the driver's seat, Carroll felt five years younger. He briefly considered buying the car on the spot. The sale price was $2,500—$1,500 more than he had received for his old clunker. Maybe he would surprise 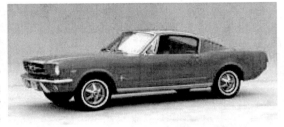 Clarice by giving her his Rambler, and he'd get another Mustang for himself.

About that time he noticed a small cigatette burn in the ceiling upholstry, in exactly the same spot as the one in *his* previous car. It took only a couple of seconds to bring him out of his dream state. This *was* his old car, and his fantasy was finished.

Softball and cars were not on Carroll's mind that day. After our usual two-out-of-three table tennis match was over, he revealed the real purpose of our meeting. A young man from Africa needed a home for the Carthage College Christmas break. Immanuel Magomolla was sponsored by the Rohrer's, members of a local Lutheran Church. He usually stayed with them during school break, but they were going out of town and needed a family to pinch hit for them. During that time, Carol and I had taken in many foster children, so we agreed to house Immanuel.

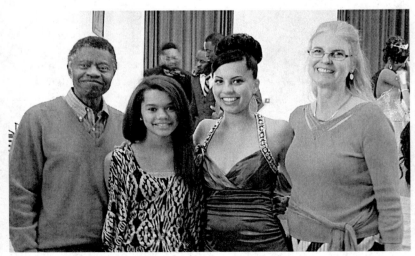

Immanueli, Makeela, Malaika, and Beth • 2011

Immanuel was from a small village outside of Arusha, a city in northern Tanzania. It is the capital of the Arusha Region, which claims a population of 1,288,088, including 281,608 for the Arusha District (2002 census). Arusha is surrounded by some of Africa's most famous landscapes and national parks. Situated below Mount Meru on the eastern edge of the eastern branch of the Great Rift Valley, it has a mild climate and is close to Serengeti, Ngorongoro Crater, Lake Manyara, Olduvai Gorge, Tarangire National Park, and Mount Kilimanjaro.

Immanuel went on to graduate from Carthage and Maharry Medical College in Nashville, Tennessee, then interned in Massachusetts and Connecticut hospitals. His father, Zakayo Magomolla, traveled from Africa to attend Immanuel's graduation from Carthage. He was a teacher at a missionary school and explained at dinner after the ceremony that he had to walk eight miles over dirt roads to reach the nearest bus that would take him to Arusha and on to the Tanzanian capital, Dar es Salaam. He was rightly very proud of Immanuel's achievement.

After graduating from medical school, Immanuel changed the spelling of his name to "Immanueli." While visiting a missionary friend in Duluth, Minnesota, Immanueli met Beth Grobe. After a two-year courtship, they married in 1985 and settled in Duluth. The long, cold winters were a shock to one who grew up living in endless summers.

In 1998 Beth and Immanueli founded a women's microloan project in his native homeland of Tanzania, East Africa, as a way to help Tanzanians out of poverty. Called "The Mothers and Children of Central Tanzania" (MCCT), the project provides $40 loans—the equivalent of about $400 in the United States—to women to invest in their business ventures. MCCT has provided hundreds of loans to women, with the goal of 100% payback. "I am so proud of the women of our project who, despite drought and economic hardships, have successfully invested their loans in business ventures," Beth says. "All are repaying their loans plus interest. They are becoming strong individuals who are learning their basic human rights and defending them in a male-dominated society."

Immanueli found that middlemen are often exploitative and take the villagers' crafts without fulfilling their promise to pay. This leaves the people with no money for food, medicine, and rent, and in debt for their production costs. Buying directly from the market at low prices can eliminate some greed and corrupt behavior.

The Magomolla's program is similar to one run by my niece and her husband, Catherine and Les Todd, in Guatemala—Atitlan Arts, Panajachel, Lake Atitlan, Guatemala. Their Web site is www.AtitlanArts.com. Catherine reports, "You might want to note that we don't just 'buy from the artists,' we work with the artists to design our own line of unique, exclusive products, and we provide benefits far beyond the cost of the work. We market their products at art fairs and museums around the Eastern USA." Similar to the Magomolla program, Atitlan Arts benefits the native women directly.

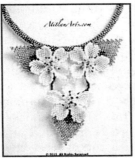 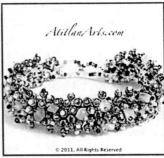

Blossom Necklace, $80 • Bead/Stone Bracelet, $18

Immanueli and Beth also established their own business, Magomolla Enterprises, which markets Tanzanian basketry and tours, in addition to

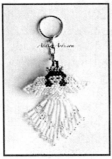 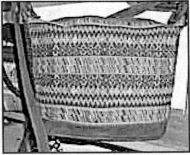

Angel Keychain, $6 • Hand-woven Bag, $20

overseeing the MCCT project. Ten percent of the business's proceeds go directly to further assist Africans. In 2001 the Magomollas received the Labovitz Emerging Entrepreneur Award, a recognition presented by the University of Minnesota–Duluth Center for Economic Development. The awards are given to small business owners deserving recognition for their contributions to the regional economy.

Leblanc, Cailliet, & KSL

Leon placed Anwar gingerly on the exam table. Yes, Anwar was named after Anwar Sadat, the Egyptian leader who led the Yom Kippur War of 1973 against Israel, making him a hero in Egypt and, for a time, throughout the Arab world. Afterwards he engaged in negotiations with Israel, culminating in the Egypt-Israel Peace Treaty. This won him the Nobel Peace Prize but also made him unpopular among some Arabs, resulting in a temporary suspension of Egypt's membership in the Arab League and eventually his assassination. Leon thought Anwar was a perfect name for his feisty, independent Siamese kitten. Leon Pascucci was vice president of G. Leblanc, the musical instrument maker. The time was 1984.

The usually placid, cooperative Anwar complained when moved, more so when I palpated his abdomen. He had been slowed by a fall a few months ago, injuring his right knee. Medication relieved some of the pain, but arthritis was setting in. In addition to a depressed appetite, Anwar had been having frequent trips to the litter box the last few weeks. "I feel a large mass near the bladder," I informed Leon. I recommend sending him to the University of Wisconsin vet school in Madison for a more certain diagnosis and treatment regime. I gave a very guarded prognosis. Leon could easily afford the cost and time away from home, but because of Anwar's age and general deterioration, decided against any radical treatment. Once off the exam table, Anwar rewarded me with a fresh urine sample. Quickly siphoned up, it was ideal for a complete urinalysis (except for culturing for bacterial growth). The UA revealed results typical for an aged tomcat.

Within a short time Leon was headed back to my animal hospital to end Anwar's suffering as humanely as possible. Anwar decided otherwise and died in the arms of Leon's friend, Mike. People without children experience the same grief and sense of loss when a cherished pet passes that parents feel when losing a child. There are no adequate words to describe the event. Happy memories can mollify the pain.

Leon's father, Vito Pascucci was drafted into the army in 1943. He applied to join the army band, and was given a spot as the band repairman. Vito became good friends with Glenn Miller while working on some of Miller's instruments. The famous bandleader came up with a plan to launch a chain of Glenn Miller Music Stores when the war was over. Miller planned to import European instruments, which were of better quality than U.S.-made ones. Vito was to scout various clarinet suppliers in France.

Glenn Miller's plane disappeared over the English Channel on December 15, 1944. Pascucci was crushed at the loss of his friend. Nevertheless, he went on with plans he and Miller had made, and arranged to visit musical instrument factories in France. At the Leblanc factory in La Couture-Boussey, he met Georges and Leon Leblanc. When he told the Leblanc's about the Glenn Miller Music Stores idea, they instead asked him to distribute their instruments in the United States. He left the factory with a duffel bag full of clarinets, and Leon Leblanc promised to meet him in the United States when the war was over.

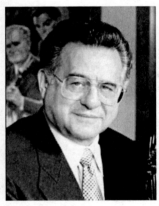

Vito Pascucci

Leblanc kept his promise and wired Pascucci to come to New York in 1946. Pascucci entered a 50–50 partnership with G. Leblanc Cie., forming Leblanc USA in May 1946. Although Leblanc had wanted Pascucci to work in New York, where the musical instrument import business was centered, Pascucci insisted on returning to his hometown. So he signed a lease for a tiny storefront in Kenosha. With the baby boom that followed the war, school music programs also grew quickly, and Leblanc USA began supplying inexpensive instruments for beginners.

In 1975 Pascucci's son, Leon (named for Leon Leblanc), joined the company, beginning as vice-president for advertising. The younger Pascucci contributed to the striking interior design of the new Leblanc headquarters, and became known for staging beautiful exhibits at industry trade shows. He seemed to have the artistry and flair that was vital to the firm's image. Leon's father, Vito, was named to the list of America's 10 Best-Dressed Men, year after year. I asked Leon what one had to do to qualify for the honor? He replied tongue in cheek, "Spend enough money at the right tailor."

"Bob," I complained, "you must want Carol on your Kenosha Symphony board of directors. She's the musician in our family."

"No," Dr. Robert Sternloff explained, "I don't need any more people with musical ability. I need a ticket salesman. After watching you sell out the Globetrotters for Kiwanis last year, I decided you're my man." Dr. Sternloff was the director of the Kenosha Public Recreation Department. As such, he was the "General Manager" of the Kenosha Symphony. The time was 1960. I'd had a very successful fundraising event for the Western Kenosha Kiwanis. Bob assured me my only job would be promotion and ticket sales, so I reluctantly accepted. It turns out the person in charge of ticket promotion is usually the first vice president, so I not only had a job, but a title as well.

Since 1940, the Kenosha Symphony Orchestra (KSO) has been a cultural cornerstone of southeastern Wisconsin and has entertained and educated thousands of music enthusiasts and local school children. The KSO was formed by the Department of Public Recreation and Kenosha Board of Education, with the support of community organizations in 1940. Its first concert was performed in 1941. Since then, the orchestra has grown in number and skill through the high standards of its music directors, and hard work of the Kenosha Symphony Association (KSA), which strives for excellence in its music selection, performances, and its outreach to Kenosha families. KSA endeavors to make quality music a part of our community. Its missions is to provide a bridge between the community and the arts, expanding a base of support for the arts in the area.

In the 1950s, with the help of G. Leblanc Company, Lucien Cailliet was installed as the conductor of the KSO. Lucien Cailliet had been educated at the Conservatory of Dijon and the Philadelphia Musical Academy, and he was a prolific composer, conductor, arranger, orchestrator, clarinetist, and educator. He studied with Paul Fauchet, Georges Caussades, and Gabriel Pares in 1935 at the Officier d'Academie in France. He arrived in the United States in 1918 and became an American citizen in 1923. He arranged for the Philadelphia Orchestra (where he was a bass clarinetist) and conducted the orchestras at Interlochen, Michigan, where he served as professor of music and the USC conductor at the Balle Russe de Monte Carlo.

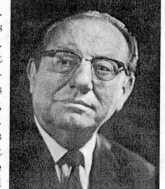

Lucien Cailliet

Cailliet also enjoyed a prolific career creating music for films. He contributed to nearly fifty films as either composer or arranger. Among the best known of these films are *She Wore a Yellow Ribbon, The Ten Commandments* (for which Elmer Bernstein wrote the score), and *Gunfight at the O.K. Corral.*

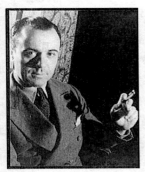

José Iturbi

At a meeting to discuss the upcoming program, Dr. Cailliet mentioned he was a personal friend and former neighbor of José Iturbi. Iturbi had appeared with Cailliet in symphony concerts. Iturbi had wanted to perform "Peter and the Wolf," a composition written by Sergei Prokofiev in 1936 in the USSR. It is a children's story (with both music and text by Prokofiev), spoken by a narrator accompanied by the orchestra. At the time, José Iturbi was a famous Hollywood actor. I couldn't imagine getting someone of his caliber to perform in Kenosha. Dr. Cailliet assured me that José would come for whatever we could afford. I've always had the suspicion Vito Pascucci may have sweetened the deal a little.

When word spread about our next concert season, tickets flew off the shelf. We not only sold out the Iturbi date, but most of the remaining tickets as well. The Kenosha Symphony League (KSL) enjoyed their best season in memory. I would like to think I had something to do with our success, but I'm sure most of the applause needs to be directed elsewhere. Just as the appreciative clapping and bravos of the audience for a great performance is directed at the conductor; the orchestra members, stage hands, board of directors, and a sophisticated public can share in the glow of a job well done. I was rewarded by being elected president of the KSL for the next two years. Sales remained good, but not as robust as when we had a star Hollywood attraction.

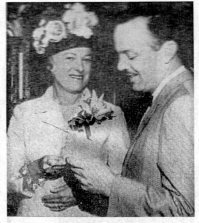

Mrs. John P. Braun, president of the Symphony League, presents a check to Dr. John Merrick, Kenosha Symphony Association president, for expenses of the past season.

Oscar Zerk Story

"Docktor, you have built the second best house in Kenosha," Oscar Zerk exclaimed after touring my almost-finished residence. It was an unexpected compliment from the man who became famous for inventing the Zerk Fitting in 1929. Oscar's house/mansion was built on 40 acres of oak woods, on the southwest side of town. Mine was on the back of five acres of oak woods, 600 feet behind my animal hospital. At the time of his death in 1968, 20 billion of the bubble-shaped Zerk Fitting lubricating devices were on cars, trucks, and planes worldwide.

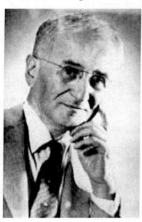

Oscar Zerk

Austrian born, the engineer/inventor arrived in America in 1924 at the age of 46. He had over 300 patents to his credit, including quick-freezing ice cube trays, shatterproof nail brushes, leg-slimming hosiery, fail-safe trolley brakes, vibration-free camera tripods, oil well–recovery systems, and automotive refrigeration equipment. He also invented a personal coffee-bean grinder for his kitchen, but thought it so unimportant that he never bothered to apply for a patent.

With the command and arrogant demeanor of a Prussian general, Oscar dominated most encounters. I'm sure he thought of himself as descended from Hapsburg noblemen. I learned early on that the only way to gain his respect was to be as outspoken as he was. Oscar's second wife, Dorothy, was a prime example. Dorothy had been a private secretary to a Wisconsin Supreme Court justice, marrying Oscar soon after the death of his first wife. Oscar was already 75 years old. Dorothy probably expected to inherit everything in a few years. This was not to be the case. She had to suffer—endure—14 years of browbeating and ridicule before Oscar passed at the age of 90.

Despite his wealth, Oscar was very frugal. In the grocery store, he would weigh each egg to make sure they were not charging the "large" price for "medium size" eggs. During World War II,

Oscar appeared before the Gas Rationing Board to apply for an increase in his gas allowance. When refused, Oscar laid on the floor like a two-year-old in the supermarket, yelled, and kicked his feet. My wife, Carol, related that Oscar would drive Dorothy to the hairdresser and wait to take her home so she could not shop for anything Oscar had not approved of in advance.

His pet of choice was a German Shepard—large, male, obedient, and surprisingly mellow. Each time he left Prince with me to board for a few days, Oscar asked for a discount or request a half-day charge for picking Prince up early. I had to be just as forceful in explaining my fees were by the night, just like a hotel charges. If I charged by the hour for a drop off, the price would be the same as a one day's boarding. Once Oscar tried a different tactic. "Perhaps I could bring his food," Oscar exclaimed. I replied that he would be welcome to bring Prince food or treats, but the price would be the same. Evidently Prince liked our establishment and personnel, for he was our routine guest. Oscar would be astonished at the charges of today's upscale "Pet Motels and Spas."

Set on 40 acres of woods on the outskirts of Kenosha, Oscar's estate, "Dunmovin," was a fitting home for this Austrian nobleman. Art objects were scattered throughout, climaxed by a third floor ballroom, later converted to hold Oscar's large collection of petrified wood and dinosaur droppings. His favorite prank involved a full sized nude statue of a young man at the foot of the winding staircase. When leading a tour that included women, Oscar would draw attention to the "beautiful Greek statue." When everyone was focused on the unclothed figure, Oscar would push a button behind the artwork to activate the "Viagra effect" on the statue's genitals. Shock from the ladies was followed by Oscar's hearty laughter.

Zerk was in the worldwide press after a daring robbery at his opulent and art-filled Kenosha mansion on February 4, 1954. Zerk was tied to a chair as the invaders stole an untold number of valuable paintings and escaped with the artworks in Zerk's personal car. The robbery was never solved.

Dorothy was never able to enjoy her riches after Oscar died. Prince was allowed full run of the house, no longer confined for any length of time to his yard and doghouse. Unfortunately, Dorothy soon became a recluse and died in a nursing home within two years of Oscar's passing.

Back on the Farm

"I've driven 50 years and never had an accident," Uncle Wendell said, just before he hit the pig.

Ginger, ten, Peggy, eight, and I were in Iowa for the weekend. Grandpa Santee had died the year before. Wendell wrote he was preparing to demolish the old farmhouse where I'd spent many happy times in my youth. I decided to make one last visit. The young girls had never seen the farm, so I decided to take them along.

After unpacking at Wendell's neighboring farmhouse, we toured Grandpa's property. He had moved in with Uncle Wendell soon after Grandmother Santee died five years previously. The 80-year-old house was showing its age—roof leaking, floors sagging, porch screens torn. It had been left open to provide shelter for sheep grazing in the yard and orchard. The rooms downstairs were a mess.

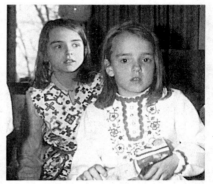

Ginger and Peggy • Circa 1970

Climbing the narrow steep stairs led to the relatively clean bedrooms. In the walk-in closet off the master bedroom, the girls delighted over the contents of an old trunk with faded postcards from long lost relatives, pictures in forgotten scrapbooks, and remnants of clothes long out of style. Being Quaker, Grandma Santee was not a fancy dresser by any stretch of the word. We next toured the fruit orchard, the scene of an accident which almost cost my right eye. Next we inspected the back yard where the large maple tree had provided for perfect climbing and swings. This was the scene of my broken arm. Trying to jump out of a swing at the back arc is bound to lead to disaster. Then to the barn, touring the empty milking stalls and the ladder climb to the haymow. Farm smells of every variety brought back a flood of forgotten happenings. The girls wanted souvenirs—an old bridle, a three legged milk stool. I took the pump from the front porch well and the old porcelain cup that hung next to it for 50 years.

When Grandpa Santee passed, Wendell called Mom and said, "I'll have to get a mortgage on the farm to give you your half." Mom replied without hesitation, "No you won't, the farm is yours, you worked it all these years." Mom just asked for a few mementos, and Wendell readily agreed. I had received the dining room furniture the year before. That and the old wall phone were my legacy from my mother. This lack of bickering over inheritance is a wonderful characteristic of the Merrick and Santee families. The farm is still in the family.

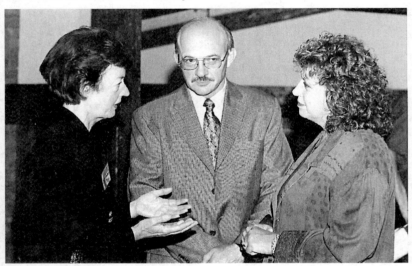

Margaret Reif, Les & Diane Santee • September, 2001

Les recently e-mailed me his current bio:
I used to sharecrop with Barry Flint (a neighbor and classmate) but now cash rent to Jack McKain, who was a few years behind me in school. I taught school in Cedar Rapids for 35 years, one year at Jefferson High School, and 34 years in middle school. I retired in 2002, but I'm currently coaching my 40th year of boys' and girls' swimming at Jefferson High School. I also coach boys and girls for Taft and Wilson middle schools.

I was the *Sports Illustrated* assistant coach of the year in 1998. They chose 15 across the U.S. for all sports. Our staff has been our conference coaches of the year several times. Two years ago I was inducted into the Iowa High School Swim Coaches Hall of Fame. I believe I am the only assistant coach in the Hall of Fame.

When Diane and I moved to our 32 acres in 1979, we farmed the tillable land around the house we were building. After five years of farming I put the land into the Conservation Reserve Program (CRP), where it has been ever since. If my bid is accepted this year, it will be in CRP for another ten years.

The Conservation Reserve Program a voluntary program for agricultural landowners. Through CRP, you can receive annual rental payments and cost-share assistance to establish long-term, resource-conserving covers on eligible farmland. The Commodity Credit Corporation (CCC) makes annual rental payments based on the agriculture rental value of the land, and it provides cost-share assistance for up to 50% of the participant's costs in establishing approved conservation practices. Participants enroll in CRP contracts for 10 to 15 years.

The program is administered through the Farm Service Agency (FSA). Natural Resources Conservation Service works with landowners to develop their application and to plan, design, and install the conservation practices on the land. County Land Conservation Departments and the Wisconsin Dept. of Natural Resources also provide technical support for the Conservation Reserve Program.

The Conservation Reserve Program reduces soil erosion, protects the nation's ability to produce food and fiber, reduces sedimentation in streams and lakes, improves water quality, establishes wildlife habitat, and enhances forest and wetland resources. It encourages farmers to convert highly erodible cropland or other environmentally sensitive acreage to vegetative cover, such as tame or native grasses, wildlife plantings, trees, filterstrips, or riparian buffers. Farmers receive an annual rental payment for the term of

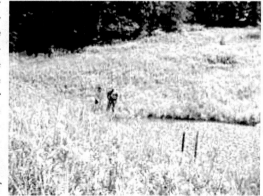

the multi-year contract. Cost sharing is provided to establish the vegetative cover practices.

After visiting Granddad's farm, I took the girls two miles north to the small town of Gibson. Never more than a tiny country hamlet, it now had lost the grocery/hardware store, restaurant, post office, grain elevator and farm equipment dealer. Only the gas station and Bank of Gibson remained. I wanted to visit Marvin Wilhite. He had owned the farm equipment dealership and recently retired. Wendell said I should stop by and say hello.

Marvin greeted us warmly and showed us into his living room/showroom. After offering hot or ice tea, he explained his collections. On one wall, covering an area 16' long, hung dozens of 6"×12" boards, each with three strands of barb wire attached. A small marker identified what type of wire, where it was made, etc. On the opposite wall an equal number of railroad spikes were hung for show. They also contained information as to type and place of production. We learned that people collect any number of artifacts of almost anything you can name. Just as my Uncle Byron collected music boxes, Marvin and his wife go to shows where farm stuff is offered for sale. I was impressed, but Ginger and Peggy seemed bored. Marvin told them the best was yet to come.

Leading the group into the backyard, Marvin proudly showed us his railroad. The rail stub to Gibson had been abandoned ten years before when the grain elevator was closed down. The single track ran directly behind Marvin's house. He had acquired a flatbed railcar and kept it next to his "station house" (bench) in the yard. He invited us to get on board and we were off. Marvin's railroad was one and one half miles long, past orchards, cornfields and pastures, and ended where the bridge over the North Skunk River had been removed. A large earthen berm prevented any further travel. This was better than any Disney ride could provide.

The following morning, Wendell declared we should go over to a friend's farm to see his Clydesdales. These magnificent horses are glorified in the Budweiser beer commercials that are seen on television every Christmas.

Traveling on the country gravel roads in Wendell's new Buick, he remarked, "I've been driving over 50 years and never had an accident." Peggy complained about the dust from the road and closed her back seat window—just in time, as it turned out. Coming over a rise at 50 miles an hour, Wendell saw a large pig in the middle of the road. He tooted the horn and slammed on the brake. Like a hesitant squirrel, the pig went one way then the other, back and forth. Wendell turned the car like a skier sliding to a stop, but not before he hit the pig broadside on the right rear of the car. Pig poop covered that side of the car. Peg would have been covered in manure. The pig, evidently not seriously injured, ran off towards home. Wendell pulled into the farmer's yard and explained the situation to his neighbor. They hoped the pig was okay and that no others had found the hole in the fence. Wendell cleaned the car with a garden hose. The visit to the Clydesdales was anticlimactic.

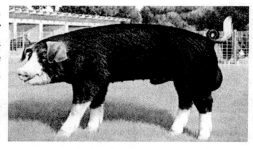

Poland China Hog

Wendell told us the following week the pig had survived with only bruises. He said he does not consider that a blot on his good driving record, as the incident involved a pig, not another car.

What Cheer, Dr. Maxwell, and Corn

In the spring of 1972 *The Chicago Tribune* did a feature story on the trials and tribulations of a typical small Midwest town. What Cheer is four miles southeast of the Santee farm. Dr. John Maxwell is the same surgeon who sutured my wounds in 1934.

The emphasis on getting ethanol from corn has dramatically helped midwest farmers in the last few years. Sadly, research shows the energy used to grow and harvest the corn crop may exceed the energy saving for automobiles. For corn, these factors, along with increased demand for ethanol, helped push prices from under $2 per bushel in 2005 to $3.40 per bushel in 2007. In January, 2011 the following story appeared in the US Ag Network:

Could Corn Price Hit $11 Per Bushel?

, 01/07/2011 — Are corn prices on their way to $11 a bushel? It looks that way, comparing Chicago futures prices this time round with those 15 years ago when stocks last got this tight. According to AgriMoney.com, the similarity in the move in corn prices is startling, says Travis Carter, a consultant at U.S. broker FCStone.

Driving through Iowa in the fall of 2011, every other field seemed brimming with corn ready to harvest. So what is limiting yield on Iowa fields?

Iowa's average corn yield was 166 bu/acre in 2006, which is just slightly above the 30-year trend line. Our highest average yield was 181 bu/acre in 2004. Iowa is increasing yield at approximately 2 bushels per acre per year; more than 60 years will be necessary to have a state average of 300 bu/acre.

Two primary factors come into play: environment and management. We can generally rule out genetics since most producers have access to the same genetics. Management factors that can be controlled include nutrients, weeds, diseases, insects, and water (through irrigation).

Indeed, many Iowa producers average 230 to 270 bu/acre by paying close attention to management. So, one

Sunday, March 19, 1972 — CHICAGO TRIBUNE

In What Cheer, Future's Bleak; Few Seem to Care

BY DAVID THOMPSON
AND DAVID YOUNG
[Chicago Tribune Press Service]

WHAT CHEER, Ia.—The name seems more and more of a misnomer as What Cheer, a tiny Iowa community of 877 persons, slowly erodes.

Nobody seems to care.

Every morning, many local residents gather in small groups around a large round table in the rear of the Chuck Wagon Cafe, sip owner Audrey Smith's coffee, and discuss corn and the weather, seemingly oblivious to the deteriorating main street outside with its score of boarded-up stores.

Vacant Houses, Stores

Abandoned railroad spurs protrude from What Cheer. South of town, beyond the shuttered Little Chicago Club and adjacent abandoned live stock pens, are the crumbling ruins of the kilns and factory that were once the What Cheer Clay Products Co. The town is dotted with vacant houses, and the nicest looking business in town is the recently remodeled funeral home.

"We just talk about day-to-day topics," said Mrs. Dorothy Baylor, head of the one-room First State Bank of What Cheer, housed on the first floor of a turreted brick Victorian building along the main drag. "We are all happy the hog prices are up.

"It seems like you make a lot of money each year, but you seem to spend it all.

"So that takes care of everything but the weather," she concluded.

"Business has really been bad," said Mrs. Raymond Newcomb, who with her husband puts out the What Cheer Chronicle [circulation 1,700]. "There's only one large grocery store left in town. There's no lady's shop; so when women want something to wear, they have to go to Oskaloosa, Ottumwa, or Sigourney."

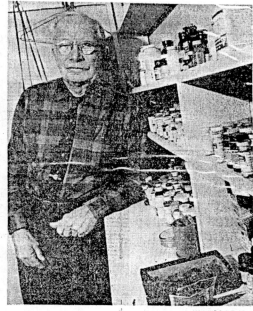

[TRIBUNE Staff Photo]

Dr. John Maxwell, 81, the only doctor in What Cheer. There is no drug store so he also acts as pharmacist.

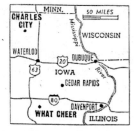

Few Young People Left

She said the town has many residents on pensions and welfare, and most young people leave town to find jobs elsewhere.

Dr. John Maxwell, 81, who is the town's only physician and who figures he will be its last, guessed he had delivered 2,500 babies since he came to town just after World War I. Last year he delivered only two.

"The rarity of a baby born around here indicates the absence of young people, who have left What Cheer in search of jobs," he said. His own two sons entered medical professions but practice elsewhere.

Dr. Maxwell, by the way, charges $1 for an office call.

Another town pillar is Carl G. Draegert, What Cheer's only lawyer and the municipal attorney. He dismissed any idea of What Cheer's getting an infusion of state or federal money to help revive it.

Attempts Made, but Failed

"They [the city fathers] would be glad to have some help from somewhere if they knew where to get it and what to do with it if they got it.

"Two or three development groups have been established from time to time, but they never got very far. After a while, they just gave up."

The white-maned Draegert likes to lean back in a chair in his modern but unpretentious office and reminisce about the historical What Cheer—a bustling coal mining town of an estimated 8,000 persons served by two railroads with daily passenger trains.

"But the coal mines played out, and the railroads eventually left," he said with a sigh.

The future? He sighed again. "All I can see at the moment is just a small community accommodating the needs of the local farm trade."

Have Opera House

The apparent rigor mortis is not complete, however. The town recently built, with a federal loan, a four-unit low-income housing project for the elderly, and many residents have high hopes for the town's civic icon, the What Cheer Opera House, Inc., a 600-seat theater within an overaged, former Masonic hall astride the main street.

The opera house, since its creation in 1965, has featured the likes of Fred Waring, Guy Lombardo, Wayne King and Stan Kenton. Kenton was considered too loud for local tastes, according to Mrs. Wanda Burriss, wife of the president of the opera association.

Her husband, Thomas, who raises 500 market hogs each year on his nearby farm, believes the opera house can continue to subsist on a diet of bands and country and western shows and may even draw attention to What Cheer. He is also contemplating luring a resident straw hat company made up of students from an Iowa college performing for credit.

Aside from Burriss, few people have any plans for What Cheer's destiny.

"It's a friendly, close little town," Mrs. Newcomb said. "I guess people like it that way."

might ask, what is limiting the yields for this group? Experts suggest that it is a higher degree of management and water.

Iowa cornfields producing 200 bu/acre of corn, sold at $6.50 per bushel (market price on October 21, 2011), will produce a gross income of $1300/acre.

I recall Uncle Wendell proudly declaring he got over 40 bu/acre in the 1930s. He would marvel at the change.

DMSO—Wonder Drug???

The next penicillin? The best drug since aspirin?

I was fascinated by a story in *Time* magazine about the discovery of DMSO's remarkable properties. Published in the mid '60s, it documented the serendipitous finding of Dr. Stanley Jacob, who was working with dimethyl sulfoxide (DMSO) in his lab when he was burned by a Bunsen burner. In reaching for a cup to get water on the burned skin, he accidentally tipped over the beaker of DMSO onto the inflamed skin. Within a few seconds, Dr. Jacob noticed the pain was lessening and the skin was less inflamed than he anticipated. Being a good scientist, Dr. Jacob asked himself, "What is going on here?" Like the discovery of the effects of penicillin—found by leaving a discarded Petri dish in a drawer—DMSO was an accidental finding.

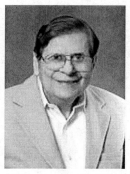

Stanley Jacob, MD 2008

The history of DMSO as a pharmaceutical began in 1961, when Dr. Jacob, head of the organ transplant program at Oregon Health Sciences University was investigating DMSO's potential as a preservative for organs. He quickly discovered that it penetrated the skin quickly and deeply without damaging it. He was intrigued. Thus began his lifelong investigation of the drug.

The first quality that struck Dr. Jacob about the drug was its ability to pass through membranes, an ability that has been verified by numerous subsequent researchers. In addition, DMSO can carry other drugs with it across membranes. It is more successful ferrying some drugs, such as morphine sulfate, penicillin, steroids, and cortisone, than others, such as insulin. What it will carry depends on the molecular weight, shape, and electrochemistry of the molecules. This property would enable DMSO to act as a new drug delivery system that would lower the risk of infection occurring whenever skin is penetrated. DMSO is a byproduct of the wood industry and has been in use as a commercial solvent since 1953. It is also one of the most studied but least understood pharmaceutical agents of our time—at least in the United States.

In the first flush of enthusiasm over the drug, six pharmaceutical companies embarked on clinical studies. Syntex Corporation was the drug company that focused on investigating DMSO's use in vet med. I contacted Syntex in early spring of 1965 and was one of over 100 veterinarians around the country recording the effects of DMSO on various ailments of dogs, cats, and horses. Since then, Syntex was purchased by Roche in 1994.

Over the next six months I treated nearly 100 dogs and cats with DMSO for ailments ranging from A to Z. These included, but were not limited to: corneal ulcers, allergic dermatitis, chronic arthritis, abrasions, pyogenic otitis, burn lesions, interdigital cysts, pannus, cellulitis, joint pain, and ligament sprain. The results were very encouraging; 90% healed within a few days. Pain was reduced in nearly all cases. I was sure I was helping advance scientific knowledge and healing my patients at the same time.

Everything changed in November of that year, 1965. It seems there had been a couple of reports of eye problems which "might" have been caused by use of DMSO.

The drug thalidomide was introduced as a sedative drug in the late 1950s. In 1961, it was withdrawn due to teratogenicity (the production or induction of malformations or monstrosities, especially in a developing embryo or fetus) and neuropathy (nerve disorders that occur with diseases that disrupt the chemical processes in the body). There is now a growing clinical interest in thalidomide. It is introduced as an immunomodulatory agent used primarily, combined with dexamethasone, to treat multiple myeloma. Its use remains controversial, including its testing in the developing world. Thalidomide is a potent teratogen in zebrafish, chickens, rabbits, and primates including humans; severe birth defects may result if the drug is taken during pregnancy.

Thalidomide was sold in a number of countries across the world from 1957 until 1961, when it was withdrawn from the market after being found to be a cause of birth defects in what has been called "one of the biggest medical tragedies of modern times." It is not known exactly how many worldwide victims of the drug there have been, although estimates range from 10,000 to 20,000.

The thalidomide tragedy led to much stricter testing being required for drugs and pesticides before they can be licensed. Remembering thalidomide, the U.S. Food and Drug Adminstration

(FDA) apparently was looking for things to stop, and they found their chance in late 1965. The FDA learned that tests in rabbits, dogs, and pigs (but not humans) had shown some problems. When quantities of DMSO equal to about ten times the maximum human dose (i.e., equal to 350 grams a day for a 175 pound man) were given every day over a period of six months, slight changes in the lenses of the animals' eyes would result—enough to produce a slight nearsightedness. The lens changes were not enough to cause dogs difficulty when running—they didn't bump into things—and in some cases, the changes disappeared after the massive DMSO doses were stopped. In no test—at that time or since—has DMSO ever caused cataracts, either in animals or in humans. Nevertheless, the FDA decided that DMSO was the "dangerous drug" it was looking for.

The first Dr. Jacob and his colleagues knew of the animal tests was on November 10, 1965. On that crucial date, the FDA sent notices to all the drug companies involved in DMSO research (Squibb, Syntex, Merck) that "administration of the drug must be discontinued and the drug recalled from all clinical investigation." In addition, the FDA put out a series of press releases, carried by media all over the world, warning of the blinding effects of DMSO, and leading people to believe that DMSO caused cataracts. But no animals had ever been blinded, and the FDA knew that. The "spin" was designed to show that once again the FDA had "saved" us.

Some 20 years and hundreds of laboratory and human studies later, no deaths have been reported, nor have changes in the eyes of humans been documented or claimed. Since then, however, the FDA has refused seven applications to conduct clinical studies, and approved only one, for interstitial cystitis, which subsequently was approved for prescriptive use in 1978.

Dr. Jacob believes the FDA "blackballed" DMSO, actively trying to kill interest in a drug that could end much suffering.

Why, if DMSO possesses even half the capabilities claimed by Dr. Jacob and others, is it still on the sidelines of medicine in the United States today? "It's a square peg being pushed into a round hole," says Dr. Jacob. "It doesn't follow the rifle approach of 'one agent against one disease entity'. It's the aspirin of our era. If aspirin were to come along today, it would have the same problem. If someone gave you a little white pill and said take this and your headache will go away, your body temperature will go down, it will help prevent strokes and major heart problems, what would you think?"

Worldwide, some 11,000 articles have been written on its medical and clinical implications. In 125 countries throughout the world, including Canada, Great Britain, Germany, Japan, and many in Latin America, doctors prescribe it for a variety of ailments, including pain, inflammation, scleroderma, interstitial cystitis, arthritis, and elevated intracranial pressure.

Several legal battles have been fought in an effort to overturn FDA labeling and help legalize the use of DMSO in the medical field. Mark Hatfield of Oregon, along with his senate colleague Wendell Wyatt, have both introduced bills into the Senate and the House of Representatives in order to help legalize the use of DMSO across the country. The result of these bills being introduced is a legislative investigation conducted by the USA into the practices surrounding the FDA and the legalization of DMSO. In fact, Florida, Louisiana, Nevada, Montana, Oregon, Oklahoma, Washington, and Texas have all legalized DMSO as a prescription drug.

Yet in the United States, DMSO has FDA approval only for use as a preservative of organs for transplant and for interstitial cystitis, a bladder disease

The news media soon got word of Dr. Jacob's discovery, and it was not long before reporters, the pharmaceutical industry, and patients with a variety of medical complaints jumped on the news. Because it was available for industrial uses, patients could dose themselves. This early public interest interfered with the ability of Dr. Jacob—or, later, the FDA—to see that experimentation and use were safe and controlled and may have contributed to the souring of the mainstream medical community on it.

In 1980 Mike Wallace featured it on *60 Minutes*. He interviewed Dr. Jacob and people who had used DMSO to bring relief to their joints. Their testimonials overwhelmingly showed that it worked.

Mike Wallace also interviewed Mr. June Jones, once a quarterback and later coach of the Atlanta Falcons pro-football team. His career almost didn't happen, he told the House of Representatives Committee on Aging in 1980, which was investigating why the FDA was still telling people that DMSO was dangerous. With a bursitis calcification in his right shoulder, he could hardly lift his arm, let alone throw a football. Since he was from Oregon, he was aware of DMSO and that Dr. Jacob had used it for sprains on thousands of others. So he went to Dr. Jacob, who gave him a shot of DMSO in the shoulder and told him that the calcification might disappear if he used DMSO for 30 days straight. He followed the doctor's instructions, and it did disappear. But

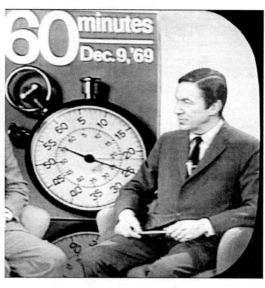

the FDA still would not approve DMSO for sports medicine.

Former Oregon Governor Tom McCall knows about DMSO. Stricken suddenly by bursitis in 1963, two daubings of DMSO on his shoulder put an end to the problem—DMSO dissolved the calcification that caused the painful condition. Stories circulated that anyone entering the locker room of professional sports teams would smell the garlic odor produce by the use of DMSO.

You'd think that DMSO would have become a household name after *60 Minutes*. But it didn't. That's because an ugly smear campaign was started by third parties who, for financial reasons, did not want DMSO to compete with other pain relievers. Others cite DMSO's principal side effect—an odd odor, akin to that of garlic, that emanates from the mouth shortly after use, even if used on the skin. Certainly, this odor has made double-blinded studies difficult. Such studies are based on the premise that no one, neither doctor nor patient, knows which patient receives the drug and which the placebo, but this drug announces its presence within minutes.

Terry Bristol, a PhD candidate from the University of London and president of the Institute for Science, Engineering, and Public Policy in Portland, Oregon, assisted Dr. Jacob with his research in the 1960s and 1970s. He believes that the smell of DMSO may also have put off the drug companies, that feared it would be hard to market. Worse for the pharmaceutical companies, however, was the fact that no company could acquire an exclusive patent for DMSO—a major consideration when the clinical testing required to win FDA approval for a drug routinely runs into millions of dollars.

Dr. Jacob continues to believe that DMSO should not even be called a drug but is more correctly a new therapeutic principle, with an effect on medicine that will be profound in many areas. Whether that is true cannot be known without extensive, publicly reported trials, which are dependent on the willingness of researchers to undertake rigorous studies in this still-unfashionable tack and of pharmaceutical companies and other investors to back them up. That this is a live issue is proved by the difficulty the investigators with approval to clinically test DMSO for closed head injury are having finding funds to conduct the trials.

I continue to use medical grade DMSO today on any bump, bruise, or cut with uniform good results.

John Myers of the *Duluth* (Minn.) *News Tribune* reports:

Tom Levar, a forestry and horticulture specialist for the University of Minnesota Duluth's Natural Resources Research Institute, developed the idea using a chemical first used to treat muscle soreness in racing horses, and later, human athletes. The benign chemical, called DMSO, absorbs quickly through animal and human skin and into the bloodstream.

Levar found out that it passes through plant "skin" as well, and then he combined DMSO with several bitter and otherwise unpleasant-tasting chemicals. A pepper concentrate offered the best combination of being easy to use, natural, and extremely effective.

"You can use it when the plant is first put in the ground or incorporate it into the soil with established plants," said Levar, adding that the plant will even emit a peppery smell. People "don't notice the smell as much, but the deer sure know what it is. It's not really clear which is the better deterrent, the smell or the hot taste. Usually it's one bite and they move on."

The pepper concentrate, called capsicum, is natural and doesn't harm the plant.

The stuff also works great to keep dogs, cats, rabbits, mice, voles, moles, and gophers from eating plants and young trees, Levar noted. In tests at an Alexandria, Minn., tree farm that had suffered huge losses of young conifer to field mice, the repellent proved 100% effective.

Michigan-based Repellex USA already has purchased the licensing rights from the university amd has applied to the Environmental Protection Agency for approval.

Repellex is currently available at garden stores. Levar notes that Repellex Systemic shouldn't be used on edible plants "unless you want your strawberries to taste like hot peppers," he joked. "You'd definitely be able to taste it."

Repellex discovered Levar's patent as they looked for a new product line. And the University's Office for Technology Commercialization negotiated the license agreement with Repellex.

It may be premature to call for the full rehabilitation of DMSO, but it is time to call for a full investigation of its true range of capabilities.

AAHA Conventions

National conventions present an opportunity for professionals to meet and greet old friends and classmates, learn current ideas and techniques, vacation with family, and sometimes just goof off. Many states require professionals, including veterinarians, to attend postgraduate training classes totaling 20 to 40 hours per year. Some states require actual class attendance; others just require proof of registration. It's a case of leading the horse to water and hoping he will drink in a little knowledge.

Carol and I attended the American Animal Hospital Association (AAHA) national convention in Washington, DC, in the summer of 1969. It afforded me a chance to attend our premier convention and visit my brother, Phil, and his wife, Francine, in their suburban DC home in Reston, Virginia.

Phil dropped me at the Capitol Hilton Hotel in downtown DC. After mall shopping all day, Carol borrowed Francine's car to come to the hotel for the dinner and speeches to follow. No one thought to tell Carol there were two Hilton hotels in DC—the Washington Hilton and the Capitol Hilton. Carol got directions to the wrong one. She was used to Chicago traffic—among the worst in the U.S.—but DC was worse. After fighting the bumper-to-bumper snarl for an hour to reach the Washington Hilton, she had to drive cross-town to the Capitol Hilton, arriving just before dinner was served.

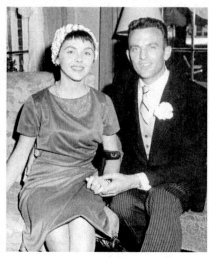

Francine and Phil Merrick

At that time Phil was a regular Army Lieutenant Colonel, working in the Pentagon under the command of General Yarborough, the Assistant Chief of Staff for Intelligence. One of Phil's duties was to guide foreign embassy attachés (spies) on a tour of U.S. Army facilities. In addition to making sure the group had plenty of food and drink, he was to impress them by showing off our latest equipment. He made sure they had some free time to explore a few "secret areas" on each base. They could then report what they had been able to discover "on their own" to their bosses at home. Of course, they knew we let them see what we wanted them to see. That's how the game was played, both here and abroad. When Phil retired 15 years later, he used this experience to start a travel business around Colonial Williamsburg and Washington, DC.

Some ten years later, the National AAHA dermatology convention was again held in Washington, DC. Combe, Inc. was sponsoring one of the principal speakers and hosting a dinner to celebrate their twenty five years in the animal health field. Ivan Combe, the president and CEO of Combe, Inc. gave a brief account of how, acting on a tip from a friend, he had acquired a pair of pet products from an Illinois veterinarian, Dr. Andrew Merrick. These products were Dr. Merrick's Scratch Powder, which he renamed Scratchex Powder, and Sulfodene Skin Medication, used to treat hot spots on dogs. Carol and I and two of our kids, Buzz and Peg, were introduced as honored guests.

The Combe Company is little known, primarily because it would rather promote its brands than its corporate name. Most of Combe's brands are, in fact, household words. As a charter advertiser on American Bandstand, the product had its commercials delivered by the popular Dick Clark. Clearasil became a household word. Men's grooming products include well-known brands Grecian Formula, Just For Men, Brylcreem, Aqua Velva, and 'Lectric Shave. In the skincare category, Combe markets the Lanacane brand. The Cepacol brand is the core of the sore throat/oral care category. Vagisil is their main brand for feminine care. In the foot-care category, Combe relies on Odor-Eaters and Johnson's Foot Soap. Sea-Bond adhesive makes up the denture care category. The man behind the Combe name was Ivan DeBlois Combe, regarded as the father of the self-medication industry.

Even as Combe was growing Clearasil and continuing to promote Espotabs, he remained on the lookout for new products. In 2002, the company acquired J.B. Williams in a deal that brought such well known brands as Aqua Velva, Brylcreem, and Cepacol mouthwash into the Combe family of products.

The Midwest Regional AAHA Convention was held in October, 1983, at a resort in Lake Geneva, Wisconsin, just 30 miles west of Kenosha, making it easy for Carol and me to attend. The celebratory speaker of the evening was Dr. Brian Sinclair from Trisk, England. For those unfamiliar with the James Herriot books, *All Creatures Great and Small,* James Herriot was the junior partner to Donald Sinclair. In the stories about rural veterinary practice in Trisk, England, after WWII, Herriot renamed Donald Sinclair and his brother, Brian Sinclair, Siegfried and Tristan Farnon, respectively. James Herriot is the pen name of James Alfred Wight, OBE, also known as Alf Wight (October 3, 1916–February 23, 1995), an English veterinarian and writer. Wight is best known for his semi-autobiographical stories, often referred to collectively as *All Creatures Great and Small,* a title used in some editions and in film and television adaptations.

Dr. Brian Sinclair joined the practice a few years after Dr. Herriot, and he became the junior partner. In the books, Dr. Tristan Farnon (Brian Sinclair) is portrayed as having a fondness for alcohol. In his evening speech, Dr. Sinclair stated, with a straight face, it was actually Dr. Herriot who had the drinking problem, and Herriot must have stolen Sinclair's stories and claimed them as his own. After a good laugh, he confessed Herriot really did author *All Creatures Great and Small.* He also stated he never in his wildest dreams imagined people would pay him money to give speeches around the world commenting on his experiences working with the famous James Herriot. He thanked Dr. Herriot for sending him on his many journeys and making retirement a joy. He was the model for the character "Tristan Farnon" in Wight's semi-autobiographical novels, which were later adapted to the big screen in two films, and to television under the name *All Creatures Great and Small.* Unlike his elder brother, who for some time saw the books as a great trial of his friendship with Wight, Brian made no objections to Wight's ne'er-do-well portrayal of him, and in fact seemed rather to enjoy the celebrity, appearing on television and lecturing at veterinary schools all over the U.K. and elsewhere.

I attended three or four conventions or seminars every year. Conventions are usually a three- or four-day affair with something for everyone—large animal, dairy, small animal and exotics. Seminars are daily meetings devoted to one subject—dermatology, ophthalmology, orthopedic surgery etc. My goal was to learn one thing I could apply to my practice immediately. Anything in addition was gravy.

Madeline Reynolds Hough

Madeline Reynolds, my wife's mother, rode the street car from her home in suburban Chicago to the Grand Chicago Theatre, where she played the huge pipe organ for silent movies. The time was 1922, and she was 18. Mad, as her two sisters called her, was a member of the "flapper" generation. The girls were known to sneak out of her bedroom window, after her parents were asleep, to meet a boy or another adventurous girlfriend. Dad Reynolds was general manager of the large corn products plant in Argo, Illinois. Thousands of workers there produced dozens of items such as Karo Syrup and Niagara Starch. The smell of roasting corn permeated the surrounding area for miles.

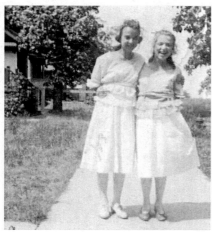

Madeline Reynolds and a classmate • 1919

The Reynolds family had the only private grass tennis court in town. This was not lost on Bill Hough, an employee in the plant and an early suitor of Madeline's. Bill (Ora) Hough had been an all-state fullback in Indiana and a member of the Arizona University football team until a torn knee ligament ended his athletic carrier.

Madeline and Bill married in 1924. In 1938 they built their dream house in Western Springs, Illinois. Carol was 7 at the time, and her older brother, Harry, 12, was in my grade-school class. Madeline loved to be a "stay at home mom." Attending a bridge club twice a month, a book club weekly, and a garden club monthly kept her busy. She enjoyed "antiquing," and eventually she became quite an expert. Only the very wealthy had two cars. Less than 25% of women worked outside the home. Kids were expected to walk to and from school. Only rural schools had regular school bus service.

If Madeline was the queen, Bill Hough was the king. With the dedication and discipline of an athlete, Bill was the undisputed master of his castle. He was up at 6:00 AM, at work by 7:15, home by 5:15, ate supper by 5:30, listened to the evening radio news at 6:00, and was in bed by 10:00. Bill was an avid gardener. I volunteered to help so I could spend more time with his daughter.

Bill taught contract bridge to friends and neighbors. Charles Goren was the master of the bridge world. Carol and I learned well enough to win a few "master points" until too many "discussions" of bridge play carried over into the night. We finally gave up our card partnership to help keep our marriage partnership intact.

Supper in the Hough household was invariably meat, potatoes, vegetable, and dessert, followed by very strong coffee. Madeline said she knew when the coffee had percolated enough—when it bubbled over the pot and put out the gas stove's flame, it's done. Madeline was a good cook, but she had no inkling about finances. Bill doled out whatever money was needed to both mother and children. After constant complaining about lack of money for food, clothes, and household items, Bill said in desperation, "If you can do better, you take over the budget." Big mistake! Madeline made no attempt to follow a plan. She used her one and only opportunity to buy all the clothes she thought everyone needed and enough food and household supplies for a small army. Her assault on the budget lasted less than a month.

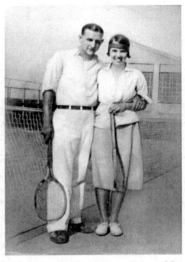

Bill Hough, Madeline Reynolds
Summit, Ill. • 1924

After another lengthy family argument over money, Madeline decided she needed a vacation. Until then, the family had always vacationed together. Sister Ruth, a high school English teacher, was the vacation expert. Ruth decided she and Madeline would spend a week touring Mexico. Their first driver was named Jesus, pronounced "hey-sus" in English phonics. Ruth related that every time "hey-sus" would speed up and down the narrow country roads, Madeline would yell, "Oh, Jesus!"

Madeline brought a beautiful drindle skirt with Spanish written all around the bottom edge. Since Madeline had forgotten to have the saying translated, Carol wore the dress to school. Her Spanish teacher laughed and translated for the assembled gaggle of girls, "Keep your mouth shut or the flies will get in." Carol never wore the skirt again.

Bill Hough died at the age of 59. After falling off a ladder while cleaning gutters on the house, he had a fatal stroke in the hospital three days later. Madeline was despondent. She had no preparation for managing a household. Carol and I had been living in Kenosha for five years by that time. She called me a few weeks after Bill died. She was in tears. She cried, "Johnny, I don't know what to do to balance my checkbook." It turned out she had never balanced a checkbook. She was unaware the bank returned her checks in a random order. I went over the procedure with her. Madeline's sisters did what they could, but Madeline's depression worsened. After a couple weeks' stay in the hospital to treat her depression, Madeline was able to put her house up for sale and move into an apartment.

Bill Hough did not provide Madeleine with much of a retirement income. Between Bill's check and Social Security, Madeline was able to live very frugally. After a couple of years she applied for a job at the local Ace Hardware. By sheer determination and will Madeline developed enough business skills to be made manager of the gift department. Her bubbly personality made her a natural saleswoman. After seven years at Ace Hardware, she retired when she moved into the Scottish Home (SH)—a retirement home for people with Scottish ancestry. Madeline had been volunteering at the SH for many years, so they overlooked her Irish heritage and decided Bill's Scottish background was sufficient.

Madeline soon became a fixture in the SH. She was in charge of the lending library and played piano every evening after dinner. Everyone gathered around to sing the songs from the '20s and '30s. Carol mentioned to her mother, "They really sang off key." Madeline replied, "It doesn't matter, they can't hear anyway." At that time it was the common practice for places like the SH to figure the life expectancy of the new arrival; multiply the yearly cost; subtract any pension or Social Security income, and set the entrance fee. Madeline had only minimal pension and Social Security income. She had no other source of income, as the house sale funds had been used up long ago. The SH asked her

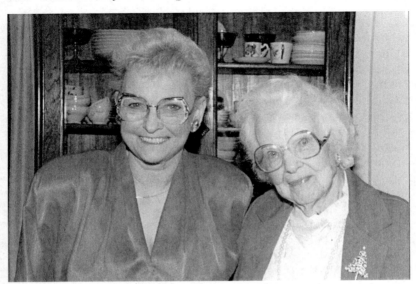

Carol Hough Merrick and Madeline Reynolds Hough
Scottish Home • North Riverside, Ill. • 1985

son, Harry Hough, and myself to make up the $500/month that Madeline was short. She was one of their youngest residents, moving in at the age of 74, so her life expectance was longer than most, which caused a higher entrance fee. Harry was unable to provide assistance. Carol and I sent $100 a month for a few months, then we had more pressing expenses, with six kids and Carol starting back to college. The Scottish Home generously allowed Madeline to stay and accepted her pension, Social Security, and an occasional check from Carol and me as payment.

Madeline remained in the SH for 12 years. She passed in 1990 at the age of 86, after a full, rewarding life. She brought joy to all who knew her. Always one to smile instead of frown, Madeline enjoyed people, and her infectious spirit was reciprocated. Fortunately, the family has a few video minutes of Madeline describing her favorite antiques, which now reside in the homes of her progeny.

Dorothy Santee Merrick

They found the young lovers in Sigourney, the county seat of Keokuk, Iowa. High school sweethearts, Dorothy Elizabeth Santee and Roland James Burris eloped and were married by a Justice of the Peace. I'm not sure if the marriage was ever consummated; Mom rarely spoke about it. Within twenty four hours the elopers were back home in Coal Creek with their Quaker parents.

This whole episode came to light 30 years later. Dorothy and Andy Merrick's 30th wedding anniversary was approaching. Dorothy decided she wanted to join the Roman Catholic faith. She had persuaded dad to celebrate by being married in the Catholic Church—at the same St. Francis Xavier that Carol and I had said our vows seven years prior. As part of her conversion, Dorothy revealed her prior marriage to the counselor, Father O'Hara. He informed Dorothy that the church still considers Dorothy and Roland married in the eyes of God. The church would have to have written proof that Roland indeed did not want to continue the relationship and would agree to end it. Imagine the surprise when a fifty-year-old Iowa farmer received that letter from the Catholic Archdiocese of Chicago. Naturally, Roland agreed to the terms, and the conversion and wedding celebration proceeded.

Young Dorothy overcame this minor setback and was the first in her family to enroll in college. Her first and second year was at William Penn College, a Quaker School in nearby Oskaloosa, Iowa. She received mostly A's and B's with a lone C in piano. She met and married my dad, Andrew Clarence Merrick, a young veterinarian practicing in Oskaloosa. I never heard what her family thought about Dorothy dropping out of college. If it was similar to Carol's parents, it was a major disappointment; however, a niece who lived with my parents for a number of months in the '50s reports the following:

> Grandma told me plenty of stories, and she told me this one more than once: Dorothy and Andy were out on a date in his Model A or Model T Ford. He, of course, was drinking. One thing lead to another and she didn't get home until the sun came up. She didn't drink (or not very much), but they were having a good time and she was very

new at dating, having been raised on the farm. This was their first date, or very early in their courtship (if there actually was one). I don't remember her saying that they had actually gone "all the way," but there was something about the back seat of the car. Of course, I remember Dorothy saying that when Andy finally took her home in the early hours of the morning, her father was furious. Out all night could only mean one thing—get married. She said she didn't know him very well at all and had to learn everything that came along with him as time went by.

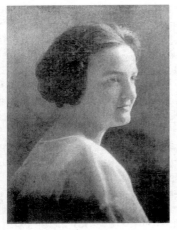 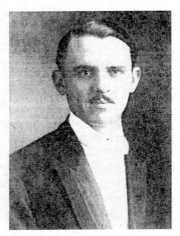

Dorothy S. Merrick
Penn College • 1923

Andrew C. Merrick
Ohio State • 1924

Times were hard on the farm in the early part of the 20th century, and 90% of the population lived on a farm. Using mostly horse and mule power, farmers struggled to make ends meet. At least most families had a large garden which supplied food that could be canned for the winter. Dorothy's mother, Viola, tended a one-acre garden—the size of two city lots. Imagine planting, weeding, watering and harvesting that big a plot. There were no paved roads, no indoor plumbing, no electricity, and few automobiles. The two children born between Wendell, Dorothy's older brother, and my mother, died as infants; one when a fierce winter storm prevented the doctor from reaching the farm in time to help. I only recently learned about the second infant mortality when visiting the family gravesite in Sixteen Cemetery near the family farm.

The Veterinarian's Son   Dorothy Santee Merrick

Life as a large animal vet in the early '30s, in the midst of the Great Depression, was equally as difficult as it was for farmers. The depression was deepening. Vets were often paid with produce. In 1933 my parents were forced to send the three kids to relatives. Margaret went to Uncle Byron and Aunt Jo in Berlin Heights, Ohio. I was sent to my grandparent's farm in Iowa. Phil began at Uncle Russ and Aunt Ann's in Freeport, Illinois, but soon moved to Uncle Ruffy and Aunt Manon's in Forreston, Illinois. Each of Andy's three brothers were veterinarians. Fortunately, all were without children in their homes. After Dad opened his first small animal hospital in 1935, we were all able to become a family again. Somehow, Dad got the financing in 1936 to build a very modern animal hospital in Brookfield, Illinois. Dad never told me directly, but the $25,000 down payment either came from a very lucky streak at the craps table or a loan from very rich clients, Mr. and Mrs. Freund. The Argonne National Lab in Naperville, Illinois was built on their property.

By 1939, partly due to his joining AA, Dad's practice was a resounding success. Mom and Dad bought their first home in Western Springs, Illinois. They paid $7,500 for a three story, 5 bedroom, 2½ bath house. It sold for $550,000 in 2008.

Dorothy was a great cook. Carol often remarked, "My mom is a good cook, but your mom really taught me how to cook." Standing rib roasts, any kind of potatoes, gravy, al dente veggies, cookies, pies, and cakes—Mom could do it all. Dad had walk-in office hours 9 AM–noon, 2–5 PM, and 7–8 in the evening, five days a week. Saturday hours were 9 AM–noon and 1–5 PM, and Sundays were 10 AM–noon. Dad came home for supper, so the meal needed to be served by 6 PM. The Sunday family gathering of the Merrick clan was a bimonthly occasions. The other two local vet brothers and their families would come over for Sunday dinner, typically served around 1–2 PM. It was following such a dinner in 1941 that we heard about the bombing of Pearl Harbor. We had celebrated my 12th birthday, and I received a Boy Scout knife. It's the first birthday present I remember receiving—ever. Our family wasn't big on birthdays then. Our Boy Scout troop met in the Western Springs Village Church. Unbeknownst to anyone at the time, the preacher—newly ordained from nearby Wheaton College— was none other than Billy Graham. If I'd have had a little foresight, I might have attended some of his talks.

Dorothy longed for a partner in marriage. Sadly, this was not to be. During the first 15 years of the marriage, Dad's alcoholism was a too-frequent problem. Andy was a binge drinker—going weeks or months without a drop, then off an a drunken spree for days at a time. This necessitated Dorothy to "keep all the balls in the air," both at home and at the veterinary practice. She became very adept at telling white lies and making excuses.

After a drunken session in 1938, two of Dad's brothers, Russ and Ruffy, checked him into the famous rehab hospital in French Lick, Indiana. Fortunately, Andy got the message and joined AA. Anyone with an AA member in their family knows the dedication and zeal they often display. He even met Bill W., one of the co-founders of the organization.

Andy hosted weekly meetings at our home in Western Springs. He accompanied others on "Twelve Step" calls to rescue, counsel, or assist other AA members.

Mother was no longer the "Chief Cook and Bottler Washer" in the Merrick family business. She longed once again to wear her white nurse's uniform and be the greeter, bookkeeper, and general manager of the Merrick Animal Hospital. Dad refused her pleas and ordered her to stay home and raise the kids.

Andy finally agreed to marriage counseling. After three visits, the psychiatrist spoke to Dorothy alone. "Your husband will never change; you can accept the fact or seek a divorce." Dorothy slit her left wrist the following day—deep enough to spill blood all over the kitchen, but shallow enough for surgical repair and future use of her arm and hand. To my untrained eye, this looked like a desperate call for help and attention.

The time was 1956. I was working for Dad after graduating from the U. of I. in 1954. Carol and I did what we could. We now had three children under the age of five. My father and I never had a serious conversation about any family problems he and Dorothy were having. I had bought a practice in Kenosha, Wisconsin, and would soon be 60 miles north of the problem.

My parents had occasionally slept in separate bedrooms. This now became their permanent arrangement. Dorothy tried her damnedest to become a drug addict—downers to sleep and uppers to start the day. Friendly druggists supplied her habit. Two or three visits to "rest homes"—read "psychiatric hospitals"—finally enabled her to stop the medications. If drugs would not kill the pain, maybe alcohol would. No matter how much Johnny Walker Black Label scotch or Canadian Club whiskey she consumed, Dorothy couldn't get drunk. She'd pass out before inebriation. Her next effort was the conversion to Catholicism and remarriage. That seemed to help for a while. In the end, they were two people living separate lives in the same house.

Andy died in 1976. Even after selling the animal hospital five years earlier, Dad "went to work" almost every day. Most clients were unaware the practice had changed hands until months later. Dad experienced a mild heart attack and died after a suffering a stroke while recovering in the hospital. Those golden years of romance and travel were not to be. Mother now faced the world alone. She had no husband to argue with, no close relatives, and no real friends to visit and gossip. She made occasional visits to children, but no trips to exotic locales.

Despite the hardships Dorothy endured, she was never mean-spirited. She always looked out for her children and their families. Dorothy and Andy put on happy faces for sister Sue's wedding in the summer of 1959.

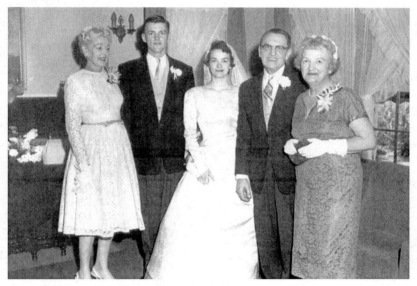

Mrs.Kinch, Jack Kinch, Sue Merrick Kinch, Andy, Dorothy • 1959

When Carol and I were engaged, Dorothy convinced—ordered—Dad to pay me $200 per month while I was in vet school. She reasoned that my schooling would have cost more if I wasn't married, so what's the difference? Rather than argue, Dad relented. Dorothy gave us her nearly new '49 Chevy coupe to take on our honeymoon trip to Yellowstone, Salt Lake, and Pike's Peak. She enjoyed visiting children and their families, often staying with our kids when we took an infrequent vacation. She told me after I had graduated that she wished she had purchased a home for us in Champaign. One of my classmates, Jim and Elaine Nadler, did that and paid their way through school by taking in roomers. It gave me the motivation to purchase a house in Madison for my two oldest kids when they attended the University of Wisconsin. My oldest daughter, Dorothy, found her calling as a realtor because of her experience in renting and managing the property.

In early December, 1976, on the occasion of my 47th birthday, I received the following letter:

> Dear Johnny
>
> Tomorrow morning at 8:30 I will be especially thinking of you —
>
> It was 9:30 Eastern Standard Time in 1929 when you first made your appearance.
>
> It sure doesn't seem that long ago —
>
> I want you to know you've been a source of joy to me always —
>
> Much love,
> and have a Happy Birthday
>
> Mother
>
> Dec. 5, 1976   xx

Dorothy sold the family home in 1980 and moved into the Scottish Home, joining Madeline Hough. When the director figured what her total bill was, taking into account her age, life expectancy, and income he said, "Dorothy your total is $100,026.00. Dorothy's immediate response, "What the hell is the twenty six for?" The director nearly fell out of his chair.

Mom had a mischievous streak. She and Madeline Hough had been living in the Scottish Home together for four years. Dorothy usually had a box of chocolates on her dresser. When Mom neglected to offer a candy, Madeline took to helping herself. One day, Dorothy left an empty box, with the lid on, in plain view. After her morning visit, Madeline announced, "Well, I'll just help myself to a candy if you're not going to offer any." Dorothy laughed all day remembering Madeline's look and outburst after seeing the empty box.

Over the years, various grandchildren, nieces and nephews have lived with my parents for extended periods of time. Margaret's two oldest girls spent summers in Western Springs in the late

'50s. My oldest son, Bill, lived with his grandparents during some of the time he was attending the University of Chicago. My second son, David, cared for Dad for a few months after returning from a hitch as a Navy diver.

Dorothy died on April 7, 1987 at the age of 81. Her cremains were buried next to Andy's on a hillside in Sixteen Cemetery, What Cheer, Iowa, three miles from her childhood home. Carol Hough Merrick joined them in July, 2006. I'll be there in the future.

Note to readers—

I sincerely wish I had started this project while my sisters, Margaret and Susie, were alive. I had started writing *Animal Stories* and received encouragement from both girls. I know they could do a better job than I of describing our parents. Sue never saw Dad drunk. She lived with them as an "only child," born eight years after the previous baby, Phil. Writing the words, "baby Phil" let me recall a long forgotten photo of Phil with long, shoulder length, blonde curly hair. He was probably 4 or 5 at the time. I'm sure each of you, my readers, will have similar remembrances as you start to put your thoughts on paper.

Carol Merrick's Special Deliveries

The birthday song rang out, loud and clear. "Happy birthday, Nurse Carlson, happy birthday to you." The cake had to wait in the corridor, outside the delivery room of St. Catherine's Hospital in Kenosha, until the candles were blown out. Then during a break in the controlled panic, Dr. Rattan asked for the cake to be brought in. "Maybe a bite of birthday cake will speed up Carol's contractions," he said. Carol was in the final stages of labor, giving birth to Margaret Manon (Peggy), the last of our six children. This was not the first time I had "assisted" in the delivery of my children. Ten years previously, I had helped the short-handed Burnham Hospital staff in Champaign, Illinois strap Carol into the stirrups for the delivery of our first-born, Dorothy Ann Merrick.

Each incident occurred in the middle of the night. Do women *ever* start labor during daylight hours? Dorothy's entry began on the coldest night of the winter of 1951 in Urbana, Illinois. Carol announced the pains were every five to ten minutes, and it was time to leave home for the ten-minute drive to Burnham Hospital. I had parked our vintage '36 Chevy facing downhill, in case it wouldn't start. Cars with a clutch could be started by turning on the ignition, getting the car rolling up to 10 MPH, releasing the clutch, and voilà—away we go. Fortunately, the Chevy turned over easily, and we were off to Burnham City Hospital, five miles away, in neighboring Champaign.

Carol had been laboring to deliver Dorothy for six hours. The pains were coming every five minutes by the time we reached the maternity ward. A nurse determined that Carol's cervix was 3 or 4 cm dilated and wheeled her into the delivery room. The room was as quiet as a library reading room. Gurneys were lined up. Delivery tables were empty and at the ready. No hustle and bustle, no monitors beeping. No other staff was around, so the nurse asked if I would help strap Carol to the table. Sixty years ago hospital protocols were not what they are today. Unfortunately, Dorothy decided to wait another 24 hours, entering the world on December 22nd instead of the 21st.

Peggy's birth in February of 1962 was a different story. Dr. Walt Rattan, Carol's OB/GYN, was not only her gynecologist, but a close family friend and frequent tennis partner and ski companion. It was 2 AM when Carol and I arrived at the St. Catherine's Hospital on Kenosha's north lakeshore. Dr. Rattan allowed me to accompany Carol into the delivery room. It was then, as now, definitely against protocol in many hospitals, but in the middle of the night, who was to know? After one hour of labor, Carol showed no signs of imminent delivery. As luck would have it, February 17 was OB nurse Carlson's birthday. The staff had brought in a cake to be eaten during a break in the action. Dr. Rattan decided now would be the time. Carol declined. So except for the happy birthday celebration, Peggy's arrival was routine. I even got to hold her after the first nurse finished cleaning, weighing and measuring. I was also allowed to cut the umbilical cord. After I commented about the length of the episiotomy, Dr. Rattan remarked facetiously, "I always put in a couple of extra sutures to tighten everything up a little." Walt and I laughed; the nurses frowned.

The next day, February 18, 1962, produced six inches of fresh snow. This usually meant most of my appointments would be cancelled, so I had my receptionist call everyone to reschedule. That left me free to take the older kids skiing at Wilmot Mountain, 15 miles west of Kenosha. Wilmot could be considered a mountain only if you had never been to Colorado. Carol was not at all impressed by my putting skiing before a hospital visit to a new mother. She never failed to bring up the subject every five or ten years, just to keep it fresh in my mind.

William Andrew (Bill), the second child and first boy, was born like his older sister, in Burnham Hospital, on July 3, 1953. In the '50s, routine post-delivery hospitalization was four or five days in a two-bed room. To Carol's surprise, she was greeted by her roommate, Mary Swanson. Unusual as it may seem, Mary and Carol were roommates 19 months earlier, after delivering their first babies. They had both been delivered by Dr. Gernon Hesselschwerdt. Specialists were still a few years distant in many areas of the country. Gernon looked like he should have been delivering calves in some dairy barn. He was stout, 6' 2", 220 lbs., with big "farm boy" hands—more appropriate for milking cows than delivering babies. In any event, he had a wonderful bedside manner and the women loved him. I asked why Dr. Hesselschwerdt's delivery fee was $105 for Bill but only $95 for Dorothy. "Boys are always $10 more," he replied, "Circumcision, you know." Remember, this was 1951 and 1953. Carol's five-day stay in the hospital totaled $105.

After graduation in 1954, I began working for my father, Dr. A. C. Merrick, in Brookfield, Illinois. We rented the "Bohemian Bungalow" behind the animal hospital owned by my dad. As usual, Carol's third pregnancy was an unplanned but happy event. My next door neighbor, Everett Carlson, and I weatherproofed the back porch to create a third bedroom for the baby.

Dr. Walt Burke had recently left Dad's practice to open his own small animal hospital in nearby Glen Ellyn. As luck would have it, Walt's older brother, John, was a board certified OB/GYN, practicing in Hinsdale, ten miles west of Brookfield. At that time (1955), specialists were just beginning to be accepted in major cities around the country. It seemed natural for us to pick Dr. Burke for Carol's delivery. Dr. Burke delivered only on Tuesdays and Thursdays, except in emergencies. That way he could avoid most of the disruptions in his schedule and ensure he and his staff would be on hand for every minute of the birthing process. This was done by calculating when the prospective mother had completed 38 weeks of her pregnancy, had no untoward complications, and was willing. Carol had no problems and was looking forward to a four-hour—rather than a 24-hour—delivery.

Since we knew the delivery date, Carol and two of her girlfriends planned a pre-birth party the night before the big event. Dick and Shirley Slouka and Bob and Dee Jones were invited over to share homemade pizza and beer. Carol didn't drink, fortunately, so she was able to get me awake the following morning to drive her to Hinsdale Hospital for her 7:00 AM appointment. True to his word, Dr. Burke delivered David John Merrick at 11:30 AM.

During one of Carol's post-delivery visits, Dr. Burke confided in us how he almost didn't make it through medical school. Grades were no problem for Dr. Burke. The trouble was his proclivity to faint at the sight of blood. Since childhood, Dr. Burke confessed that he passed out almost every time he was exposed to bleeding. After fainting in surgery as a third year med student, he was held up between two classmates for the next semester until he finally was able to put "mind over matter."

That was at about this time that Carol and I decided to look to starting our own practice. I purposefully say "our," not "my" practice, for as any young professional knows, it usually takes both husband and wife to kick-start a successful career. Dad had let me know that I would be given the practice upon his retirement, some ten to twenty years in the future. He also made it clear that he would never have a partner. His previous experience when selling Sulfodene soured his outlook on partnerships. It may also have been due his tendency to "forget" to enter all receipts in the ledger. Sometimes cash payments went into his pocket instead of the cash box, which might pose difficulties with a partner and the IRS.

Fourth born, Byron Robert (Buzz), was the first of three kids Carol delivered at St. Catherine's Hospital in Kenosha, Wisconsin. Buzz arrived on November 17, 1957, three days before Carol's 26th birthday. Carol's birthday celebration was in her hospital room this time. We had been worried Byron might have problems due to Carol's midterm illness. A flare-up of her chronic atopic dermatitis resulted in Carol's hospitalization for a two-week period in the summer of 1957. My mother, Dorothy, served as the substitute mom during that time. Fortunately, Carol recovered in time to deliver a healthy baby boy. We had recently moved into our first house. That, plus the burden of three kids under six years of age, probably contributed to Carol's illness.

Virginia Elaine Merrick arrived on September 28, 1959. She was named after Carol's cousin, Virginia Reynolds, and best friend, Elaine Carlson. After her divorce, Virginia retook her maiden name and changed her first name to Ginger. She mentioned to me once that whenever Mom called her Virginia, she knew she was in trouble.

In 1959 ultrasounds were not available to determine gender before birth. Even if they had been, Carol and I decided we would rather be surprised. Dorothy, by then the eight-year-old big sister to three brothers, pleaded with Carol to bring her a little sister—please!

Lightning struck again. After Carol had been ensconced in her private room in St. Catherine's, she found out her next-door neighbor was once again Mary White. One hears about this happening in twins or sisters, but to different people in different states and eight years apart? Mary had been Carol's roommate after Buzz's delivery. She had recently been promoted to Head Dietitian at the hospital, so Carol's food was excellent during her recovery.

Married at 18, Carol gave birth at ages 20, 22, 24, 26, 28, and 30—a seemingly regular production line. Each child, though, was unplanned and very welcome. We had always talked about a big family—four to six kids. "The Pill" was now available, thankfully, and Peggy was the end of the line.

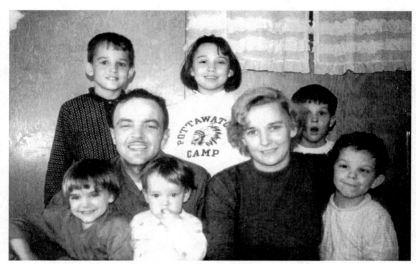

John and Carol Merrick, surrounded by their six children.
Clockwise, from top left: Bill, Dorothy, David, Buzz, Peggy, Ginger
Kenosha, Wisconsin • 1963

Mrs. Charles Roberts

"That damned Carter—again!" "That damned Jimmy Carter," Mrs. Roberts screamed, "He wants all my money!"

I didn't make many house calls in the '60s, but when Mrs. Roberts called, you bet I was out to her estate in a flash. She had been a bailiff in the Cook County, Illinois, courts for 20 years when she met Mr. Roberts on a Caribbean cruise. Mr. Roberts was the recently retired VP of Northwestern Mutual Life, a large insurance company based in Milwaukee. His wife had recently passed, and he was smitten by Mrs. Roberts on the cruise. Mrs. Roberts had the regal bearing of a Kennedy or a Bush—attractive for her middle 50s age. No "Trophy Wife," she was more of a "No Nonsense Wife." They lived in the then-fashionable Beverly Park area on Chicago's south side, with a home in Miami Beach and a large farm a mile south of Kenosha. The Roberts lived the happy life of the idle rich until Mr. Roberts died of a heart attack five years later.

Mr. Roberts had built a mini-mansion on the farm and employed a staff consisting of a cook, a cleaning lady, a gardener/chauffeur, and a part-time secretary/bookkeeper. The farming was share-cropped with locals.

The downstairs marble floors were practically covered with oriental rugs so that their many adopted dogs running around wouldn't get cold paws. Most of the smaller ones were kept in playpens during the day, but a couple of the middle-sized ones had full run of the house. Mrs. Roberts current favorite was a Kerry Blue Terrier, "Irish." Irish went wherever he pleased.

As I entered to do some routine vaccinations, I heard Mrs. Roberts swear. "Damn Carter! That damned Carter!" Mrs. Roberts never swore, so I surmised the then-president Carter had declared war on some country or done some other dastardly deed. Being a good Republican now that she was rich, Mrs. Roberts was very concerned that she pay no more taxes than the law allowed. She was, however, the most generous person I've ever met. The first duty of her bookkeeper, on the first day of every month, was to write some 20 to 25 checks to various charities and individuals Mrs. Roberts deemed worthy of assistance. Anyone who thought Mrs. Roberts was an easy mark, soon learned what 20 years in the Cook County court system taught her about recognizing a scam when she saw one.

When I asked for an explanation or reason for her wrath, she replied, "That damned Carter has gone and spent all my money. The IRS says I underpaid my estimate for the quarter by $25,000. I guess I'll have to sell some stock!" The insurance business must have been pretty good that year.

Mrs. Roberts was also very generous to local charities. She was the major donor that helped fund the Vet Aid program I started a few years later. She later purchased and donated land near the Kenosha Humane Society for a pet cemetery.

Mr. Roberts had been a 32nd degree Mason who despised Catholics. Mrs. Roberts had no particular religious affiliation, but after Mr. Roberts passed away, she was influenced by the TV programs of Archbishop Fulton Sheen, among others. She decided to give the farm and house to the Carmelite Sisters and help build them a Mother House on the front of the property. She had her will rewritten to allow her to stay on the property as long as she lived. In time, the sisters would inherit the entire estate. True to their word, the nuns cared for Mrs. Roberts until she passed in April, 1985.

I learned after her passing that Mrs. Roberts's brother, whom she hated, got the bulk of her money that was not tied to the property or specifically gifted. Funny how life works in strange ways. Mr. Roberts must be spinning in his grave with the current use of his farm. Mrs. Roberts may also be doing a slow turn after seeing what happened to all her money.

That's not the end of the story by a long shot. Checking with the Carmelite Sisters in Kenosha, I learned it was Dominicans, not Carmelite order, that inherited the estate. Sister Edward informed me The Dominicans were splitting up and could not keep the property. It was sold to the Franciscans who in turn sold it to the Greek Orthodox St. John Chrysostomos. Sister Edward stated. "Doctor, you won't believe what they built after tearing down the Dominicans's Mother House and Mrs. Roberts's home. It's a huge mega church, with minarets and all."

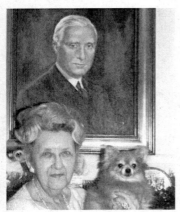

Mrs. Charles Roberts, Charles Roberts (in portrait), Precious

St. John Chrysostomos
Greek Orthodox Monastery

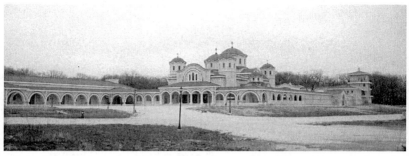

Phase I: 32,926 sq.ft. • Phase II: 31,629 sq.ft. • Phase III: 66,254 sq.ft.
Completion Date: 2003 • Roula Associates Architects, Chtd.

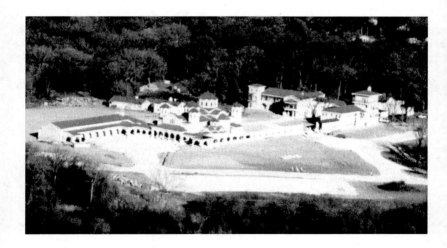

Vet Aid

Carol and I were lucky—or just plain unlucky, depending upon your point of view. With six kids, three boys and three girls, born in ten years, from 1952 to 1962, we enjoyed (endured) most of the '70s with three or four teenagers in the house. As many of you recall, those were difficult times for adults, teenagers, and the country as a whole.

I have been very thankful to have a profession where I could gainfully employ (teach and motivate) my children outside the home. I'll wager that few children reached adulthood without spending time doing household chores. In addition, our youngsters got to clean kennels, do yard work, and answer the office phones. Hard work and motivation is one thing; it's quite another to teach about poverty, welfare, and unemployment.

The dinner table was crowded, as usual. Supper was the meal where the entire family was together for food and discussion. My wife, Carol, related a story in the Kenosha News about families on welfare receiving food stamps and surplus foods to fill out their monthly budget. "I never heard of bulgur," she commented. "I'm sure we could never get by on food stamps and surplus stuff."

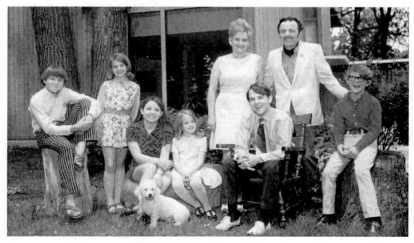

David, Ginger, Dorothy, Peggy, Carol, Bill, John, Buzz • 1969

After a spirited discussion, the family voted to try a "welfare diet" for one month. The vote was seven in favor, one against (Ginger, 11 at the time). She was sure we would all starve. Ginger related to me years later she and Peggy, then nine, hid cans of food in their bedroom, just in case.

The director of Kenosha County welfare office, Paul Hickey, was a client. An initial phone conversation elicited his enthusiastic support for our one-month trial on a "welfare diet." The Kenosha News reporter was also excited to have a follow-up to her original story.

The meeting with Mr. Hickey got us the necessary paperwork to pick up one month of free supplies: one large bag of bulgur, five pounds of peanut butter, flour, rice, a large box of dried milk, spaghetti, etc. We provided our own "food stamp" money—$198.00, as I recall, for a family of eight.

Despite some grumbling, we made it through the month with $1.05 to spare, mainly because of Carol's abilities as a cook. I was congratulating everyone when Ginger asked, "What about Fritz," (our 105 pound Lab/Shep mix) "and the two cats? Did you count their food that you bring home from the animal hospital?" Then it hit me: If I had to choose between feeding my family and my pets, who gets left out? It's easy to say, "You would chose your family, of course." But many pets *are* family. What do people do who are laid off or unemployed? How do they manage when their pet is sick or injured and needs veterinary care? I'm sure most vets, including me, do a lot of charity or *pro bono* work. In the past I've wondered why "these people" couldn't pay something for their pet's care. Now I know.

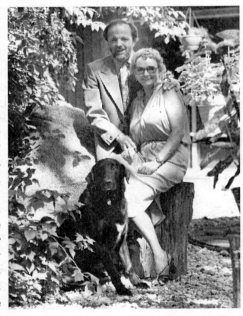

John, Carol, and Fritz • 1978

The story in the paper of our family adventure drew mixed reviews, ranging from sympathy and understanding to disgust and condemnation. Nevertheless, it did serve as an agenda item for discussion with the three other animal hospital owners in Kenosha. I had proposed starting a program, "Vet Aid," to raise funds to care for sick and injured pets of Kenosha County welfare recipients. The clients would be asked to contribute 50% of the routine costs and the program would try to cover the rest. If the client couldn't or wouldn't pay, Vet Aid would bear the entire burden. I was happily surprised when two of the three hospital owners agreed to try the program for one year.

Various individuals and civic groups contributed approximately $1,000 during the first year. I had vastly underestimated the demand once the program was announced to the welfare recipients. To qualify, one needed a card verifying he/she was receiving assistance from Kenosha County. We were soon spending about twice our income, even though half of the clients paid something toward their bills. A story in the AVMA journal in the summer of 1973 brought a positive response from the profession, especially from student chapters of the AVMA. I was invited to speak at the student VMAs at the University of Minnesota, Purdue University, and Tuskegee University.

Lady Luck, Good Fortune, God's Grace—whatever you call it—smiled on us one bright summer day. Mrs. Charles Roberts, one of my few "very rich clients" called with the distressing news that her favorite dog (of over a dozen) was very sick. Her chauffeur brought Mrs. Roberts and "Irish," a 10-year-old Kerry Blue Terrier, to the animal hospital. I diagnosed acute pancreatitis and gave Mrs. Roberts a very grave prognosis. Similar to many people with money, she practically ordered me to cure her baby, knowing full well that some conditions are almost untreatable. Finally, she blurted out, "Dr. Merrick, if Irish lives through this ordeal, I'll give you $1,000 a month for your Vet Aid program as long as I live." Take your pick—Lady Luck, Good Fortune, God's Grace—Irish pulled through, after many a sleepless night, to regain most of his normal functions and survive for another three years. Mrs. Roberts not only sent us $1,000 a month as promised, but a check for $10,000 upon her death three years later. I closed the program at that time for lack of another benefactor.

In researching this story, I contacted my son, Dr. William Merrick, in Madison, Wisconsin. He sent me the following message:
Funny how things link together...
Mrs. Roberts was the only reason I ever started college, and that resulted from this very same experience.

That dog must've been blessed with some very good karma for so many people.

The year was 1971. The summer was hot, and as Dad pointed out, we kids were always able to not only find guaranteed employment outside the home (well, the phrase "outside the home" has to be taken with a bit of poetic license), we were fortunate to be able to know very well what our dad did at his job (how many of our friends could say the same, even if they could say what their dad's job title was and maybe even know where he worked, most had no real clue what that work actually entailed on a day-to-day basis, unlike what we knew!)

That (standard-sized) Kerry Blue Terrier, one of two she had, did have this terrible disease that Dad diagnosed. Part of the treatment plan was to have someone stay with the animal all day and all night, and administer regular IV feedings and watering, take and test many samples, and tend to it intensely as we nursed it back to health. I'll never forget Mrs. Robert's offering, "If dad was to find someone to sit up with her doggie all through the night, and help nurse it back to health, she'd pay the princely sum of $100 per night."

"Interested?" Dad asked me that afternoon. "Are you kidding!?! $100 a night!?! Count me in."

So for three nights, I did just that. I fed the dog little bits at a time. I gave it water as needed. I took samples as Dad directed, and I tried to retain my sanity from being up through the wee hours of the morning. As I recall, our regular kennel man, Melvin, was working days at that time, and he had the daytime shift responsibilities. The dog was in the cage in the "treatment room" (the one just past the swinging door, where we had the dogs recovering from surgeries and had the elevated tub for shampooing the dogs after grooming).

Yes, doggie did recover. Very nicely, too.

Melvin and I drove the dog home to Mrs. Roberts's estate (on Cooper Road, if memory serves me correctly). We dropped him off after Mrs. Roberts's butler initially greeted us at the door. Boy, was Irish glad to be home. And Mrs. Roberts, the most stately, elegant woman I could have ever imagined, was oh, so glad to see her honey. As she and the dogs bounded about together so happy to be reunited after this ordeal, she handed me an envelope, saying, "Thank you for your hard work. I know you've earned this, and I'm so glad to have him back all healthy."

I daren't open the envelope until after we'd left the drive. But inside, as I shortly thereafter discovered, were three new, crisp $100 bills.

I was overcome with bliss! "Ahh! Wealth, power, prestige! All mine, all mine, all mine!" I muttered to myself, under my breath. I could do so much with that money—much more than any I'd seen before in my entire life. What could I do? What should I do with it? I could get that new sound system I've been coveting. Or I could put a down payment on a good car. Okay—on a car. Or, maybe I should be responsible. Hmmm. Now that's a thought. What does college cost?

Dad and Mom had already made it clear that with six kids, they would do what they could, but I would have to help if I was to go beyond high school. When they asked me what I was planning on doing after I graduated (just a month or two before, in May or June, 1971), I said I didn't really know, but thought that maybe I'd go to college. They said something like, "Well, that's good. But how are you going to pay for it?" I must admit... I never really thought about that part before.

I called UW–Parkside the next day. Classes cost $30 per credit, I was told. "Hmm, lessee... That means that I could take three classes, and have money left over to boot (I forgot about costs for fees and books, of course). Well, best to 'invest' this in me. I'll never be able to save that much again—not anytime, soon, anyway."

The next day, I enrolled in Philosophy 101, Psychology 101, and an advanced philosophy course, Eastern Philosophy. I figured I'd try to load the dice and take my best chances at courses I was pretty sure I could do well in.

I was right. I was lucky. In more ways than one.

I will forever be in Mrs. Roberts's debt for this act of kindness.

— William A. Merrick, PhD

I know all the individuals and animals are grateful to our benefactors: Mrs. Roberts; James Watts, DVM; James Nordstrom, DVM; and Jan Wolf, DVM.

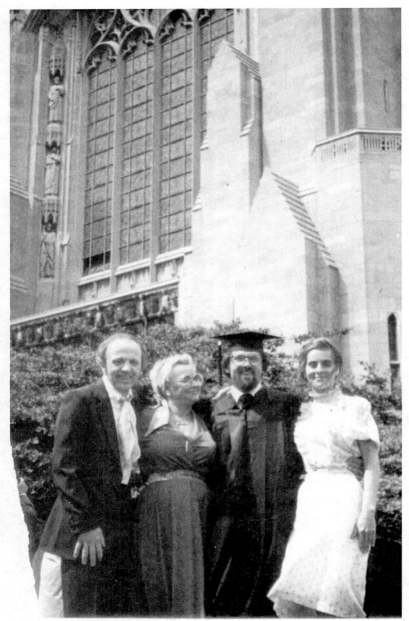

John, Carol, Bill, and Marianne • Bill's PhD graduation
Rockefeller Chapel, University of Chicago • 1989

Minneapolis to Tuskegee

Following the publication of the Kenosha Vet Aid program article in the *Journal of the AVMA,* I was invited to speak to the student AVMA national convention, which was held in the summer of 1975 at the University of Minnesota Veterinary School. Jack Antyles, DVM, from New York City gave a wonderful presentation on the psychological aspects of vet med. I followed with a slide show depicting the Vet Aid program and its benefits to the community. The talk was well received. Dr. Antyles invited me to speak to the New York City Veterinary Medicine Association (VMA). I also received invitations to speak to the student VMA at Purdue and Tuskegee Universities.

This was my first visit to New York City. Dr. Antyles asked if there was any particular hotel I liked. I told him I'd rather stay with him, if he had room, so we could visit and see his animal hospital. He agreed. After a hearty breakfast, we toured Dr. Antyles's hospital. It was nothing like I had imagined—just an average clinic on a neighborhood business street. I had visions of an ultramodern place. Dr. Antyles had two associates helping him manage a very busy practice. As you could imagine, the cost of building a modern 5,000 square-foot hospital with parking for 20 cars would run in the millions of dollars in New York City. The lunch, however, was something special. A few blocks from Dr. Antyles's clinic was Antonio's, a modest neighborhood restaurant. Dr. Antyles introduced me to the owner, Tony Mizzerelli, as a very good client. The lunch was marvelous—soup, small salad, and entree—served by Tony himself. Jack had two glasses of wine; I didn't drink. Tony presented the bill—$65.00—and I about fell out of my chair. In Kenosha, the bill for lunch would not have exceeded $25.00 at the best place in town. I learned in a hurry the perils of big city living.

My presentation to the New York Veterinary Medical Association was politely received. Many, however, were skeptical as to how it would work in NYC. Purdue and Tuskegee would be visited later in the year. Both presentations were given in more humble settings, but to very enthusiastic audiences.

My presentation to the vet students at Purdue was a repeat of the Vet Aid program in Kenosha presentation I had given to the national student AVMA. Students asked probing questions and wondered how they could establish similar programs when they started in practice.

Carol and I then flew from Indianapolis, Indiana, to Montgomery, Alabama. Dr. J. A. Clinkscales met the plane and drove us 40-some miles to Tuskegee. He must have just finished clinics, as he was wearing his white lab coat and name tag. On second thought, it may been his way of showing airport personnel he was a professional—not just a chauffeur. This was 1975 Birmingham, Alabama—still not accepting of Negros as professionals.

Bad news: Carol's luggage didn't make the flight. Fortunately, Carol was carrying her small case with makeup and a few essentials. "Never fear," I told Carol on the ride to Tuskegee, "we'll find a nice dress shop in Tuskegee and get you all fixed up." "I'm afraid you won't find any dress shops in Tuskegee, at least not any Mrs. Merrick would want to patronize," Dr. Clinkscales said. "We'd have to go back to Montgomery." Off the expressway and onto country roads, we passed through a very desolate countryside. Carol remarked, "It looks like those chicken coops and hog houses are about to fall down." "Those aren't chicken coops, Mrs. Merrick. People live there," Dr. Clinkscales said.

Members of the student VMA met with us for supper at the Howard Johnson motel. Upon hearing of Carol's lost luggage, two of the girls offered Carol clothes. Carol mentioned that if anyone had a sari, she was used to wearing one when she teaches yoga at the University of Wisconsin. One also doesn't have to worry about the size, since most are adjustable to any size. With that knowledge, many of the students asked Carol to give a yoga class that afternoon while I was lecturing. She readily agreed. One woman mentioned her student/husband was also very interested in yoga, and asked if Carol would give another lecture after the meeting was over. Word spread like wildfire. This was the mid '70s and yoga was very popular on college campuses. Her first class had ten or twelve attendees—the second, nearly fifty. Carol looked right at home in her borrowed sari.

I was a member of a four-vet panel discussing pet-oriented psychotherapy. They covered the use of companion animals in a specific psychiatric population, in a VA therapeutic setting, working with disturbed children, and preparing vet students to participate in the programs outlined. I talked about the role of the

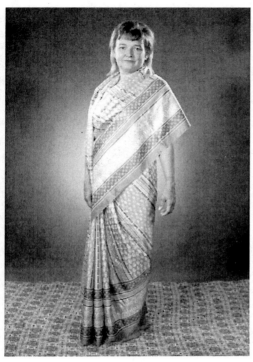
Carol Merrick • 1975

practicing veterinarian in a pet psychotherapy program. I counseled the students that while wild animals don't survive if they show any illness—real or psychological—pets and their owners do. Clinicians need to be aware they may be asked to diagnose imaginary illnesses in animals brought in for treatment. Many pets serve as therapy for lonely or depressed individuals. All vets have heard clients remark, "My pet is more of a comfort to me than my kids." Recommending the appropriate pet is one of the best things we can do for clients. We can explain and show how to avoid selecting an aggressive pup or an introverted one.

The trip was an all-around pleasant experience. Carol received more letters of thanks than I. I told her it was because she looked so great in the borrowed sari. United Airlines called to say they had Carol's luggage in Birmingham and asked if she wanted it delivered. Since we were about to leave for the airport, she thanked them and explained that she would pick it up in an hour. She also requested they keep it in sight until we get there.

Super Family—Pfarr Excellence

Jerry called himself the "clean" Pfarr brother. As sports editor of the *Kenosha News,* he was the youngest and the only one of the five Pfarr boys not to follow in his father's footsteps—that of service station owner and mechanic. I reminded him there wasn't much difference between automobile grease and newsprint. He didn't buy my argument.

We had met on the golf course. Jerry introduced me to his family soon after. His dad, Jerry Sr., started the business in 1932 and, together with the four older brothers, ran the Sinclair service station on the north side of town.

Each of the living Pfarrs has a unique story. Bob, the eldest, was a cyclist. He rode with the Olympic team in Rome in 1960 and won four national championships. He won a gold at the Pam-Am Games in 1959 and represented the USA on many goodwill

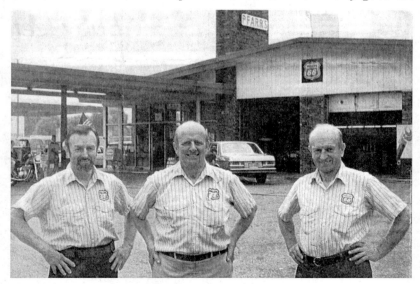

Earl, Ralph, and Bob Pfarr • 1985

tours around the globe. Until his passing in 2006, Bob rode almost every day.

Before and after retiring from the automotive business, Ralph was part-time professional magician. His hobby and passion has kept Ralph occupied for 50 years. He still entertains at veterans' and children's hospitals. Ralph founded the Automotive Technicians of Southeast Wisconsin—a very good learning experience for the multitude of new systems on today's cars.

An experience of being attacked by a drunk on a family camping trip lead Earl to his avocation. He and his five sons studied karate under Rev. William Foster at the local youth foundation. Earl earned his black belt in 1970 and began teaching a credit karate class at the University of Wisconsin–Parkside, in Kenosha. He retired from teaching in 2006, but he continues to work out three or four times a week. Earl's son, Reid, has taken the torch just as Earl and his brothers took the flame from their father. Buddhists believe our spirit affects everyone we encounter. Never was this more true than in the Pfarr family.

George, the youngest brother in the auto business, died from a brain tumor at the age of 51. He was the comedian, although all the boys had a good sense of humor. You would have to be of good cheer to work for 30 years with your brothers. George was a good friend, wonderful father and husband, and better-than-average table tennis player—especially against yours truly.

Wikipedia reports:

> All stations in New Jersey and Oregon offer only full service and mini service; attendants are required to pump gas because customers are barred by statutes in both states from pumping their own gas. New Jersey banned self-service gasoline in 1949 after lobbying by service station owners. Proponents of the ban cite safety and jobs as reasons to keep the ban. Likewise, the 1951 Oregon statute banning self-service gasoline lists seventeen different justifications, including the flammability of gas, the risk of crime from customers leaving their car, the toxic fumes emitted by gasoline, and the jobs created by requiring mini service. In addition, the ban on self-service gasoline is seen as part of Oregonian culture.

It seems most service stations are mini-marts or add-ons to Kroger's. Hoping for a return to "The Good Old Days" is as likely as the return of buggy whips. Those of us who were fortunate to have lived through this remarkable era remember the maxim:

"When you find a good, honest auto mechanic, treasure him—they are a rare species." I received the above photo and following letter from Earl Pfarr:

HISTORY OF PFARR'S SUPER SERVICE

By Earl Pfarr (4th son)

My father, Gerald (Jerry) Pfarr started Pfarr's Super Service on 50th st. and Sheridan Rd. in 1932. He worked there with his sons until the day he went to heaven, at 81 years.

His three sons Bob, Ralph, & George worked full time with their father. I worked part time with them from the time I was in high school.

My five sons, Reid, Randy, Brian, Steve, and David worked for us part time while they attended high school.

When my father retired in 1958 my brothers offered me a full partnership to come into the business. I was still working with them part time, but I had a full time job at Fansteel Metallugical Corp. in North Chicago as a Mechanical Draftsman. After their constant urging me to take their partnership, and becoming tired of driving to North Chicago five days a week, I weakend & accepted their offer.

We had a four bay building for our repair service. My brother Bob did the brake work and bookkeeping. Ralph did the tune ups, electrical work and carburetion. George did the exhaust work and lubrication. George passed away at the age of 51 and I inherited his jobs along with my tire repairs and tire sales.

Our business was a full sevice station at the gas pumps, including the checking of oil and fluid levels, tire pressure, and cleaning windows. Our part time help mainly took care of the gas pumps service.

My brothers Bob & Ralph retired in 1987 and then we decided to sell the business. We had no trouble selling it and the new owner hired me for I wasn't yet ready to retire.

After three years the new owner sold the station to a Quick Stop business. I then retired from full time work at that location.

Irish Wolfhounds, Gentle Giants

They arrived at my animal hospital in the back of a large station wagon. Stretched out in the space usually reserved for six people was an expectant Irish Wolfhound, Queen, and her proud consort, Duke. The stout, middle-aged "grandparents" introduced themselves as Mr. and Mrs. Alfred Churchill. "No relation to Winston," but implying they were equally important. She exuded upper class haughtiness, as if to say, "Aren't you fortunate to have been chosen to care for our precious children." They had traveled 30 miles from the resort town of Lake Geneva to Kenosha because of a friend's recommendation for a prenatal exam of their prize bitch. Allow your mind's eye to picture Horace Rumpole and his wife, Hilda, the English characters in the drama, *Rumpole of the Bailey,* about an eccentric British lawyer. This will give one a good picture of the couple, except the roles were completely reversed. Mrs. Churchill was the dominant partner; Alfred was Mr. Milquetoast indeed.

Prenatal exams were infrequent in 1970, usually limited to a few breeders of prized bitches or expectant mothers who had experienced a difficult previous whelping. Queen was a first-time mom; Duke was an experienced producer. Everything was normal until I palpated a dozen or more golf ball–size embryos in Queen's elongated bicornate (two-horned) uterus. It was difficult to determine exactly how many lumps were presented, so I made an educated guess of 14. Better to err on the high side. I could always explain the missing ones were absorbed during the gestation.

Bred as hunting dogs by the ancients, who called them *Cú Faoil,* the Irish continued to breed them for this purpose, as well as to guard their homes and protect their stock.

During the English conquest of Ireland, only the nobility were allowed to own Irish wolfhounds, the numbers permitted depending on position. They were much coveted and were frequently given as gifts to important personages and foreign nobles. Wolfhounds were the companions of the regal, and were housed themselves alongside them. King John of England, in

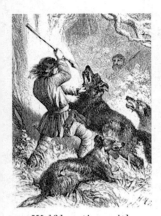
Wolf hunting with wolfhounds.

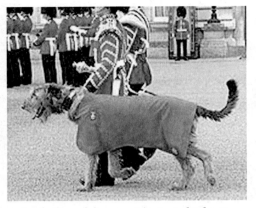
Irish Guards' mascot in parade dress.

about 1210 presented an Irish hound, Gelert, to Llewellyn, a prince of Wales. The poet, the Hon. William Robert Spencer, immortalized this hound in a poem.

As the Churchills were boosting the clumsy canines into their wagon, Mrs. Churchill let it be known that she expected me to deliver the offspring when the time came. Expense was no object. She insisted I be present for the delivery. I assured her that giant breeds like Saint Bernards and Wolfhounds had very little birthing problems. Dystocia (difficult delivery) was relatively rare in giant dogs, due to the large number of embryos and therefore proportionally smaller pups. She would not be dissuaded. We decided on an appropriate fee and an approximate delivery date, five weeks in the future.

I thought back a few years to the birthing appointment for the delivery of our third child, David. Carol's obstetrician, John Burke, MD, happened to be the older brother of Dad's associate, Walt Burke, DVM. Dr. Burke scheduled deliveries on Tuesday or Thursday—take your pick. (See the full story on pp. 241–245.)

Over a month went by and the due date came and went, as did the next three. Mrs. Churchill was nervous but understanding, especially for a middle-aged woman who had never experienced childbirth herself. Wednesday was my normal afternoon off; Carol and I usually played 18 holes of golf. We could make a quick visit to examine Queen and have plenty of time to play one of the many courses surrounding Lake Geneva. We arrived at the Churchill's castle shortly after noon on a bright, sunny day. The house, which today one would describe as a mini-mansion, stood on 20 acres of prime land on the south side of beautiful Lake Geneva. A massive, open, iron gate revealed the tree-lined, curved, 100-yard drive to the house. Beyond the house, at lakeside, a large pier featured a mailbox where the daily mail boat delivered the U.S. Mail. Two doors east, about one quarter of a mile away, was the Wrigley estate, owned by the family of the chewing gum magnet and then-owner of the Chicago Cubs. Immediately south of the property was the estate of William Grunow, previously mentioned in the "mob" story. William Grunow's son turned the Lake Geneva vacation property into a ski resort with the unlikely name of "Majestic Hills." Bulldozers had turned a sloping hill into a mini-mountain. Rope tows carried people to the top. My family learned to ski at Majestic Hills and nearby Wilmot "mountain."

I couldn't believe my luck. Queen had started labor one hour earlier. Mrs. Churchill had been calling but unable to reach me, as this was decades before cell phones.

Grandmother Churchill proved to be a very competent practical nurse. The birthing area was prepared according to my instructions—a "Queen-sized" bed, underpinned with a copious supply of newspaper, in a room off the library. Untouched water and food were nearby. Vaginal palpation determined that Queen would need no oxytocin to induce labor. A head-first pup was already in the birth canal. Over the next four hours Queen delivered 14 live, wiggling, beautiful bundles of joy. I couldn't believe my good fortune. My guess of 14 had proven correct.

Queen proved to be an excellent mother. Duke tried to help out, but Queen shooed him away with a low growl. Despite extra nursing, the runt died the next day when Queen pushed it aside and refused to care for it. I explained to the grieving family that many of these abandoned pups have heart or other organ problems and have a very small chance of reaching adulthood. That may or may not have true, but it was my best guess at time.

The house was divided into four levels. The dogs occupied what was the guest's or maid's quarters—two rooms and a private bath. The problem of selling the 13 pups is another story. As you can imagine, Mrs. Churchill had trouble finding prospective buyers who were good enough for her "grandchildren." I heard via the grapevine that she parted with the last one, at 4 months old, only after Mr. Churchill threatened to move to a hotel and not return until all the pups were gone. She had already convinced him to keep their "favorite" pup to add to their family.

Finished and exhausted by 6 PM, we were too late for golf, but ready for a martini followed by a fish dinner—the perfect ending to a remarkable day.

All's well that ends well.

Majestic Hills and Checker Limos

How are you gonna keep 'em down on the farm after they've seen Paree? Midwest skiers modified that catchy World War I song to say, "How are you gonna keep them on these bumps on a pickle after they've skied Colorado?" This was the common lament when Midwest skiers visited real mountains for the first time.

Majestic Hills and Wilmot Mountain were the ski areas of choice for Chicago and Milwaukee skiers in the '50s, '60s, and '70s. One of my first clients after moving to Kenosha was Dr. Bob and Kay Sternloff with their Springer Spaniel, Lady. Bob was the director of recreation for the city of Kenosha, an unusual position for a city of 50,000. Our family started skiing with the Sternloffs and Bob's sister, Lois, from nearby Lake Forest, Illinois. Lois's husband, Norm Abplanalp, was to become a close friend and our architect in the future. Norm's stories are featured in a later chapter in the book.

William Grunow, Sr. was a partner in the Grigsby-Grunow Company, manufacturer of "Majestic" brand radios—the first model to combine receiver and speakers into one unit. Although the company went bankrupt during the Great Depression, it was re-formed into the Majestic Radio & Television Corporation and General Household Utilities, producing radios, phonographs, and refrigerators. Majestic was one of the first radios which used alternating current rather than messy, expensive batteries. Both he and his partner, B. J. Grigsby, became wealthy within two years. Grunow built a palatial home at 915 Franklin in River Forest, Ill., in the 1920s. It later became the home of reputed mob figure Tony Accardo (previously mentioned in this book).

When the Grigsby-Grunow Company failed, William Grunow was able to keep control of a home in Phoenix, Arizona, as well as his Wisconsin home, Majestic Lodge, on a 60-acre property near the Wrigley estate on the south shore of Lake Geneva, Wisconsin. Grunow constructed an 18-hole, nine-green private golf course and had a huge horse stable purchased from a Kentucky farm and shipped to Wisconsin.

Dr. "Pinky" Jordan, Purdue University Ag Specialist in chicken-raising methods, captivated Grunow. Grunow sold the Phoenix, Arizona, estate to finance a poultry-raising venture, Val-Lo-Will Farms, Inc., of Lake Geneva, Wisconsin. In short order, the horse barn was occupied with batteries of rolling cages. Other chicken coops were established over most of the golf course. By 1940 the Val-Lo-Wil chicken farm—named that after his children, Valerie, Lois, and William—with its half-million birds, became the world's largest commercial chicken farm. As with his earlier ventures, Grunow sought to combine value with economy. He brought scientists and engineers together to design a cutting-edge facility for the raising and processing of chickens. He also decided to market chicken parts individually, to meet consumer preferences. In its heyday, Val-Lo-Wil sent out 40,000 broilers each week and operated 28 stores that sold fresh and rotisserie chicken products and chicken pot pies. The chicken enterprise came to an end when Bill Grunow, Sr. died in 1951.

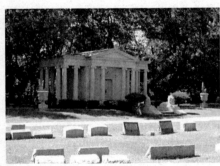

Grunow, William C.
Born April 30, 1893, Chicago, Illinois.
Died July 6, 1951, Chicago, Illinois.
Buried in Forest Home Cemetary.

Grunow's classical mausoleum of white granite is the second largest at Forest Home Cemetary. It is perched above the east bank of the Des Plaines River; only a few feet behind it the ground drops away sharply. The Grunow mausoleum features columned porticos on either side. Within each is a statue; one represents commerce, the other communication, the two areas which dominated Grunow's life.

Bill Grunow, Jr., after graduating from the University of Wisconsin, searched for a way to parlay his passion for skiing into a business. He and his future wife, Melita, scoured the area between Chicago and Milwaukee for the best place to open a ski hill. Following in his father's footsteps, Bill decided to build one in his own back yard. The following article appeared in the *Chicago Tribune* in the fall of 1957. This was exactly one year after I had started practice in Kenosha, 30 miles to the east.

If you could put on your own ski boots, you were able to accompany our family to the hills. Buzz was able to con his baby sister,

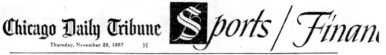

$500,000 Ski, Skate Center a Glide Away

Chicken Farmer Raises Hill and 'Grows' Snow

BY ROBERT CROMIE
(Chicago Tribune Press Service)

Lake Geneva, Wis., Nov. 27 — One of the most scenic areas in the midwest hopes to begin catering to the blade and slalom set Friday, Dec. 6, when Majestic Hills, a new half - million dollar winter sports center, opens at Val-Lo-Will farm, South Shore rd., on Lake Geneva, 6 miles west of town. An open-house will be held next Sunday to provide a preview of the new area.

William Grunow, 26 year old vice president of Val-Lo-Will, the world's largest chicken farm, will be director of the 25 acre center, which will offer six toboggan runs, three ski areas—for beginning, intermediate and advanced riders—and three skating rinks.

Three Skating Rinks

These will consist of the figure skating rink, 80 by 100 feet; a 300 by 150 foot practice rink, and an Olympic rink, 602 by 229 feet, the use of which will be turned over to the Olympic committee Dec. 22 in a formal ceremony. National speed skating events and Olympic tryouts also will be held there.

The work of building a tremendous hill for skiing enthusiasts, and cutting toboggan runs thru the timbered slopes is completed. Grunow, a former varsity tennis player at the University of Wisconsin, directed the moving of almost 500,000 tons of earth, uncovering a fine natural spring—for which he has no use—and an ancient tree trunk, buried deep in the clay, which geologists, now examining it, believe was deposited by a glacier some 30,000 years ago.

The new center, situated on what once was a private golf course built by the elder Grunow, overlooks Lake Geneva and is within easy view of Yerkes observatory. It is only 84 miles from State and Madison in Chicago's Loop.

Grunow has two reasons for building what should turn into a Mecca for the snowmad. First, of course, he hopes to make a profitable business venture of it. Second, or maybe this really should have been first, he loves to ski, and thinks nothing of traveling 400 miles into Northern Wisconsin to indulge in the sport.

Plans for Future

Majestic Hills, he believes, will be sporty enough to save him the trip, and if enough folks feel as he does, there are plans for the future which include sleigh-rides, hay-rides, and perhaps some sheets of ice for the rapidly growing sport of curling.

Grunow's aim is to make Majestic Hills one of the largest winter sports centers in the nation. And he's confident that despite the location, the project will not lay an egg.

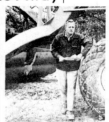

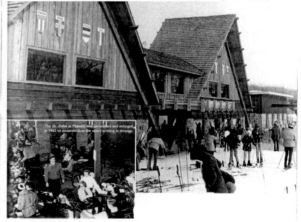

Majestic Hills Chalet • Remodeled 1965
(No longer "fancy chicken coops.")

Ginger, into helping him with his shoes until he started first grade, but ski boots were different. Everyone learned by the age of five.

When Majestic Hills opened, the rope tows were operated by ropes around auto tire rims. It would be many years before chair lifts were installed. The rope moved constantly; one needed to stand next to it and gradually tighten your gloved hands until you started on your journey to the top of the hill. The first time or two, people tended to tighten too quickly and were pulled forward, flat on their face. I taught each child, starting out between my legs and allowing them to get the feel before riding solo. Buzz started in perfect style, but his gloves were wet and stuck to the frozen rope. At the top of the hill Buzzie didn't slip out of his gloves, and he was pulled into the air toward the upper rotating pulley. The emergency cutoff stopped the rope before Buzz was in any real danger; now he just had a eight-foot fall though my arms into a snowdrift.

Carol and friends would often join to carpool to the hills. Julia Finch and two of her kids combined with our six for a day at nearby Wilmot Mountain. Despite parental warnings about skiing the bunny hill (beginners) for the first half hour, Bill proceeded to the expert run in front of the chalet. The second time down the hill his speed caused him to lose control, plow into skiers and stacked skis, and fracture his ankle. Needless to say, that ended the day on the hill for everyone. Ginger and Peggy were still getting ready in the chalet. Dorothy, Dave, and Buzz were already on the hill. Somehow the older three got word of Bill's accident and avoided "capture" for nearly an hour.

I had purchased a Checker Limo, with jump seats in back and a window between the driver and passengers. Just the ticket, Carol and I decided, to allow a little peace and quiet on long family trips. This was before mandatory seat belts, so we could pile all six kids in back. Eight pairs of skis on the roof and we were set for a day on the hills.

One glorious snow day, Carol, Julia Finch, and Kay Sternloff sat in the front seat with six youngsters in back. Unbeknownst to the adults, the three older girls had secretly placed a microphone in the front seat, wired to a speaker in the rear. It took 30 to 40 minutes of hilarious laughter from the back before the moms figured what was going on. Fortunately, this was before the time of easy recording devices. Each in turn tried to recall exactly what they had said, hoping no real damage had been done.

We bought a family pass to Alpine Valley Ski Resort when it opened near Burlington, Wisconsin, in 1968. I paid $200.00 for all eight—Carol, myself, and the six kids—for the whole year. What a bargain! At that time it cost around $50.00 for two adults and six kids for a day on the slopes. Alpine Valley also featured night skiing—too cold for most of us adults, but the kids could care less.

The Checker Limo suffered a "fractured leg" after six years of dedicated service. Driving the Checker to Parkside College, Bill skidded on an icy road and ended up in a ditch. By this time I only had casualty insurance, so the Checker was totaled. I salvaged only the recently purchased battery.

Homer the Hospital Cat

Churches welcome new worshipers with greeters. Wal-Mart has "Senior Greeters." Cities like Paris and Chicago have "Greeter Programs." Animal hospitals have "Hospital Cats." These ambassadors of good will are expected to brighten the customers' day and exude good cheer. Most feline greeters do their job very well and without complaint.

Over the years we've had many cute, cuddly, vivacious, lazy, sometimes aloof cats roaming and ruling our establishment. One spring morning I arrived to find a very noisy box lying by the front door. Inside were two eight-week-old male kittens, loudly proclaiming their need for breakfast. Gina, our vivacious receptionist, remarked, "They sound like Homer and Jethro." The names stuck. Jethro was soon given to a family whose beloved cat had been hit by a car. Homer, a medium-haired orange tabby, was left in charge—a role he happily accepted.

Popularized by Morris from the 9-Lives cat food commercials and the ever-so-comical Garfield, orange tabby cats are not considered a breed but are just a colorization of the tabby cat. If your heart is set on a female orange tabby cat, it might take you some time to find one. Orange males outnumber females by about three to one.

Arriving early in the morning, Gina would let Homer outside for his daily rounds. Visiting three or four neighbors to see who had left food for him or would invite him in for a rub and a treat, Homer would return around 10 AM, in time for a tongue-bath and nap on the front desk counter. By now the morning "rush" had passed and fewer disturbances would be expected. In a dead sleep, Homer appeared to some new clients as a stuffed toy. It was much to their surprise when the "toy" stretched out a paw or "meowed" a greeting.

Homer had a special way with most dogs. Canines were astonished and taken aback at Homer's fearlessness. This usually translated into the patented "bewildered dog" look or a renewed respect for sharp cat claws. Occasionally, a particularly chatty Chihuahua or excitable Shepard would send Homer scurrying off the counter, with an admonition to the offender from Gina. But just as often, the angry growl of an annoyed hound would be greeted with no more than a bored look from Homer, or worse yet, a yawn followed by the dreaded full frontal stretch!

Clients, especially children, would inquire about Homer's whereabouts, health, and activity if he were not in the reception area. So it was a major crisis when Homer disappeared.

Having recently been written up and pictured on the "metro page" of the *Kenosha News,* Homer quickly became a local celebrity when he joined me on a visit to a local school for career day. As a matter of practice, I always took the "hospital cat" along with me when speaking at schools, to encourage involvement and spice up the entertainment value. Homer was the center of attention in any classroom.

Upon word of his disappearance, teams of employees fanned out. We looked in all his favorite hospital hiding places, checked with neighbors, and called the local Humane Society. No Homer. We placed an ad in the paper and called Debbie Metro, the reporter who covered this story (and who just happened to be a client). Still, not hide nor hair of Homer. Three days later, Gina took a call from a lady in Racine, a city ten miles north of Kenosha. "Were we missing a orange cat?" the woman asked. "Yes!!!" came Gina's excited reply. When he was castrated four years prior, I had Homer "chipped," just as a precaution.

Microchips have been available for animal identification for many years. They provide pet owners peace of mind, knowing their animal will be returned if found and taken to any animal shelter. All shelters have scanners which ID the number implanted between the shoulder blades. It also provides proof of ownership for animals such as Black Labradors, who all look alike. Microchips are required for entry into many countries and are good for the life of the pet. Once registered, the information is available worldwide.

Gina and I left immediately for Racine. Homer was lounging on the sofa with another cat, acting like he was one of the family. Sure enough, the chip reader beeped a positive confirmation. The famously vanished feline was found! Thousands of missing pets have been returned to their owners through this modern miracle—some from half way around the world. We'll never know the exact story, but what we surmise is intriguing. One day, Mr. George Carlson, who worked the second shift at the Kenosha Chrysler plant, left to drive home to Racine around 11 PM. On the side of the road between the cities, George spotted a cat ambling along the roadside. Fortunately for all concerned, George stopped, opened his door, and was surprised when Homer jumped right in beside him. George took Homer home to live with his mother and two cats. Homer fit right in with the bunch and would have stayed forever had it not been for Mom's concern for Homer's prior family. Checking the Racine and Kenosha newspapers' lost-and-found ads resulted in Homer's safe return.

Our best guess is that Homer jumped into a client's car while at the hospital. Arriving at their home on the north side of town, Homer somehow got out of the car and headed in the wrong direction trying to find his home base. We'll never know.

The metro editor was impressed enough to send out photographer and write another story about the lost cat—this time aptly entitled, "HOMER'S ODDESSY."

Homer was the spitting image of Morris, the TV cat. Many clients assumed his name was Morris. "Morris the Cat" (voiced by John Erwin) is the advertising mascot for 9-Lives brand cat food, appearing on its packaging and in many of its television commercials. A large orange tabby tom, he is "the world's most finicky cat," and prefers only 9-Lives brand, making this preference clear by means of humorously sardonic voice-over comments when offered other brands. Every can of 9-Lives features Morris's "signature." He also appears as a "spokescat," promoting responsible pet ownership, pet health, and pet adoptions through animal shelters.

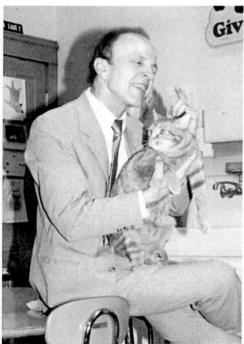

Dr. Merrick and Homer • 1987
Bain School 2nd Grade Class

Homer lived to be 18 years old. He diedpeacefully in his sleep and was buried in our back yard.

Celebrities

Politicians, movie stars, presidents, generals—even traitors and assassins—are celebrities. With the advent of the Internet and YouTube, ordinary people can get their "fifteen minutes of fame." I've met a few celebrities. Actually, it was more of an encounter.

In the 1972 presidential campaign, Jimmy Carter stopped in Kenosha and addressed a few hundred people at the Christian Youth Center (CYC). It was early in the morning, and Carol and I had gone to hear what he had to say. After his usual stump speech, Carter asked for questions from the audience. I asked for his policy on immigration. Carter gave a well-reasoned response that drew applause from the assembled, mostly union members. Standing a few feet behind me, Sam Donaldson, from ABC News, commented to a fellow reporter, "That was a planted softball question."—implying that I was a member of Carter's staff. I had no connection to the future president's staff, but I didn't have the guts to challenge Donaldson's comment. Carter went on to win the election and served as the 39th President of the United States (1977–1981) and was the recipient of the 2002 Nobel Peace Prize.

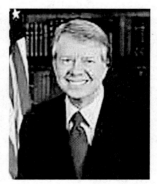
Jimmy Carter • 1978

Returning from a meditation retreat in Barre, Massachusetts, in the late fall of 1968, I changed planes in Washington National Airport (now Reagan National). Entering the men's room, I heard a voice I instantly recognized as belonging to Bob Hope. He was standing at one of the two urinals and talking to another middle aged man. Hope said, "Do you think we'll be able to catch any of the 'skins game?" The second man (Robert Cooke, owner of

Bob Hope • 1964

the Washington Redskins NFL team) said, "There shouldn't be any traffic at this time. My driver will get us there before the second half." Hope, zipping up and turning around toward me, said, "It's all... ahh... no, I can't say that." Flashing that Hope smile, he and his companion left me to finish my task.

Bob Hope, KBE, KCSG, KSS (born Leslie Townes Hope; May 29, 1903–July 27, 2003) was a British-born American comedian and actor who appeared in vaudeville, on Broadway, and in radio, television and movies. He was also noted for his work with the U.S. Armed Forces and entertaining American military personnel in numerous USO shows. Throughout his long career, he was honored for his humanitarian work. In 1996, the U.S. Congress honored Bob Hope by declaring him the "first and only honorary veteran of the U.S. armed forces." Bob Hope appeared in or hosted 199 known USO shows.

In 1961, Jack Kent Cooke purchased a 25% interest in the Washington Redskins after team owner and founder George Preston Marshall became incapacitated by a stroke. He became majority owner in 1974 and sole owner in 1985. While owner of the Redskins, Cooke's team won three Super Bowls—in 1982, 1987, and 1991—under head coach Joe Gibbs. It was the franchise's first championships since the 1940s.

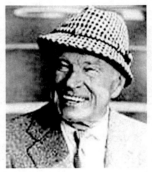

Jack Kent Cooke

The LPGA (Ladies Professional Golf Association) tour event in 1954 was played at Tam O'Shanter Country Club in suburban Chicago, Illinois. Carol and I attended to see the great women players of the day. As luck would have it, two of our favorites, Patty Berg and Babe Didrikson Zaharias, were paired. Missing a three-foot putt for a birdie, Babe turned around, straddled the ball, lifted her long skirt and tapped the ball into the hole backward. Carol commented facetiously, "Nice putt." Babe responded, "I should play backwards more often."

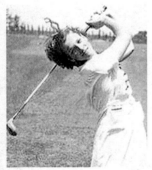

Babe Didrikson Zaharias

Wikipedia reports that Didrikson gained world fame in track and field and All-American status in basketball. She played organized baseball and softball and was an expert diver, roller-skater, and bowler. She won two gold medals and one silver medal for track and field in the 1932 Los Angeles Olympics.

Mildred Ella "Babe" Didrikson Zaharias (June 26, 1911– September 27, 1956) was an American athlete who achieved outstanding success in golf, basketball, and track and field. She was named the 10th Greatest North American Athlete of the 20th Century by ESPN, and the 9th Greatest Athlete of the 20th Century by the Associated Press. Zaharias was diagnosed with colon cancer in 1953, and after undergoing cancer surgery, she made a comeback in 1954. She took the Vare Trophy for lowest scoring average, her only win of that trophy, and her 10th and final major with a U.S. Women's Open championship, one month after the surgery and while wearing a colostomy bag.

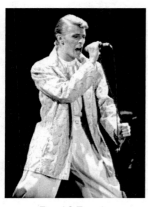

David Bowie

Carol and I met David Bowie after he performed the lead in *The Elephant Man* in Chicago. Carol and I made it a regular habit to see three or four theatre shows yearly. This one was a must see.

The actress Concetta Tomei was to play the female lead in the show when it hit Chicago. Her parents had been clients for many years. This was an opportunity I didn't want to miss. Calling Concetta's dad, I learned *The Elephant Man* was scheduled for a four-week run. He promised to tell Concetta we would be in the audience next week. She said she would be happy to introduce us to David Bowie. Our kids were very jealous.

The show was wonderful. David Bowie was fantastic; Concetta was marvelous. They more than lived up to the excellent reviews given by New York and Chicago critics. David was very gracious when we visited with him and his agent after the show. He commented, "I have never met a 'real' John Merrick before."

We would usually attend a Wednesday matinee, followed by supper at one of Chicago's nicer restaurants. I offered to take Concetta with us, but she declined, as she had another show at 8 PM. Leaving by the theatre's back door into an alley, we encountered 15 to 20 "groupies." They assumed we must be "somebody." We waved and smiled as if it were true.

David Bowie, born David Robert Jones on January 8, 1947, is an English musician, actor, record producer, and arranger. A major figure for five decades in the world of popular music, Bowie is widely regarded as an innovator, particularly for his work in the 1970s, and is known for his distinctive voice and the intellectual depth of his work. Bowie took the title role in the Broadway theatre production *The Elephant Man,* earning high praise for an expressive performance. He played the part 157 times between 1980 and 1981.

Concetta Tomei was born on December 30, 1945, and raised in her hometown of Kenosha, the only child of a policeman. She made her debut on Broadway in 1979, replacing Carole Shelley in *The Elephant Man,* playing the actress/grande dame Mrs. Kendal. She continued in her role when a subsequent tour went out starring David Bowie. She later starred in the ABC television series, *China Beach,* as Major Lila Garreau, U.S. World War II veteran and career-Army commanding officer.

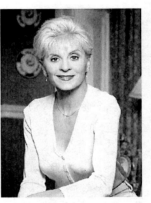

Concetta Tomei

Elephant Man

"John Merrick" said the cashier at the bookstore, "You must be related to the Elephant Man." That happens once or twice a year. I usually explain that I was named after an uncle and our family is Irish, not English as was that John Merrick.

Actually the correct name for the Elephant Man is Joseph Carey Merrick. Early biographies inaccurately give his first name as "John," and this name was used in the 1980 film *The Elephant Man*. Joseph Merrick (1862–1890) was an Englishman with severe deformities who was exhibited as a human curiosity named "The Elephant Man." He became well known in London society after he went to live at the London Hospital. He was so deformed he wore a hood and cape whenever out in public. The protrusion from his mouth had grown to 8–9 inches and severely inhibited his speech and made it difficult to eat. He was operated on at the Leicester Infirmary and had a large part of the mass removed.

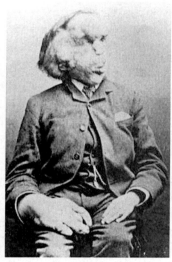

Joseph Merrick (1862–1890)
"The Elephant Man"

Until the stage play, the name was familiar only to historians. In 1979, a Tony Award–winning play, *The Elephant Man,* by American playwright Bernard Pomerance, was staged. The character based on Merrick was played by Philip Anglim, and later by David Bowie. In 1980 David Lynch released *The Elephant Man* film, which received eight Academy award nominations. Merrick was played by John Hurt, and Frederick Treves was played by Anthony Hopkins. The movie starring John Hurt followed the next year. In 1982, U.S. television network ABC broadcast an adaptation of Pomerance's play, starring Anglim.

Ever since Joseph Merrick's days as a novelty exhibit on Whitechapel Road, his condition has been a source of curiosity for medical professionals. One of the doctors present at the meeting was Henry Radcliffe Crocker, a dermatologist who was an authority on skin diseases. After hearing Treves' description of Merrick and viewing the photographs, Crocker proposed that Merrick's condition might be a combination of dermatolysis, pachydermatocele, and an unnamed bone deformity, all caused by changes in the nervous system

In 1909, dermatologist Frederick Parkes Weber wrote an article about von Recklinghausen disease (now known as neurofibromatosis, type I) in the *British Journal of Dermatology*. He gave Merrick as an example of the disease, which German pathologist Friedrich Daniel von Recklinghausen had described in 1882. Symptoms of this genetic disorder include tumors of the nervous tissue and bones, and small warty growths on the skin. Neurofibromatosis, type I, was the accepted diagnosis through most of the 20th century, although other suggestions included Maffucci syndrome and polyostotic fibrous dysplasia (Albright's disease).

In a 1986 article in the *British Medical Journal,* Michael Cohen and J. A. R. Tibbles put forward the theory that Merrick had suffered from Proteus syndrome, a congenital disorder identified by Cohen in 1979.

Unlike neurofibromatosis, Proteus syndrome affects tissue other than nerves, and it is a sporadic disorder rather than a genetically transmitted disease. Cohen and Tibbles said that Merrick showed the following signs of Proteus syndrome: "macrocephaly; hyperostosis of the skull; hypertrophy of long bones; and thickened skin and subcutaneous tissues, particularly of the hands and feet, including plantar hyperplasia, lipomas, and other unspecified subcutaneous masses."

In a letter to *Biologist* in June 2001, British scientist Paul Spiring speculated that Merrick might have suffered from a combination of neurofibromatosis, type I, and Proteus syndrome. A Leicester resident named Pat Selby was discovered to be the granddaughter of Merrick's uncle, George Potterton. A research team took DNA samples from Selby in an unsuccessful attempt to diagnose Merrick's condition. The results of these tests proved inconclusive, however, and therefore the precise cause of Merrick's medical condition remains unknown.

Merrick's death was ruled accidental and the certified cause of death was asphyxia, caused by the weight of his head as he lay down. Treves, who performed an autopsy on the body, said that Merrick had died of a dislocated neck. Knowing that Merrick had always slept sitting upright out of necessity, Treves came to the conclusion that he must have "made the experiment" of attempting to sleep lying down, trying to sleep like other people.

> 'Tis true my form is something odd,
> But blaming me is blaming God;
> Could I create myself anew
> I would not fail in pleasing you.
> If I could reach from pole to pole
> Or grasp the ocean with a span,
> I would be measured by the soul;
> The mind's the standard of the man.

—Poem used by Joseph Merrick to end his letters, adapted from "False Greatness" by Isaac Watts.

Ping Pong to Acupuncture

Wikipedia reports, "The U.S. Table Tennis team was in Japan in 1971 for the 31st World Table Tennis Championship when they received, on 6 April, an invitation to visit China. From the early years of the People's Republic, sports had played an important role in diplomacy, often incorporating the slogan 'Friendship First, Competition Second.' On 12 April, 1971, the team and accompanying journalists became the first American sports delegation to set foot in the Chinese capital since 1949."

Thus began the introduction of acupuncture to the United States. Henry Kissinger soon followed the American athletes, setting up Nixon's visit with Mao in February, 1972. Soon reports of alternative Eastern medicine were all the rage in the Western press, including acupuncture and moxibustion (heat to acupuncture points). The National Library of Medicine currently classifies alternative medicine under the term "complementary therapies." This is defined as therapeutic practices which are not currently considered an integral part of conventional allopathic medical practice. They may lack biomedical explanations, but as they become better researched, some, such as physical therapy, diet, and acupuncture, become widely accepted, whereas others, such as humors or radium therapy, quietly fade away, yet are important historical footnotes. Therapies are termed "complementary" when used in addition to conventional treatments and "alternative" when used instead of conventional treatment.

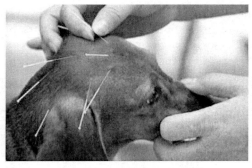

Spurred by the reports of acupuncture's anesthetic effect, I traveled to Aurora, Illinois, weekly during the winter of 1974–75 to learn the secrets of acupuncture from a Korean specialist, Dr. Kim Park. I was especially eager to learn anesthetic techniques after seeing the television reports of acupuncture in China. At that time, anesthesia in dogs and cats over 12 years of age was a risky undertaking. If I could achieve a low-risk alternative way to prevent pain during surgery, I was all for it.

Over the next 16 weeks I learned how and where to apply the small, painless needles. Acupuncture "points" are the same in humans and animals. These are points on 14 meridians which course through the body. There are 172 points on the meridians and 26 outside the meridians. Over centuries of trial and error, practitioners have learned to stimulate certain points to relieve various ailments in animals and people. There is always the suggestion that the beneficial effects from acupuncture treatment is due to the "placebo effect." Indeed, some studies show that to be true. However, there can be no placebo effect with animals undergoing surgery with acupuncture anesthesia, since the patient can't know in advance what is going to be done.

An assistant constantly twirls the needles to prolong the anesthetic effect on the patient. Anesthesia was the most dramatic application of acupuncture in my practice. Older animals were a definite anesthetic risk. This was years before I had access to the methods of cardiac monitoring we have today. I successfully removed golf ball–size mammary tumors from a fourteen-year-old terrier with a chronic heart valve disease using only light sedation and acupuncture.

Over the next few years, I treated many animals with a variety of conditions with acupuncture. Clients were given the choice: acupuncture or routine Western medicine. Most who chose acupuncture did so because regular medicine was not working. Many of the patients I treated were suffering from chronic lameness. Others included skin conditions, intestinal problems, and weight issues. Many animals showed improvement. Whether they would have improved without acupuncture is unknown.

The drawback to acupuncture is the very time-consuming treatment. Most routine office visits last 15 to 30 minutes. Acupuncture therapy usually took twice that time. I eventually decided it wasn't worth it. Newer, fast-acting anesthetics had been developed. EKG machines now monitor heart and lung function.

In the last ten years alternative medicine has become more popular and acceptable in both human and veterinary medicine. Holistic veterinarians now use acupuncture, chiropractic, herbal medicine, homeotherapy, and massage to treat various conditions in both large and small animals.

Research studies on the effects of alternative medicine therapies on animals have not yet been performed. These are proven scientific "double-blind" studies involve treating similar groups of animals—half with the test material or treatment and half with a placebo that's similar in all respects to the real thing. The key part is that the people in charge of administering the treatment have no idea whether they are giving the "real" treatment or the placebo. Some animals will improve when given the fake (placebo) treatment. Mother nature works in strange ways. I told my receptionists, only partly joking, "Make sure you get any sick animal in right away, before they heal themselves. I want us to get the credit." All medical professionals are sent out of school with the words of Hippocrates two thousand years ago, "Above all, do no harm."

Anecdotal information suggests alternative medicine may be helpful in certain conditions. I have doubts about the therapies and await double-blind studies to settle the question.

Admissions—Then & Now

The feminizing of the veterinary profession was in the distant future when I first applied to vet school in the spring of 1948. I sent an application to my dad's alma mater, Ohio State; my home state, Illinois, was still two years away from accepting their first veterinary class to admit non-veterans. I received a nice letter from Ohio commenting on my excellent pre-vet grades, but stating they were only accepting in-state veterans of WWII. I was disappointed because this was the last year of the five-year veterinary degree. After that, one would need six or more years in college to obtain the degree. I proceeded to finish my two years of pre-vet studies at Lyons Township Jr. College. At that time the entire junior college only occupied part of the third floor of the high school.

I submitted my application to the University of Illinois vet school for admission in the second class, but I was again turned down because of the veterans-only policy. The rejection was soon followed by an offer of employment in the vet school as a "lab assistant." Three other non-veterans were also offered jobs and were told we were on a waiting list. What a surprise to everyone except my dad, Andy. Dad had been very involved with the founding and early funding of the vet school at the U. of I. A number of politicians were clients. This included Park Livingston, President of the University of Illinois Board of Trustees.

The admission board had been informed it would be in the interests of the vet school to find a way to admit John Merrick in the class of 1950. It turned out I had the fourth best grade point of the fellows on the waiting list. The vet school somehow found room for all four. To this day I'm not sure that Stan, Al, and Bob know they owe their acceptance to the gentle push of my dad and his friends. The first two classes were limited to 28; the class of 1954 would graduate 32. I learned this from a communication from Park Livingston that I received several years after graduation. The old story is true: "It's not what you know, but who you know."

My year working for the vet school was spent in the autopsy lab—the best experience a young vet student can have. Working under the direction of Dr. Joe Alberts, Dr. Lloyd Bailey, and other fine clinicians, I learned what the inside of dozens of animals of many different species looked like. It was, and still is, the practice of farmers to bring in one or two sick or dying animals from a herd or flock exhibiting illness. They hope that close visual and microscopic inspection would reveal clues to the disease and a cure could be instituted before many more animals are infected.

There were no women in the first five classes at the U. of I. Two were accepted in the graduating class of 1956. Thereafter only a few females got into vet school until Title IX was passed in 1972. Things have really changed over the last 30 years. Title IX originally applied to schools receiving federal funds being required to treat men's and women's sports alike. This led to an equalization of admissions in all areas of the university. The sciences were affected the most. Women's numbers have gradually risen in all professions over the last 30 years.

Today's vet schools routinely get ten applications for each student they admit. In 2011, Illinois accepted 80 in-state applicants out of the 500 who applied. Only 30 out-of-state individuals were accepted from a pool of 400. The incoming freshman class now totals 110. Most vet schools currently admit about 75% women.

Another myth concerns acceptance into medical school if you don't get into vet school. As a general rule, it's equally difficult to get into either school. There is no evidence that many students are able to transfer from vet school to med school. It sounds good and boosts our ego, but sorry to say, it's not true. The only evidence to the contrary is the fact that there are 160 medical schools and only 29 schools to study veterinary medicine.

There are about 90,000 vets in the U.S.; 2,600 graduate each year and 1,000 retire, providing 1,600 to fill the needs—especially in large animal practice, lab animal medicine, public health and biomedical research. Medical schools admit 23% of out-of-state applicants and 77% of in-state applicants, which is about the same as vet schools. Women make up 47% of incoming medical students while males comprise 53%. Vet schools accept a higher percentage of women, but the gaps are narrowing.

Dean Herbert E. Whiteley recently described the admission process for the University of Illinois Veterinary class of 2016:

> The clock starts October 1, and from there, it's about a 10-month journey, every year, to arrive at the final make-up of the next incoming class of veterinary students.
>
> Illinois received 955 applications last fall. After all were reviewed to ensure that they were complete and met the baseline academic criteria, 459 applications moved

forward for review by members of our admissions advisory committee. Three reviewers who had not seen the grades and GRE scores evaluated each application on non-academic merit, and this evaluation determined the 337 applicants who have been invited for a personal interview, which will take place February 13.

The final half of the journey to admission at Illinois plays out over the spring and summer as admitted students elect to join the 120 students in the Class of 2016.

Of course, the admissions cycle is just one leg of the much longer journey toward becoming a veterinarian, a journey that may begin in childhood and last a lifetime. As we look forward to hosting prospective students and interview team members on February 13, I take this opportunity to salute all of you who participate in the making of veterinarians: mentors, teachers, clients, and colleagues.

My experience has been that women make as good or better veterinarians than men. Women have more natural empathy due their historical role as nurtures. The problem is their natural desire to start a family while they're still young. The average woman graduates from vet school around age 26 to 30. Some may take a sabbatical for a few years to begin their family. It's amazing how much knowledge and skill can be lost when away from one's profession for even two or three years. Some women choose to work for a few years until they hear their biological clock ticking ever more loudly. Either way, if they leave the profession for any length of time, they are at a great disadvantage upon returning.

Many years ago I hired a woman associate vet who had taken time off to raise her two boys. When the youngest was two, Dr. X returned to practice. She had been an assistant biology professor at the university prior to attending vet school. After graduation she worked in a multi-doctor small animal hospital for two years to allow her husband to finish his business degree. Dr. X was great with clients—a natural born teacher. Her surgical and diagnostic skills were another matter. An ovariohysterectomy, which would take me 15 to 20 minutes, would take Dr. X the better part of an hour. She was unsure of what new meds were now used to treat various conditions. In the five years she was away, vet med had changed in many ways. She was like a new graduate, needing to start all over to become familiar with her profession. Surgery is like any learned skill; the more you practice, the better the results.

In his excellent book, *Outliers: The Story of Success,* Malcolm Gladwell examines the factors that contribute to high levels of success. Throughout the publication, Gladwell repeatedly mentions the "10,000-Hour Rule," claiming that the key to success in any field is, to a large extent, a matter of practicing a specific task for a total of around 10,000 hours. At 40 hours per week, this equates to five years of work devoted to surgery, golf, music, or whatever. Talking with other professionals, there was general agreement that it took about five years for one to feel comfortable in his work, to know what you "didn't know," and know when to refer to an expert. I saw Gary Player respond to a golf fan who commented on Gary's "lucky" shot from a deep bunker into the hole for a well-deserved birdie. Player responded, "I found that the more I practice, the 'luckier' I get." Another Hall of Fame golfer, Lee Trevino, put it another way: "Don't talk to me about 'luck' until you've hit 200 golf balls every day for six months—then I may listen."

So what's the answer to the "women's dilemma" of how to combine profession and family? I believe we will see an increase in the corporate practices where women can work varied hours and not have to think about owning a practice. Job sharing will increase. Multi-doctor practices will offer "on site day care" as an inducement to both male and female employees. Computer programs will allow veterinarians to hone their skills from home.

Recent graduates have shown a disinclination to purchase a practice and become the business owner. Women reveal a higher percentage, but males also are becoming less willing to assume the burdens and possible rewards of ownership. This does not bode well for veterinarians approaching retirement.

Women in Vet Med—The Title 9 Effect

In 1960, *Seventeen* magazine surveyed teenage women to see what professions best grabbed their attention. They were shocked to find veterinarian in third place, close behind wife and teacher. Animal stories soon became a staple in *Seventeen*.

I wonder how many of the millions of young educated women in today's society know the influence of Title IX ("Title Nine") on their lives and fortunes? Wikipedia states,

> Title IX of the Education Amendments of 1972, now known as the Patsy T. Mink Equal Opportunity in Education Act in honor of its principal author, but more commonly known simply as Title IX, is a United States law enacted on June 23, 1972 that states: "No person in the United States shall, on the basis of sex, be excluded from participation in, be denied the benefits of, or be subjected to discrimination under any education program or activity receiving federal financial assistance." Although the most prominent "public face" of Title IX is its impact on high school and collegiate athletics, the original statute made no reference to athletics.

Essentially, this act opened the door to professional schools all over the country, from architecture to vet med. During the last 36 years, women's participation in the professions has grown exponentially.

Athletics has created the most controversy regarding Title IX, but its gains in education and academics are notable. Before Title IX, many schools refused to admit women or enforced strict limits. Some statistics highlighting the advancements follow:

- In 1994, women received 38% of medical degrees, compared with 9% in 1972.
- In 1994, women earned 43% of law degrees, compared with 7% in 1972.
- Women comprised 13% of graduates with engineering degrees in 1983, rising to 21% by 2002. I would surmise it's closer to 30% today.

The practice of dentistry and veterinary medicine are similar in many ways. Most individuals are self employed, with many owning their own building and equipment. Among male professionally active dentists, more than two-thirds (68%) were 45 or older. Among female professionally active dentists, almost exactly two-thirds (67%) were under the age of 45. Again, I would imagine the stats are similar for the veterinary profession.

Title IX Stats

Year	Doctorate Degrees		
	Male	Female	% Female
1972	28,090	2,688	9%
1982	22,242	10,483	32%
1992	25,557	15,102	37%
2002	23,708	20,452	46%
2008	27,000	28,800	52%

Source: National Center for Educational Statistics

Back in 1948 when the University of Illinois enrolled their first class of veterinary students, only male veterans of WWII were accepted. It was five years later, 1953, before two women were enrolled; 2007 marked the 50th anniversary of their graduation. Illinois vet school enrollment is now 75% female. As the Chinese might say, women now hold up more than one half of the veterinary sky.

It is fairly well known that women today outnumber men in American colleges. In 2003, there were 1.35 females for every male who graduated from a four-year college and 1.3 females for every male undergraduate. That contrasts with 1960, when there were 1.6 males for every female graduating from a U.S. four-year college and 1.55 males for every female undergraduate. What brought about this switch? I believe the introduction of "The Pill" a few years earlier also enabled women to better control their own destiny. Daughters of the first "Pill generation" are taking over many of the professions previously dominated by males. How close did America come to electing a female president in 2008?

So, what is the effect of the feminizing of our profession? Are we failing to produce enough vets to care for the needs of our livestock industry? The trend toward small animal practice has been going on for over 50 years. I can't speak with any authority on this subject. Farming has radically changed over the last 50 years. My guess is women are doing as well or better than their male associates in large animal or equine practice. Has the quality of individuals accepted into vet school slipped? I would venture it's better now than in my day.

Will this generation of women have the entrepreneurial desire to start or purchase a practice? The trend seems to suggest not. Corporate practice would seem to appeal to young female vets. Sharing a full time position is becoming more common. Many practices now incorporate maternal leave in their employee policies.

I can imagine the modern animal hospital of the future replacing, or adding to, the boarding and grooming center with an in-house daycare facility. What a great way to attract and keep both female and male associates and staff. No doubt there are already a number of farsighted practice owners who have incorporated daycare into their facility.

I have seen the future of veterinary medicine, and it's wearing a pantsuit or a dress.

The '70s: Great Books, Protests, Sensitivity, & Dress Codes

"The Good Old Days." "Rubbish," as the British would say. Many people seem to have very selective memory about the not-too-distant past. Actually, some of the past days of our lives were pretty good—or at least we thought so at the time.

The late '60s and early '70s were a time of great turmoil and awakening in America. The war in Vietnam was becoming ever more unpopular. "Women's Lib" (liberation) and women's rights were big issues. Carol and I attended a talk by Gloria Steinem at the University of Wisconsin–Parkside in Kenosha that convinced me once and for all to become involved in the antiwar movement sweeping the country. We even joined a local group picketing the Kenosha post office on April 15th, to dramatize the cost of the war in Vietnam.

As a general background, beginning in 1970, with our six children born between 1952 and 1962, we had three teenagers in the house for the next six years. I complained to Carol, "I wish we'd hear more about our kids' schoolwork instead of this constant nagging about the length of their hair or their short skirts. Dorothy, then 18 years old, was sent home because she wore culottes. They were not part of the dress code, even though they were much more modest than dresses

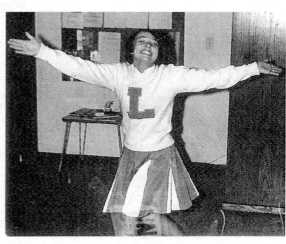

Dorothy at Lance Jr. High • 1965

six inches above the knees. In protest, 17-year-old Bill went to the Goodwill store and paid $1.00 for a man's suit—many sizes to large—and wore it with a dress shirt and tie. He was sent home for... Well, I've forgotten the reason.

Bill and a few of his friends published an underground newspaper. They were suspended for giving it away on the public sidewalk next to the high school, and all of the papers were confiscated.

This was the time of "sensitivity training" classes. Our local Episcopal minister, Peter Stone, sponsored a weekend seminar. He and his wife had just returned from the Esalen Institute in Big Sur, California. I thought it would be a good exercise for my staff to bring us closer together and help us empathize with our clients and patients. We all survived the "falling backwards blindfolded" exercise which, as seen in the popular insurance commercial on TV, is designed to build trust. When our dinner was served without any utensils—expecting us to eat with our fingers—Robbie, a 40-year-old Southern Baptist and my long-time receptionist, got up and left in a huff. I think she was bothered by the event taking place in a church meeting room. I never found out, since Robbie refused to discuss the weekend. I never told her about the "nude" group therapy sessions Rev. and Mrs. Stone attended at Esalen.

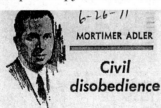

6-26-11

MORTIMER ADLER

Civil disobedience

Dear Dr. Adler:
What do the great writers have to say about civil disobedience?

J. W. Merrick
Kenosha, Wisconsin

Dear Mr. Merrick:

To understand what civil disobedience is, one must first unerstand what law is, and why it binds.

The classical definition of law in the great books is the one stated by Aquinas: "an ordinance of reason made for the common good by one who has care of the community, and promulgated." Thus a law commands obedience and respect on three grounds: (1) by virtue of its end—the common good; (2) by virtue of its source—the duly constituted authority; and (3) by virtue of its content—conformity to the dictates of reason.

If therefore a law does not serve the common good, or conflicts with the dictates of reason, according to Aquinas, the individual may disobey the law provided he prudently judges that the disruption of society caused by his disobedience does not do more harm than would obedience to the law.

These points are clarified and expanded into a doctrine of civil disobedience by John Locke. Locke was mainly concerned with conflicts that arise between what one takes to be Divine law and the civil law, but the principles he lays down apply equally to any conflict between the laws of the state and the moral principles of the individual.

In those few cases in which the positive law commands performance of an act that violates a moral principle, or forbids an act the individual feels morally obliged to perform, one can conscientiously refuse obedience to the law provided one accepts the civil penalties attached to such disobedience. "For the private judgment of any person concerning a law enacted in political matters, for the public good," Locke explains, "does not take away the obligation of that law, nor deserve a dispensation."

If the disobedience is made on grounds other than grounds of conscience, or without a willing submission to the law's penal sanction, then the disobedience is not civil but criminal.

This clear doctrine was confused by Thoreau, who coined the phrase, "civil disobedience," when he rejected the first requirement (namely, that the law disobeyed be one the individual regards as intrinsically unjust), yet still regarded disobedience as civil rather than criminal if one accepted the penalty for infraction. Later, Gandhi tried to justify Thoreau's mistake by "offensive" civil disobedience.

Those who have adopted the later conceptions of Thoreau and Gandhi now condone in the name of civil disobedience a wide variety of unlawful actions, provided these actions serve to dramatize and publicize protest against other laws, institutions, or policies of government deemed to be unjust.

Dr. John Merrick Adler column winner

Dr. John W. Merrick, 6717 French Dr., Kenosha veterinarian, is the winner of this week's Adler column gift.

His winning topic, "Civil Disobedience," which appears on the editorial page of today's Kenosha News, was submitted about a year ago.

He became interested in that topic during a period of civil disorder when his own children questioned the difference between civil disobedience and peaceful protests. Following a family discussion of what the Constitution allows in the way of protests, he decided to request Dr. Adler to devote a column to the views of the great writers on that subject.

Formerly a member of a local Great Books Club, Dr. Merrick enjoys the varying points of view expressed by the great thinkers and encourages his children to express their own ideas even if they don't agree with the current trends.

Particularly important, he believes, is helping each child develop a positive attitude about himself and an idea of his own worth and dignity.

Concern about the problems of welfare recipients and minority groups led him to drop most of his club affiliations three years ago to devote more time to the poor and their problems.

A native of Western Springs, Ill., Dr. Merrick moved to Ke-

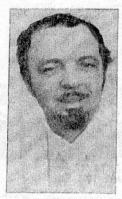

Dr. John W. Merrick

nosha about 15 years ago to take over the veterinary clinic on French Dr. He was graduated from the University of Illinois school of veterinary medicine.

He and his wife, Carol, are the parents of six children, Dorothy, 19; Bill, 18; David, 15; Byron, 13; Virginia, 12, and Peggy, 9. The boys are employed at the clinic during vacations and after school.

Unlike most other winners, Dr. Merrick already had a set of the Britannica Great Books of the Western World which is awarded each winner. Instead, he will receive a set of encyclopedias as his prize.

Carol and I joined a "Great Books" discussion group. Started by Mortimer Adler as an adjunct to the Great Books collection, it was a structured method of picking a subject and reading what the great writers thought about it. Four or five couples would meet for dinner, followed by about an hour of discussion. As with most groups, three or four of the people did 90% of the talking.

During this time Mortimer Adler wrote a weekly newspaper column published in the *Kenosha News*. He invited people to send in questions as to what the Great Books authors had to say about any current subject. In June he answered my question, "What do the great writers have to say about civil disobedience?"

In the newspaper story accompanying Dr. Adler's answer, it was noted that, unlike most other winners, Dr. Merrick already had a set of the Britannica "Great Books of the Western World," which was awarded to each winner and that, instead, he would receive a set of encyclopedias as his prize.

How times have changed in the 40 years between 1971 and 2011. The entire encyclopedia and Great Books series can now be placed on one CD. Despite that fact, many people find the books easier to read than a computer screen. When Carol and I downsized our house and moved to Georgia, we gave our Great Books set to the Park School in Baltimore, Maryland, where our grandchildren, Sheridan and Philip, attend. I asked my son, Buzz, if they are really using the books. He replied, "Yes they are. They are being used to replace the ones on the shelves as they are retired due to age and/or use. The entire set was placed in the librarian's office section in its own place so they could have them all in one spot. They told me it was wonderful, as there were several of the books that had been damaged due to years of student use, so the books you donated would help them keep their stock in good order." Mortimer Adler would be proud.

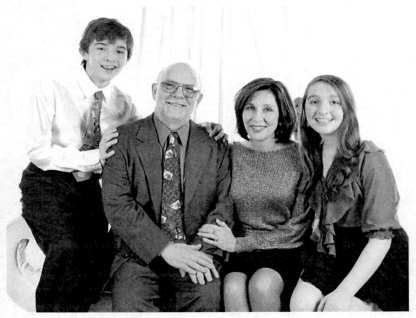

Buzz Merrick with his wife, Karis, and their children, Philip and Sheridan • June, 2012

Ray Robertson, MD

Ray Robertson entered our family life in the "Sensivity Seventies." Carol and I had participated in group sessions involving Catholic family life, leadership training, and sensitivity sessions. We heard through the local Episcopalian minister a talk about Esalen Institute being held at a church in Hinsdale, Illinois. This was only a couple of miles from our family homes, so we made plans to attend.

Wikipedia describes Esalen as follows:

> Esalen Institute, commonly just called Esalen, is a residential community and retreat center in Big Sur, California, which focuses upon humanistic alternative education. Esalen is a nonprofit organization devoted to activities such as meditation, massage, Gestalt, yoga, psychology, ecology, and spirituality. The institute offers more than 500 public workshops a year, in addition to conferences, research initiatives, residential work-study programs, and internships.

Esalen was founded by Michael Murphy and Dick Price in 1962. Their goal was to explore work in the humanities and sciences, in order to fully realize what Aldous Huxley had called the "human potentialities." Esalen soon became known for its blend of Eastern and Western philosophies, examined in experiential and didactic workshops. Over the years Esalen hosted a notable influx of philosophers, physicists, psychologists, artists, and religious thinkers.

Ray had invited the world-renown Dr. Fritz Perls to do a Gestalt demonstration at a local hotel near Hinsdale, Illinois. Carol and I signed up to meet and listen to his therapy.

Wikipedia describes Dr. Perls and Gestalt:

> Friedrich (Frederick) Salomon Perls (July 8, 1893, Berlin–March 14, 1970, Chicago), better known as Fritz Perls, was a noted German-born psychiatrist and psychotherapist of Jewish descent.
>
> Perls coined the term "Gestalt therapy" to identify the form of psychotherapy that he developed with his wife Laura Perls in the 1940s and 1950s. Perls became associ-

ated with the Esalen Institute in 1964, and he lived there until 1969. His approach to psychotherapy is related but not identical to Gestalt psychology, and it is different from Gestalt Theoretical Psychotherapy.

The core of the Gestalt Therapy process is enhanced awareness of sensation, perception, bodily feelings, emotion, and behavior, in the present moment. Relationship is emphasized, along with contact between the self, its environment, and the other.

Perls has been widely cited outside the realm of psychotherapy for a quotation often described as the "Gestalt prayer." This was especially true in the 1960s, when the version of individualism it expresses was prevalent.

"I do my thing and you do your thing.
I am not in this world to live up to your expectations,
And you are not in this world to live up to mine.
You are you, and I am I,
And if by chance we find each other, it's beautiful.
If not, it can't be helped."
(Fritz Perls, "Gestalt Therapy Verbatim," 1969)

After introductions, Fritz asked the group to divide into groups of two. For the next five minutes we should talk to each other in "Baby Talk." No actual words were allowed, but expressions were okay. Then we spent another five minutes telling our partner whom we felt during the exercise. Two other exercises followed which were designed to relax the group. Dr. Perls requested everyone sit in a rough circle; 40 or 50 individuals made up a large circle, with Fritz in the 12 o'clock position. He asked the members if they had any special problems. One of the first was a woman in her 40s who complained in a nasal voice that her friends said she was a complainer, her kids called her a nag and her husband called her a whiner.

Fritz had a two-word answer: "You are." I learned much later that her husband, a principal in a local middle school, was having an affair with one of his teachers, a friend of Carol's from childhood.

In private conversations later, the minister and his wife revealed they had participated in a "Nude Therapy" session when they attended Esalen the previous summer. They said it was similar to going to a nudist resort, with discussion groups in hot tubs. Nothing occurred that was sexually suggestive.

We learned that Dr. Robertson was doing family counseling. Over the next few years Carol, I, and some of our older children

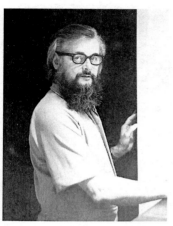

Ray Robertson, MD

sought his help in dealing with various family issues. Dr. Robertson's therapy consisted of listening to the client's stated problems and asking probing questions designed to allow the client to work through their issues and come to a reasonable solution. Dr. Robertson rarely offered advice.

Dr. Boyd Horsley was a friend, tennis partner and our family internist. After one checkup in which I said I was worried about Carol's occasional depression, Dr. Horsley said, "John, I think you should consider going into counseling." I responded, "I've thought about it, but it would take too long for me to get any credentials." "No, John, that's not what I meant," Boyd said. "I think you should *get* counseling." I was surprised and momentarily taken aback. Upon further review, I saw the wisdom in Boyd's advice. I mentioned we had a good friend in Dr. Ray Robertson and I would call him for an appointment.

Carol and I had attended Marathon weekends in the spring of 1971. Marathons begin Friday evening and ran straight through to Sunday noon. The idea was to break down inhibitions and allow individuals to freely express hidden thoughts and emotions. In the fall of 1971, I joined a therapy group meeting every Wednesday evening from 8 to 11 PM. In the first year, the meetings often lasted well after midnight. Ray would allow everyone who wanted to be heard to have their turn.

Dr. Robertson encouraged verbal expression of anger, rage, sadness, or joy. Individuals were given a tennis racquet to swat a pillow, to release inner feelings.

The group of 12 to 14 people consisted in part of a lesbian who thought she was really bisexual, an elderly (60s) Chicago bank executive who had an addiction to wearing women's clothes, his wife of 30 years who rarely spoke, a middle aged (40s) couple—he had sexual issues and she was in love with Ray, the office manager of a medical clinic who tuned in on everyone's problems but hers. The group called her "Mary the Good."

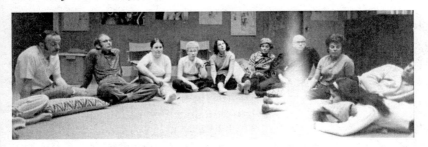

Group therapy • 1971–1973 • I'm seated on the pillow, far left.

Except for the traditional psychiatrists' holiday in August, I meet weekly with the group for the next two years. I admit—the longer I was in therapy, the better Carol became.

Someone in our group brought up the Esalen experience of groups meeting in hot tubs in the nude. It was decided we would meet the next week and disrobe as soon as everyone was present. The session proceeded as usual, sans the tubs. Fewer problems than usual were brought up for discussion. Eventually the session ended with backrubs all around.

I had been out of the group for a year when I happened to be in the general area for a vet meeting which had been postponed. I thought, "Why not visit my old group and say hello to everyone?" I arrived at Ray's office 30 minutes after the usual starting time. Hearing voices in the large meeting room, I entered as usual without knocking. Everyone greeted me warmly, but to my surprise and shock, they were all nude. By now my inhibitions were minimal, so I disrobed and joined the group. It was just like old times.

Both Carol and Bill spent months with Ray as interns. Carol spent the summer of 1975 with Dr. Robertson before getting her Masters in Guidance and Counseling. I asked Bill to relate his experience. His story follows:

> The year was 1969. I first met "Ray" in a family counseling session with Mom, Dad, and Dor, when Dor and I were summoned to Ray's private office. Mom and Dad thought that we might benefit from some of Ray's insights.
>
> Ray was a tall man (6'3" or 6'4", to my recollection), but he had a gentle spirit. His guru-like, salt-and-pepper full beard (all the fashion in those days) was soft on the face when he hugged you. And that was often; hugging was a part of Ray himself. What struck me most about Ray was his easy-going manner and polished sophistica-

tion. He spoke softly, but it was obvious that also carried a big intellectual stick. He had a way of conveying messages with multiple meanings layered over each other. Ray carried himself in self-assured way, too. He was knowledgeable and worldly, yet open to new experiences and learning lessons about and from life.

I was perplexed. "What am I even doing here?" I wondered. But since Mom and Dad said I should come and meet and talk with Ray, I obeyed (as any good Catholic son does when commanded from on high).

In our first session, Dor and I talked about our relationship with Mom and Dad. As I remember it, I felt relatively nonplussed about being there, but it didn't take Dor much prodding before a floodgate of tears opened up. She talked about her hopes and dreams, her expectations (both met and not), and she seemed to have a catharsis from letting Dad know that she missed having him more in her life. For the first time in my life, though, looking back on it now, I became aware of an emotional life that could be described with words and connected to experience. Thanks, Dor. Thanks, Mom. Thanks, Dad.

During this and other sessions, Ray mostly sat quiet, but clearly listened attentively and intently. He waited for just the right moment to interject some idea or question or re-wording—whatever seemed to be called for by the moment. He was as Spartan in his word volume as he was loquacious in his elocution and elegant in his timing—a virtual Ralph Lauren of psychotherapists.

Forward to 1973...

Two years after I graduated from high school, and two years after my own initial steps and missteps trying college at various campuses, I learned that Ray offered a three-month, private "internship" program. I was granted one of the positions as an intern. The position required that we interns (there were three of us at the time) participate in individual, marital, and most often, group counseling sessions during the day. These sessions were held both in his office and at one of the several psychiatric units in local hospitals. On weekends we participated in encounter groups in his office. These started at 6:00 on Friday, and we stayed up through the night and all of the next day, Saturday. On Saturday night we'd have dinner about 7:00, and then we were allowed a night's sleep before we met again on Sunday (all day).

One day, after seeing a couple of patients in the hospital, Ray asked me to escort the patients back onto the unit where they stayed. I did as I was asked, and then, finished with my assigned duty, asked a nurse to let me out so I could go join Ray again. "Oh, c'mon, now," she said. "You know I can't do that!" "Why not?" I queried. She told me that this was a locked unit, and patients were not free to come and go as they pleased. "But I'm Dr. Robertson's intern," I explained. Undeterred, she summoned two husky psychiatric aids and asked them to "show the new patient back to his room." I remember feeling slightly panicked as they sauntered toward me, determined that if I got rowdy with them, they could get just as rowdy back. I'm sure my face expressed the increasing panic I was feeling. Eventually, somehow, I managed to convince someone that I was indeed, an intern, and not just "the new patient." Boy! Did seeing that door close behind me when I left feel good!

Forward to 1981 and beyond...

Matriculating at the University of Chicago, I remembered Ray's soft-spoken manner and intellectual prowess. I tried to emulate him in my interactions with fellow students (although I have to admit, I had to be a bit more vocal with other students), so Ray's characterological effect on me was undeniable. That effect carried through after I graduated with my doctorate, and into my practice as a clinical psychologist. In my work with child, adolescent, and adult patients, I tried to ask more questions than provide advice. I saw my primary objective in counseling people was, first and foremost, to simply understand them as people, to understand their lives from their personal perspective. People's lives make sense, and the decisions people make are rational. I came to understand that when people make irrational decisions—decisions that have a negative effect on them or their loved ones—they do so for some emotional reason. My time with Ray was crucial for my understanding that people's emotional lives are separate from but related to the decisions they make. Thanks, Ray.

Drugs—Legal and Illegal

A visit from the police, like one from the IRS, is usually unpleasant. Such was not the case when Lt. Tom Carlson of the Kenosha Police Department brought Mandy in for her yearly checkup. Tom's wife, Cynthia, picked out this hunting dog for her husband's birthday four years prior. Mandy became a surrogate for the kids the couple could not have. Her hunting activities were limited to searching for food and a soft spot to nap.

I commented on Tom's ever expanding waistline and what a benefit it would be if both he and Mandy took daily walks or jogs. "Think how much Mandy will love it," I said. "Think about how you're adding years to her lifespan, and yours too." As usual, after our discussion started out on ways to limit Mandy's food intake and increase her outdoor activity, it turned to solving the problems of the world in general and Kenosha in particular. I had recently written an op-ed piece published in the (see p. 300). Tom allowed he agreed with the gist of my proposal, but getting a tax increase through the state or national government would be a very hard sell. When I mentioned my next plan to push for legalizing drugs—especially marijuana—Tom exclaimed, "My God, Doc, don't do that. It will put me out of a job. Half of the Kenosha Police Department is involved in the 'war on drugs'." That may have been a little exaggerated, but the message was clear. Millions, no, *billions* of dollars were involved here.

In my 1979 article, I stated that the nationwide cost of alcohol was $44 billion. Balance this number with the $9.1 billion collected by local, state, and federal governments.

By 2008 this number has risen. Alcohol problems are among the most common and costly health conditions affecting Americans: over 17 million adults have alcohol abuse disorders, either alcoholism or other, less severe, problems. The cost of these problems to the nation's economy is enormous—$185 billion yearly. Yet despite widespread public awareness of the scope of alcohol problems in U.S. society, research shows that business leaders and policymakers remain largely in the dark about its heavy economic costs. Many businesses have not examined the costs of undetected and untreated alcohol problems on their bottom lines.

In My Opinion

If We Taxed Alcohol at Rates Proportionate to Problems It Causes, We Could Slow Abuse

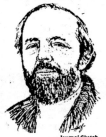

—Journal Sketch
Dr. John W. Merrick

Americans have seen the statistics so often we should know them by heart.

1. 10% of all Americans who drink are alcoholics — at least 10 million.
2. Alcohol is a factor in more than 50% of all highway traffic deaths — 28,000 deaths per year, 77 per day, three die every hour due to drunk driving.
3. Alcohol cost $20.6 billion in lost industrial production 1976.
4. Alcohol is associated with two thirds of all child abuse and wife beating complaints.
5. Alcohol accounts for over one third of all suicides.
6. Alcoholism is the "hidden" factor in 40% of all the staggering costs of welfare assistance programs.
7. Alcohol ranks behind only heart disease and cancer as major fatal diseases — even through the illness is treatable.
8. Alcoholism and alcohol abuse are a major problem to law enforcement officers and our court systems, and are responsible for overburdening our jails and penal institutions.
9. For every person who is dependent upon some other drug — six are alcoholic.

I believe Americans are not aware of the enormity of the total cost that alcohol abuse places on society. There is a vast discrepancy between what alcoholism costs us and the taxes on alcoholic beverages collected by local, state and federal governments.

Studies by Berry and Borland on the "Economic Cost of Alcohol Abuse," sponsored by the National Institute on Alcohol Abuse and Alcoholism, show that in 1976 alcohol abuse cost more than $44 billion. In lost production the cost was $20.6 billion; in direct health care costs, $11.9 billion; in fire losses, $.4 billion; in auto accident losses, $6.6 billion; in cost of violent crime, $2.1 billion, and in cost of social response, $2.7 billion.

The study points out that these figures are calculated on the low side — some estimates have been twice that amount, nearly $100 billion a year.

The other side of the coin is the amount of revenues collected from the sale of alcoholic beverages. In 1975: federal reveues were $5.5 billion; state revenues, $3.8 billion; and local revenues, $4.3 billion, for a total of $9.67 billion.

The $9 billion tax seems like a very substantial sum until compared to the $44 billion alcohol abuse cost. Clearly, $9 billion in revenues will not pay for $44 billion in problems.

I propose that the tax on alcoholic beverages be raised at least five times the amount it is now. The price of a $5.55 fifth of brandy now taxed at $2.90 would be taxed at $14, raising the toal cost to $16.65. The price of a $1.50 six pack of beer — now taxed at 34 cents — could be taxed at $1.70, raising the total price to $2.86.

The new tax would accomplish two important tasks.
1. Money would be collected in more proportionate amounts to cover the actual costs of alcoholism.
2. The public would be reminded of the scope of the alcohol problem every time a drink was purchased.

Many government programs are supported by the taxes paid by those people benefitting from the service — gasoline taxes help build and maintain highways, the postal service is supported by money collected in postal fees, etc.

Other methods of preventing the problem of alcoholism haven't worked. Young people still associate maturity with the ability to legally buy booze and get drunk. They seem totally unaware that 10% of them are destined to become alcoholics.

Very little money is spent to show the disastrous effects alcohol can bring to an individual and a family — there is no "product" to sell or profit to be made in preventing highway deaths, divorce, rape, murder, child abuse and industrial production losses.

Only when people are made aware of the real costs can we hope to stem the tide of alcohol abuse.

I believe a substantial new tax on alcoholic beverages is the best method to bring the alcohol abuse problem to the attention of the public.

DR. JOHN W. MERRICK

> Dr. John W. Merrick of Kenosha is vice chairman of the Kenosha County Social Service Department and the Kenosha County Comprehensive Mental Health Board.

> I wrote this more than 30 years ago. Prices have gone up, but the message is the same.

Two arguments need to be discussed. The tax needed to cover the costs of alcohol on society, and the legalization and taxation of marijuana. Most polls show Americans favor legalizing and taxing marijuana.

Driven by the drug war, the U.S. prison population is six to ten times as high as most western European nations. The United States is a close second only to Russia in its rate of incarceration per 100,000 people. In 2000, more than 734,000 people were arrested in this country for marijuana-related offenses alone.

The U.S. "war on drugs" places great emphasis on arresting people for smoking marijuana. Since 1990, nearly 5.9 million

Americans have been arrested on marijuana charges, a greater number than the entire populations of Alaska, Delaware, the District of Columbia, Montana, North Dakota, South Dakota, Vermont and Wyoming combined.

Once all the facts are known, it becomes clear that America's marijuana laws need reform. This issue must be openly debated using only the facts. Groundless claims, meaningless statistics, and exaggerated scare stories that have been peddled by politicians and prohibitionists for the last 60 years must be rejected.

ANNUAL AMERICAN DEATHS CAUSED BY DRUGS:
- Tobacco 400,000
- Alcohol 100,000
- All legal drugs 20,000
- All illegal drugs 15,000
- Caffeine 2,000
- Aspirin 500
- Marijuana 0

Source: National Institute on Drug Abuse, Bureau of Mortality Statistics

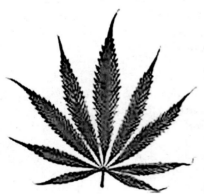

Like any substance, marijuana can be abused. The most common problem attributed to marijuana is frequent overuse, which can induce lethargic behavior, but it does not cause serious health problems. Marijuana can cause short-term memory loss, but only while under the influence. Marijuana does not impair long-term memory. Marijuana does not lead to harder drugs. Marijuana does not cause brain damage, genetic damage, or damage to the the immune system. Unlike alcohol, marijuana does not kill brain cells or induce violent behavior. Continuous long-term smoking of marijuana can cause bronchitis, but the chance of contracting bronchitis from casual marijuana smoking is minuscule. Respiratory health hazards can be totally eliminated by consuming marijuana via non-smoking methods, i.e., ingesting marijuana via baked foods, tincture, or vaporizer.

Why Legalizing Marijuana Makes Sense
By Joe Klein • *Time Magazine* • April 2, 2009

A fantasy, I suppose. But, beneath the furious roil of the economic crisis, a national conversation has quietly begun about the irrationality of our drug laws. The hypocrisy inherent in the American conversation about stimulants is staggering.

But there are big issues here, issues of economy and simple justice, especially on the sentencing side. As Webb pointed out in a cover story in *Parade* magazine, the U.S. is, by far, the most "criminal" country in the world, with 5% of the world's population and 25% of its prisoners. We spend $68 billion per year on corrections, and one-third of those being corrected are serving time for nonviolent drug crimes. We spend about $150 billion on policing and courts, and 47.5% of all drug arrests are marijuana-related. That is an awful lot of money, most of it nonfederal, that could be spent on better schools or infrastructure—or simply returned to the public. At the same time, there is an enormous potential windfall in the taxation of marijuana. It is estimated that pot is the largest cash crop in California, with annual revenues approaching $14 billion. A 10% pot tax would yield $1.4 billion in California alone. And that's probably a fraction of the revenues that would be available—and of the economic impact, with thousands of new jobs in agriculture, packaging, marketing and advertising. A veritable marijuana economic-stimulus package!

So why not do it? There are serious moral arguments, both secular and religious. There are those who believe—with some good reason—that the accretion of legalized vices is debilitating, that we are a less virtuous society since gambling spilled out from Las Vegas to "riverboats" and state lotteries across the country. Obviously, marijuana can be abused. But the costs of criminalization have proved to be enormous, perhaps unsustainable. Would legalization be any worse?

As of the summer of 2011, sixteen states and the District of Columbia have legalized marijuana for medical use. Similar legislation is pending in ten other states. In the very near future over one half of Americans will be able to get the benefits of marijuana use. The ensuing taxes will also add to the nations coffers.

How has legalization and taxation worked in other countries? This edited version follows:

Why Rick Steves believes marijuana should be decriminalized and regulated

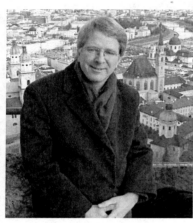

Rick Steves

With my work on the ACLU-produced TV program *Marijuana: It's Time for a Conversation,* support of NORML (a group working to decriminalize marijuana in the USA) and willingness to talk at Seattle's Hempfest as well as at other events, some people are wondering what's motivating me. Let me explain:

I support the decriminalization of marijuana among responsible adult users in the USA. "Decriminalization" does not mean unfettered use; it simply means *not* mandating that use is a criminally punishable offense. I do *not* support the legalization of hard drugs.

Like most of Europe, I believe marijuana is a soft drug (like alcohol and tobacco), not a hard drug. Like alcohol and tobacco, it should be treated as a health issue rather than a criminal issue. Crime should only enter the equation if it is abused to the point where innocent people are harmed.

I do not support children using marijuana (or alcohol or tobacco). In fact, I don't advocate smoking marijuana at all. I believe, however, that if mature adults want to smoke marijuana recreationally in the privacy of their own homes that is their own decision. That's why Nadine Strossen, president of the ACLU, Norm Stamper, former Seattle police chief, and I serve together on the board of directors of NORML.

Last year over 800,000 Americans were arrested on marijuana charges—a 100% increase since 1980. Well over 80% of these arrests were for simple possession. Many of these people were sentenced to mandatory prison time. Our courts and prisons are clogged with nonviolent people whose only offense is smoking, buying, or selling marijuana. While our nation is in a serious financial crisis, it spends literally billions of dollars annually chasing down responsible adults who are good, tax-paying citizens in all regards except for the occasional use of marijuana.

The propaganda war our government wages against the use of marijuana is not only expensive in terms of money, but it erodes its credibility among young people in regards to other more serious drugs. The White House even runs ads during the Super Bowl (between all the beer ads) claiming that marijuana causes teen pregnancies. With the tenor of our country right now, dealing with the prohibition on marijuana is considered political suicide for most elected officials. Teachers I know tell me they will put their jobs in jeopardy if they question the deceitful (and generally considered somewhere between ineffective and counterproductive) DARE program which indoctrinates children about the evils of marijuana. Average Americans embrace this big lie because it is scary to question it. The credibility of parents, teachers, police, and our government is important if we are to help our children resist the temptation to mess their lives up with drugs. Credibility on all counts suffers with the current "war on marijuana."

We've been there.

Prohibition on alcohol (1920–1933) finally fell apart in our grandparents' age because Americans came to realize that the criminalizing of alcohol did not reduce its consumption, but it did succeed brilliantly in:

- filling jails with unlucky drinkers who got caught;
- creating a stubborn network of "underground distribution" crime where none had existed before; and
- diverting enormous government resources to violate people's personal privacy.

Prohibition was a classic example of a hoped-for cure that brought more harm to society than the problem it was designed to tackle. It was Big Government at its worst. And our grandparents courageously stood up and said, "stop this waste!"

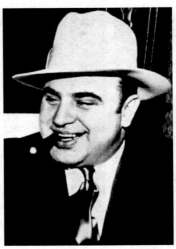

Al Capone • 1899–1947

In the early 1930s, our society didn't say booze is good. It concluded that criminalizing it only made the problem worse. Looking back, we know that was the right conclusion.

With the prohibition on marijuana, we are dealing with a similar problem today. In the name of life, liberty and the pursuit of happiness, we'll all be better off when we let our police officers, courts and prisons deal with real criminals and start taxing marijuana rather than arresting those who enjoy using it.
—Rick Steves

I must not forget one of the most potent arguments for the decriminalization of marijuana. It would dramatically lower the price, which would in turn:
1. Put the Mexican and Columbian drug cartels out of business. They will spend millions fighting the legalization;
2. Save thousands of lives, including many innocent bystanders, in the "war on drugs" in the United States and around the world;
3. Employ thousands of healthcare workers to treat—instead of imprison—people.

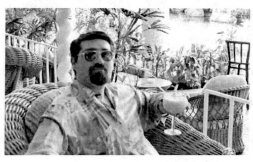
Pablo Emilio Escobar Gaviria

Pablo Escobar was the most notorious and violent drug lord of the Medellin Cartel. Escobar was killed by the Search Bloc, a group of Colombian police devoted to capturing Escobar, on a Colombian rooftop in 1993. By this time, the cartel had already been severely damaged, but, there would be no rest. After Escobar's death, the Medellin Cartel fragmented and the cocaine market soon became dominated by the rival Cali Cartel until the mid-1990s, when its leaders, too, were either killed or captured by the government. "Don Pablo" traded in a job recycling tombstones to form the Medellin drug cartel, which would control 80% of the world's cocaine supply by the end of the 1980s, making him the seventh richest man in the world, according to Forbes. But to get where he did, he left hundreds of corpses in his wake, including 101 passengers on a commercial airliner and a candidate for the Colombian presidency.

Finally—a personal story. I have never smoked or tasted, to my knowledge, marijuana. I can't say for sure if one of my teenage children might have snuck a few "California Cookies" on Carol and me 30 years ago. Since giving up cigarettes and alcohol 40 years ago, I had no desire to try this weed. I'll admit I was a little tempted after reading Carlos Castaneda's books on the effects of various "spiritual drugs," however.

My youngest daughter, Peggy, developed breast cancer in 2005. She found a small lump and immediately had it removed. Unfortunately, it had already developed into stage four. Peggy was a fighter; she never gave up. Five years of chemotherapy gave her the opportunity to spread the word about breast self screening to young women in high schools around the Atlanta area through the group she cofounded: BRA—Bikers Riding for Awareness.

The cancer finally spread to Peg's bones and liver. She came home to hospice care, still determined to beat the disease. Sadly, she was unable to eat. Even the sight of food made her nauseous. I knew she and her husband, Don, had occasionally used marijuana.

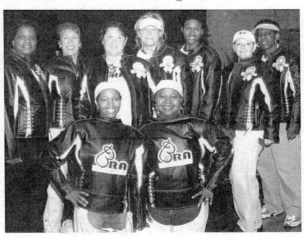

Peggy is on the back row, second from the right.

I asked Don if he had any. He replied that they had given it up years ago. It didn't take but a phone call to a friend to locate a supply, including a pipe. Peggy had not eaten for five days. Don prepared the pipe and Peggy smoked the dried leaves for a few minutes. She drifted off to sleep. Waking after 30 minutes, she sat up in bed and exclaimed, "I'm starved. Doesn't anyone have any breakfast for me. Am I an orphan, or what?" Her last days were a complete turnaround—less pain and nausea, some appetite, and a much better quality of life.

I asked the hospice nurse about using marijuana in hospice. She replied, "I can't recommend it because medical marijuana isn't legal in Georgia. I can say that 99% of my patients get positive results, just as Peg experienced."

I wonder how many years America will continue to ignore the obvious. George Santayana said it best, "Those who cannot remember the past are condemned to repeat it." Demand always drives supply. Prohibition has never worked. I hope America wakes up sooner rather than later. It may be that the frightful cost of prisons coupled with the vast tax revenues available will finally open people's eyes. I hope I live to see it.

Remembering Sensei

During the late '60s Carol and I began attending various churches so our six children could experience different religions. Pope John Paul XXIII had recently advised Catholic families to visit local non-Catholic churches to strengthen our faith in Catholicism. The minister of the Unitarian Church of Racine, Wisconsin, was on vacation. Rev. Gyomay M. Kubose replaced him at the Sunday services. For the first time in my adult life, I agreed with every word a minister said. Carol felt the same, so we decided to visit Kubose's church (temple) in the Uptown area of Chicago. Our family has been following the teaching of the Buddha since that day.

Carol and I were well acquainted with Uptown. We had been to the area many times as teenagers when we played table tennis tournaments all over the Chicago area. The Uptown Table Tennis Emporium was only four blocks from the temple. A typical middle class neighborhood at the time, by the late 1960s the Uptown area of Chicago had started to decay. It would be another 30 years before gentrification took hold.

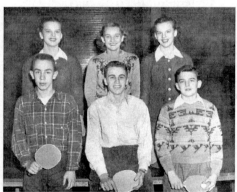

Top: Cheryl Van deHouten, Carol, Joan Van deHouten; Bottom: Unknown, Unknown, John

Visiting with Sensei (teacher) and Minnie Kubose, we mentioned our recent visit to the House on the Rock and Frank Lloyd Wright's Taliesin East Studio near Spring Green, Wisconsin. Rev. K. said he would really like to see those places, so we made plans to travel there after Labor Day.

Jane Smiley wrote this about the House on the Rock complex in 1993:

> Though most people outside of the Midwest have never heard of it, the House on the Rock is said to draw

more visitors every year than any other spot in Wisconsin. Also in the Wyoming Valley, but on top of a huge monolith, the House on the Rock reveals the spirit of its builder, Alex Jordan Jr., to be as single-minded and eccentric as Wright's, but in substance almost absurdly opposed.

... And it is hard not to be overwhelmed by the House on the Rock. The sheer abundance of objects is impressive, and the warmth most of the objects exude, the way that the toys ask to be played with, for example, makes the displays inherently inviting. But almost from the beginning, it is too much. The house itself is dusty. Window panes are cracked. Books are water damaged. The collections seem disordered, not curated. In fact, there is no effort to explore the objects as cultural artifacts, or to use them to educate the passing hordes. If there were informative cards, it would be impossible to read them in the dark. Everything is simply massed together, and Alex Jordan comes to seem like the manifestation of pure American acquisitiveness, and acquisitiveness of a strangely boyish kind, as if he had finalized all his desires in childhood and never grown into any others.

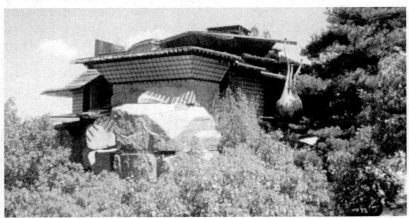

House on the Rock, Spring Green, Wisconsin

The "house" itself is atop Deer Shelter Rock, a column of rock approximately 60 feet tall, 70 feet by 200 feet on the top, which stands in a forest nearby. Additions were made to the original 14-room structure, with other buildings added over the course of several decades. When we toured in the '60s, visitors climbed ladders and navigated narrow catwalks to reach the "house." Both Kuboses expressed amazement at the magnificent structure constructed above the tree line—ohh's and ahh's at every turn.

The complex now features "The Streets of Yesterday," a re-creation of an early twentieth century American town; "The Heritage of the Sea," featuring nautical exhibits and a 200-ft. model of a fanciful whale-like sea creature; "The Music of Yesterday," a huge collection of automatic music machines; and what the management bills as "the world's largest indoor carousel," among other attractions. During the winter, the attraction features a Christmas theme, with decorations and a large collection of Santa Claus figures. The bathrooms, as well, are decorated with strange objects, including mannequins and flowers.

Lunch was taken at the Spring Green Restaurant. Located near Taliesin, this restaurant was designed in 1953 by Wright. Work began in 1957, although it was unfinished at Wright's death in 1959. The restaurant opened in 1967, somewhat altered from the original design. Today it serves as the Frank Lloyd Wright Visitor Center. The structure is very long—about 300 feet—along the side of a hill. The building is raised up above the Wisconsin River on masonry piers. A row of porthole-like windows line the length of the building on the river side. Approaching the restaurant from across the Wisconsin River at night gives one the appearance of a large ship steaming down the river.

A short distance south of the restaurant, I pulled off the highway onto the narrow gravel road leading into Taliesin East—the

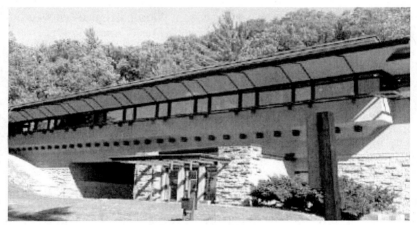

Spring Green Restaurant, Spring Green, Wisconsin

summer retreat of the famed architect. On this early September day the leaves had not started to turn, but the area, 30 miles west of Madison, Wisconsin, was uncommonly beautiful and serene.

Entering into the Taliesin parking lot, we encountered a barricade with a "Closed For The Season" sign attached. Rev. Kubose. said, "Pull around, I see a truck up ahead. I will talk to them." In his most broken Japanese-English accent, Rev. Kubose explained to the workers that he had previously met Frank Lloyd Wight and was most sorry he would not be able to see the facility. Without any hesitation, one of the men said, "Wait here. I'll be right back."

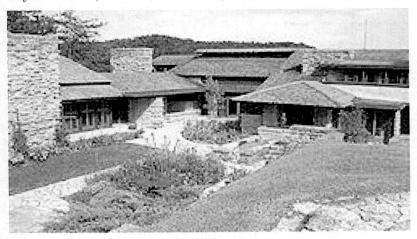

Taliesin East Spring Green, Wisconsin

Soon the workman returned with a young oriental fellow who spoke to Rev. Kubose in Japanese. Kubose apologized to the young man for pretending to be more "foreign" than he really was, explained we had driven from Chicago, and were sorry to have bothered him if he was busy. He and Rev. K. shared a good laugh. The young man explained he was an architectural student recently arrived from Japan to study with the Wright group. He had been one of those left behind to gather up everything for the trip to their winter quarters in Arizona. Needless to say, we were given a grand tour of the facility. The student eventually graduated and joined a large architectural firm in Chicago. The scene is as fresh in my mind as if it were yesterday—Rev. K. making the best of any situation, always looking for the sunshine, expecting everything to work out, but willing to accept whatever happens.

Fast forward to 2011. In researching for my book, I came across a full-page article in *The Chicago Tribune* describing Minnie Kubose and the Tea Ceremony. I mailed it to Kubose's daughter, Joyce Prosise—herself a Tea Ceremony teacher—and received her email in reply. It read, in part:

> The article about visiting the House on the Rock and Spring Green with my parents was a joy to read. An interesting part of the story that I'd like to share is that in the mid-90s, a Japanese gentleman, Mr. Hori, who was an architect, contacted me about studying tea ceremony, which he did for a year or so. He lived and worked in Evanston. At one point, he told me the story of how he met my father, and he relayed the story that you wrote about!! Mr. Hori was the Japanese gentleman who was at Spring Green that day when you and Carol and my parents visited!! How about that for a very small world?! So now I've heard that story from both sides! Isn't that something?! Thank you so much for sharing your memories! (Mr. Hori decided to return to Japan a few years later after studying with me. He was selling his furniture and things from his office and condo and actually, I'm sitting on his office chair right now as I write you!)

Born in 1905, Kubose was three years old when his parents divorced. He was sent to Japan to be raised by his grandparents. He returned to the United States at the age of 17, enrolling in grammar school to learn English. After graduating from high school, Kubose started a landscape business to help pay for his college studies.

Kubose's life was turned upside down after reading a book by Rev. Haya Akegarasu, a famous Jodo Shinshu minister. Kubose was able to act as interpreter when Rev. Akegarasu toured the U.S. in 1929. Kubose married Minnie Taniguchi in 1936, and the couple went to Japan for five years of Buddhist study. Before leaving Japan, Rev. Akegarasu advised Rev. Kubose to start an independent

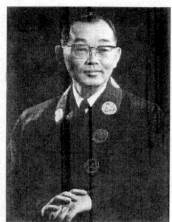

Rev. Gyomay M. Kubose
1905–2000

temple in the U.S. so that he could freely present the Dharma teachings in a way that would be understood by Americans. Rev. Kubose and Minnie returned to the United States in July, 1941, just prior to the start of World War II. After a brief stay in Los Angeles, the family was interned for two years in the Heart Mountain Relocation Camp in Wyoming. Rev. Kubose came to Chicago in 1944 and established the Buddhist Temple of Chicago. Reverend Gyomay passed away at the age of 94 in St. Joseph's Hospital in Chicago—the one and only time he had ever been hospitalized.

Kubose wrote many books, the most famous being *Everyday Suchness*. A classic collection of short stories, *Everyday Suchness* is considered one of the most significant American books on Buddhism. Buddhism teaches one to live in the moment, like a child, being open to any and all experiences. Both Rev. and Minnie Kubose (she taught Tea Ceremony), exhibited the ability to show real amazement and interest in every passing moment. Sights and smells of flowers, sounds of music, tastes of food varieties—all were "new" to the Kuboses.

Kubose liked to say, "Buddhism is a 'no' religion. No sin, no heaven, no hell, no right, no wrong. The Buddha taught there is no use wasting energy speculating about things we cannot know, such as heaven and hell. These are man-made concepts. In a similar manner, he recommended right (appropriate) speech, right (appropriate) action, etc." Rev. Kubose's son, Rev. Koyo Kubose, carries on his father's tradition, running (with the help of his wife, Adrienne), Bright Dawn Center for Oneness Buddhism in Coarsegold, California. My son, David, was recently inducted as a Lay Buddhist Minister.

Lucky Friday the 13th

"I'll bet the Queen of England never had this kind of luck," Paul Jaeger said after his Welsh corgi, Jubilee, delivered the last of 13 puppies on Friday the 13th.

Adult corgis are usually about 10 to 12 inches in height and weigh between 25 to 30 pounds. They are herding dogs that perform 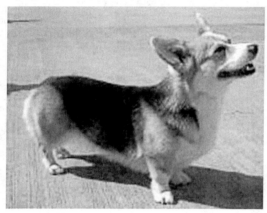 their duties by nipping at the heels, and they are agile enough and small enough to avoid being kicked. Although they specialize in herding cattle, corgis are also used to herd sheep and Welsh ponies. They are also one the few breeds able to herd geese.

Queen Elizabeth II of the United Kingdom usually keeps at least four corgis at all times. There have been no reports of unusually large births in the royal kennels. Animal lover Queen Elizabeth II (she's also an expert equestrian) has elevated the literally lowly corgi to icon status by being photographed with her dogs and stopping to chat at public events with fellow corgiphiles. Her father, King George VI, brought the breed into the family in 1933, but recent evidence suggests that the royal fondness extends even further. In 2004, archaeolo-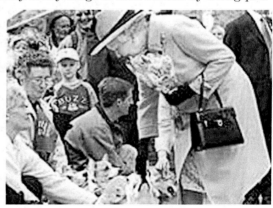

gists at a dig in Wales where the queen's ancestors lived during the ninth century discovered a leg bone from a corgi-like dog.

Thirty-five bomb-sniffing dogs were used to check the guests' parade route at the wedding of Prince William and Kate Middleton in the spring of 2011. None were reported to be Welsh corgis.

I knew Jubilee looked heavy, and I was able to palpate numerous embryos on her prenatal exam. I told the owners to expect a large litter. Little did I know it might be a world record.

She was bred to another purebred, Leetwood Bootblack, a corgi from Leetwood Kennel in nearby Union Grove. Elwin and Glee Leet, owners of the kennel, also spent the night in the "delivery room"—Jaeger's living room. Everyone was busy helping Jubilee clean her babies and encouraging them to nurse.

Bitches normally eat the afterbirth. This ensures they will remove the placenta from the head and allow the newborn to breathe. It also is chock full of hormones which stimulate uterine contractions and milk production, similar to the hormone injection I would give Jubilee around midnight.

Upon arriving at the Jaeger's home around 11:00 PM, I could palpate many more in Jubilee's uterus, but none close to the cervix. She had delivered eight pups by then and they were all nursing or sleeping next to Mom. The first pup was born at 4:30 PM Thursday and the final one at 5:12 AM Friday, February 13, 1981. The first eight pups had been had been delivered at a rate of one every 45 minutes.

I told Mr. Jaeger, "Corgis usually give birth to five or six. A litter of 13 is very unusual. The odds of this happening on Friday the 13th would be around one in a million." Large breeds such as Saint Bernards often deliver 12 to 16 pups. I had delivered a litter of 17 Saints the year before. I found out the record live births is over 20. Jubilee's delivery was one of the lead "Friday the 13th" stories in that day's *Kenosha News*.

Jubilee gave birth to ten male and three female healthy pups. The owner of the father will often get the first pick of the litter. The Leets had not immediately decided on a male or female, preferring to wait until the pups were six or seven weeks old. Mr. Jaeger said he will keep the pups until they are about eight weeks old before selling them, and they will likely sell for more than $100 each. The entire litter will be registered as a purebred with the American Kennel Club. When the pups are sold, each new owner can obtain an individual registration with the pup's name and AKC number.

Herschel and Dominique

Sports fans need no last names for stars with first names like Babe, Bronko, or Tiger. For the uninitiated, Wikipedia supplies the following bio's:

> **Babe** was George Herman Ruth, Jr. (February 6, 1895—August 16, 1948), best known as "Babe" Ruth, the home run slugger of the New York Yankees baseball team in the '20s and '30s.
>
> **Bronko** was Bronislau "Bronko" Nagurski (November 3, 1908—January 7, 1990) was a Canadian-born American football player with the Chicago Bears in the 1930s. He was also a successful professional wrestler, recognized as a multiple-time world heavyweight champion.
>
> **Tiger** is Eldrick Tont "Tiger" Woods (born December 30, 1975) is an American professional golfer whose achievements to date rank him among the most successful golfers of all time.

Herschel Walker and Dominique Wilkins fit that description for people who follow the football exploits of the University of Georgia Bulldogs or the Atlanta Hawks in the National Basketball Association.

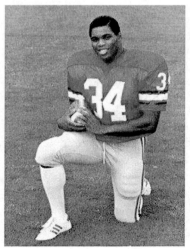

Herschel Junior Walker (born March 3, 1962) is a former American football player. He played college football for the University of Georgia Bulldogs and earned the 1982 Heisman Trophy. He began his professional career with the New Jersey Generals of the United States Football League (USFL) before entering the National Football League (NFL). In the NFL he played for the Dallas Cowboys, Minnesota Vikings, Philadelphia Eagles, and New York Giants. He was inducted into the College Football Hall of Fame in 1999.

Jacques Dominique Wilkins (born January 12, 1960) is a retired American professional basketball player who primarily played for the Atlanta Hawks of the NBA. Wilkins was a nine-time NBA All-Star, and one of the best dunkers in NBA history, earning the nickname "The Human Highlight Film." In 2006, Wilkins was inducted into the Naismith Memorial Basketball Hall of Fame. Source: Wikipedia.

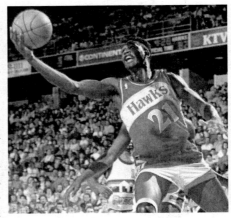

After retiring to Peachtree City, Georgia in 2001, I joined the local Kiwanis Club. Combined with my years in the Kiwanis Club of Western Kenosha, over the next few years I managed to accumulate 40 years of "perfect attendance." By 2008 I had been actively involved in Kiwanis for 50 years. Sponsoring golf tournaments are one of the many ways clubs raise money to support their local charities. In Kenosha my task was to write dozens of pro golf stars requesting donations of items to be given as prizes to the players attending our event. The Peachtree City Kiwanis had been sponsoring a golf outing for many years before I joined in 2001. I volunteered to help gather prizes for the upcoming event.

My oldest daughter, Dorothy, was a broker for The Condo Store in Atlanta, marketing dozens of condominiums around the Atlanta area. She called me one day saying, "Dad, I need some help." I replied, "Of course, I've had some experience in real estate, having owned apartments in Madison and Kenosha and..." Dorothy interrupted, "No Dad, I mean on the phone." Business was so good in 2002 she couldn't afford to have a Realtor tied up answering the Condo Store phones, but someone like "yours truly" would fit the bill very well. The ten bucks an hour at least paid for my gas. In no time I was acquainted with every major street in metro Atlanta. Over the next five years, I worked nearly one hundred sites in and around Atlanta. After a few months I managed to pass the Georgia Real Estate exam and obtain my license as a Realtor.

Herschel Walker and Dominique Wilkins happened to own condos in La Chateau, a condominium located in the upscale Buckhead area of Atlanta.

I had an opportunity to meet and visit with both men when I worked at the site on weekends. I inquired if they would be willing to sign a football and basketball respectively for our next Kiwanis Golf Outing. Both immediately responded affirmatively. I purchased balls at our local sports store and gave them to the building manager to deliver to Herschel and Dominique, since both men were out of town on business. The next weekend I picked up the basketball signed by Dominique, but Herschel had left town the night before and forgotten to sign the football. Our Kiwanis golf tournament was the following Wednesday. The building manager said, "Don't worry, Herschel told me to remind him, and I forgot. I'll call him in Athens." Herschel's reply was surprising. "UPS the ball to me overnight. I'll sign it and send it to Doc at my expense." Sure enough, the signed football arrived 24 hours before the Kiwanis event. Both balls brought in generous donations when purchased.

The rap on sports stars in general is they are selfish, egotistical, uncaring individuals who, without their magnificent physical skills, could not make a decent living in today's world. Herschel and Dominique are testament to the fact that "Nice Guys Can Finish First."

Carol in Kindergarten

While looking through family pictures to gather material for this book, I came across the following letter from my wife, Carol, to our oldest granddaughter, Alena Merrick. It is very reminiscent of the letter I received a few years before from my grandson, Adam Robinson. This must be a common class project in the lower grades.

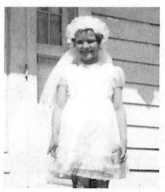

Carol Hough
8 years old • 5/12/1940

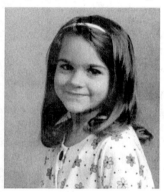

Alena Merrick
7 years old • 9/14/1992

December 26, 1991
My Darling Alena,
Thank you for the lovely letter requesting information for your kindergarten class in regard to the unit project called the "olden days." I was a little confused when I received this letter the day before Christmas, 1991, because the letter was dated November 20, 1990.

What was interesting was that November 20 is my birthday. On November 20, 1991, I turned 60 years old and feel as though this "look back" is fun and perhaps some of this information may be fun for you too.

So, my darling granddaughter, here goes all you asked for and most likely much more than you care to hear, as the expression goes.

What did you do when you were 5 or 6 years old?
The year would be around 1937 or 1938.

Where did you live?
I lived in Western Springs, Illinois, which is 130 miles south of Madison. It is a suburb of Chicago with 5,000 residents. Western Springs does not get any larger because the better-known suburbs of La Grange and Hinsdale are located on either side.

Did you go to kindergarten?
Yes, I went to Grand Avenue School, which was eight blocks from our house. The school had grades K–5. It is still there, and my cousin, Virginia Sheen, has taught 4th grade at Grand Avenue School for the past 20 years. She moved to Western Springs soon after she got married. Your grandfather and I moved to Kenosha, Wisconsin, six years after we were married, so your father went to kindergarten in Kenosha, Wisconsin.

The kindergarten your father attended is only one (1) block from where we, your grandparents, still live. You might have seen his school while you were visiting us for Christmas.

I remember my kindergarten very well, indeed. There was a large double door with ten (10) steps leading up to it, which was just the "kindergarten" door. Since my birthday was November 20th, my father had me tested, and I was allowed to enter at age four years, ten months. The usual date was September 1 when a child had to be five in order to enter school.

Do you remember any favorite games, songs, stories or books?
My favorite games were jump rope, king of the mountain, kick the can, drop the handkerchief, musical chairs, kick ball, hopscotch, trading baseball cards, "mibs" (marbles), baseball, swinging on a swing, bike riding, and ice and roller skating. My father put up a "chinning bar" for my brother and a chalkboard for me in the basement. I liked the chinning bar best and my brother liked the chalk board best.

Songs: My mother, Madeline Hough, was a piano teacher. She had played the piano for silent movies at the Chicago Theatre while she was in high school. My piano and dance lessons started when I was five years old. I clearly remember my kindergarten room as it was very large and pretty. It had very large windows. I remember singing "The Farmer in the Dell," "Ride a Cock

Horse," all the Christmas songs, "Easter Parade," musical chairs, and learning the "Virginia Reel."

Favorite stories and books: I liked stories about airplanes, sports, or about gardening. My father loved history, so we had a lot of books that told about American history. My brother and I loved to listen to "stories" on the radio while lying down on the floor, while we made scrap books.

The kinds of toys I liked best were the chinning bar, paper dolls, and my "Bo Peep" marionette (a doll on strings). Actually, I liked to ride my bike, ice skate, roller skate, play baseball, paddle ball, and "jump." My father had put a large steel pole in cement with what they now call a "tether ball" set. We played badminton when the weather allowed. My dad also built us stilts, which I still remember (clear as day) learning to walk all over on them and "jumping the cracks" of the sidewalks. He also built my brother and me a long jump pit where we learned long jumping and hurdling. He made a pole so we could pole vault and high jump also.

We lived in this house until I was in the fifth grade. At that time my parents had a house built for them but it was still in Western Springs where I continued to live until I was married to your grandfather in 1950.

My favorite toy was actually the chinning bar. My brothers' friends did not always want me to play baseball in the lot across the street, so I would go home and "chin."

What kind of transportation did you use?

My father always drove a Buick. I never rode a bus until I got into college. However, my mother and I took the Burlington train from Western Springs into Chicago to shop once a month. This was a one hour "commuter" train trip.

Did you grow much of your own food?

We tried, but the rabbits always ate it up. We did have a garden in our yard. We grew green beans, onions, and carrots. Maybe more, but I remember those well. My father loved the garden and we had a large flower garden. We had a trellis separating the first part of the back yard from the part that was on the side of the garage. We grew morning glories on the trellis and roses lined the two sides—one to where our garage was and the other went to the other side of our property. Our "jumping pit" was in the field behind the house and garage.

How did we preserve our food?
Now that I think back, we did have an "ice box," and ice was delivered once a week. I remember our getting a refrigerator and how happy that made my mother.

Did you have electricity?
Yes, we always had electricity and all the conveniences. However, my dad did have a coal stove in our first house where we lived until my 5th grade in school. I remember the coal deliveries and my father getting up in the night to "stoke" the furnace.

Thank you, Alena, for asking me to become more a part of your life, and I hope this unit turns out fun for all of you. Your teacher has selected an interesting topic, even though it is hard to consider myself as having lived in the "olden days.'
Love,
Grandma Merrick, 12/26/91

Afterword: January 4, 2011—
I quoted the letter to Alena in its entirety. It's striking, but not surprising, that Carol only had one mention of "girly" items, but many mentions of physical activity. This was a foretelling of her pursuit in learning which lead to her obtaining her Master's Coaching Certificate and teaching yoga at the University of Wisconsin–Parkside for 10 years. Carol also was a Vocational Counselor and Psychotherapist. She signed her letters, "Carol H. Merrick, MA, NBCC"

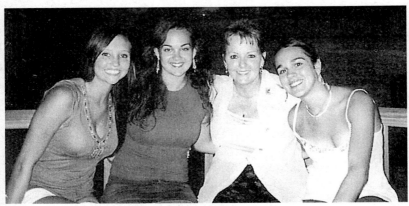

Cc, Kristina, Peggy, Alena • 2005

Torn Toenails at Midnight— Emergency Clinics

Many medical professionals create partnerships or hire staff to share or delegate their emergency calls. Dad, Dr. A. C. Merrick, was a firm believer in the common practice of sending his assistants out on Sundays or evenings. He rarely took any calls unless from a close friend. I can't say I blame him. The animal hospital was open seven days—a total of 60 hours—a week. As a rule, Dad did not answer the home phone. That way one of the kids or Mom could tell a white lie: "Dr. Merrick's not here right now. No, I don't know when he'll be back. Please call another vet." Actually, he was probably napping, reading, or listening to the White Sox on the radio.

In the two and a half years I worked for Dad, I was happy to take emergency calls, since I got to keep half of the fee. Living next door to the hospital made for a quick commute. The only drawback: I was often the only vet within 20 miles to see patients at all hours of the night. I'd tell myself, "Remember, you're not in some farmer's barnyard delivering a calf."

The first 20 years in Kenosha, I was a solo practitioner most of the time. I had my share of late night calls—usually a real emergency, but sometimes a case that could have easily waited until the next day. Rarely, the dreaded "no show." It could take more than an hour for me to get from whatever activity I was in to my hospital. The client would call my home, Carol would then call me on the golf course, someone would hurry out to the links to contact me, and I would drive to the animal hospital. There had to be a better way, especially for the animal's sake.

Around 1980 I read an article in one of the veterinary journals describing an emergency clinic started by a group of vets in San Francisco. It described how they started with self-staffing—each vet taking one night every two weeks—until they could hire outside professional help. Two things really piqued my interest—to be on call only twice a month, and not at all after a couple of years. It also mentioned the original clinic was sold for a $20,000 profit and a new modern one built to replace it. Serendipity struck. The vet who was managing the emergency clinic in Frisco was scheduled to speak to the Milwaukee VMA the following month.

Within a week I had contacted every vet in the three-county area south of Milwaukee, organizing a meeting at my recently remodeled animal hospital. The invitation read in part, "No More Midnight Torn Toenails." Of the 15 vets attending the meeting, thirteen signed on to establish the TriCounty Animal Emergency Clinic. Most of the group had read or heard about ECs starting up around the country. Ours was the first in Wisconsin. We elected officers, hired an attorney to draw up papers, and started looking for an appropriate site. Within six months we were in business. It took almost four years to hire two full-time emergency vets. Until that time, each owner would pull one shift every two to three weeks.

Most of the week nights were uneventful. If you were lucky, the phone would not ring after midnight, and you could sleep until dawn. The older vets often paid younger vets to work their shifts. Within eight years the TriCounty EC was getting too busy for the remodeled house we started in. A new clinic was built one mile north of the original. We had hoped to have specialists from Chicago or Madison in dermatology, ophthalmology, and cardiology utilize the clinic during the day. While this has been the trend in many areas of the country, Kenosha has yet to achieve this goal. At last report, most of the original investors have retired and sold their interests with a good profit. This provides a excellent example of a win-win solution to a long-term problem—providing immediate, good-quality care for the animal at a reasonable price and dependable availability. It gives the local vets a work week closer to 60, rather than 80 hours, and makes EC specialists available to the local clients and their pets.

The Animal Emergency Center (AMC) in Milwaukee, Wisconsin, started soon after the TriCounty EC in Kenosha. Under the excellent direction of Dr. Rebecca Kirby, the center now occupies a 14,000 sq. ft. state-of-the-art facility. The staff of 60 includes specialists in emergency and critical care, internal medicine, dentistry, oncology, radiology, and surgery.

Commensurate with the level of expertise available to pet owners for the care of their sick and injured pets is the rise in fees. Fortunately, many clients have purchased pet health insurance, which can pay for up to 80% of the cost. Many diagnostic and treatment procedures can run into the hundreds or thousands of dollars. Our grandfathers, dealing with livestock, would not believe the prices people willingly pay to provide their pets the best quality care. The AMC estimates approximately 15% to 20% of their clients have pet insurance. Unlike human hospital insurance, the client pays the vet in full and then collects from the pet insurance company. Since most bills are approved in advance, there are rarely any problems in receiving payment from the pet insurance company. You can now pick up an application for insurance for your beloved pet at Kroger.

There are now many veterinarians who work full time filling in for practitioners who are sick or on vacation. A recent newsletter of the Wisconsin VMA listed 21 veterinarians available for relief work in Wisconsin alone. I believe this trend will continue as more women enter the veterinary workforce.

Nowadays, when one hears that "medicine has gone to the dogs," it's a compliment.

Pet Spas

"Doggie Day Care," I told my colleague, Jan Wolf, "that's the coming thing in vet practice." Jan agreed, "...as long as the boarding and grooming are separate from the medical facility." We were on our way to visit the American Pet Resort in Lincolnshire, Illinois, fifteen miles north of O'Hare Airport. If the "Old Money" lived in Lake Forest, the "New Money" resided in Lincolnshire. The joke going around was that Lincolnshire was so exclusive that the police department had an unlisted number and the fire department doesn't make house calls. Carol and I had a car problem when driving through Lincolnshire a few years earlier, and the kid from the local garage came to pick us up in a new Cadillac. This was the area served by the American Pet Resort.

Robert X. Leeds had built the first pet motel in Florida in 1972. One of his partners was Ray Kroc. Yes, the Ray Kroc who made billions selling McDonald's hamburgers. They disagreed on policy, so Leeds moved to Illinois to start his own operation. Dr. Wolf and I were trying to figure a way to combine our practices. Maybe if we started with a pet boarding, grooming, day care facility, we could eventually add veterinary services—kind of like putting the cart before the horse. Mr. Leeds greeted us like long-lost brothers. With the zeal of a car salesman, he showed us around his large facility. There was room to board 100 dogs and 50 cats. He was in the process of adding another 100 kennels/suites. There were single and double kennels, condos for cats, private areas for birds and reptiles, and various exercise areas. His hope was to establish American Pet Resorts around the country. He was very disappointed by his experience working for Ray Kroc. I wasn't sure just what to believe. Before we left, Robert gave us an autographed copy of his book, *All the Comforts of Home.* Mr. Leeds has since retired to Las Vegas to write his autobiography, *The Last Knight Errant,* describing the adventures he encountered in over 70 years of service as an American Knight-Errant. Since we were going to build 40 miles north—out of his client base—he happily shared his knowledge with us. I was interested in his "insurance plan" for boarders. Every animal admitted to the kennel was assessed a $3.00 insurance fee. This would cover any reasonable medical problems encountered up to two weeks after the animal's stay at APR. He related that only one animal in 300 ever took advantage of the insurance. He covered all vet bills—some obviously inflated—without question. The plan had made a $12,500 profit the previous year.

In answering the question about the cost of boarding and grooming, The Association of Pet Boarding and Grooming states the following on their Web site:

> Just like motels, this varies between different locations and the standard of accommodation offered, such as luxury suites. Unlike people motels which charge per night, generally boarding rates are charged per day. Standard boarding rates for dogs start from around $14 to $22, and cats from $12 to $20, with luxury suites varying from around $35–$70. Other costs to consider are for additional services such as hydrobaths, playtime, extra care with medications, special feeds, and holiday pricing. Some of these are included and some are extra.

The American Pet Products Association reports that in 2008, 62% of U.S. households owned a pet—up from 56% in 1988. This equals 93.6 million cats, 77.5 million dogs, and 15 million birds. Sadly, Jan Wolf's sudden, unexpected death at age 50 put an end to our dreams; however, the pet boarding/daycare/spa movement has carried on. In the last 20 years market forces created a ever-expanding need for their services. Women now make up 55% of the workforce. Stay-at-home moms are a vanishing commodity. The market for pet services will continue to expand as the trend to consider pets "family" continues.

The Waggin' Tails Doggie Dude Ranch and Pet Lodge in Madison, Wisconsin, offers the following services: day boarding, daycare, geriatric and hospice care, play groups, grooming, swimming, and training—a cornucopia of choices for the pet owner. They also offer reduced rates for monthly guests.

The Park Pet Retreat in suburban Atlanta, Georgia, offers the ultimate in pet boarding and daycare. The following is taken from the Park Pet Resort brochure:

Sleepovers at The Park are Fun!!

> Once you and your pooch experience 24-hour cage-free attended care, you will never return to your old concrete-and-cage facility.
>
> Most cage-free boarding facilities are only cage-free during the day and your pet is left alone in a cage during

the night. Being away from you is stressful enough for your pooch without the added stress of being left alone in a cage.

If your pooch is boarding overnight with us at the Park Pet Retreat, there will be a Park Ranger on duty throughout the night to ensure their safety and wellbeing.

In the evening, we will serve dinner, have a little play time, and then take everyone outside for an evening stroll in the meadow. As the hour grows late, we will turn down the lights, put out plenty of beds, and turn on soft music. Then, just like at home, each doggie will find their own spot to sleep through the night. Should we have any night-owls wandering around looking for playmates, the Ranger will be able to move them to another part of the park until they get drowsy.

Your pet will never be put into a cage or kennel or left alone.

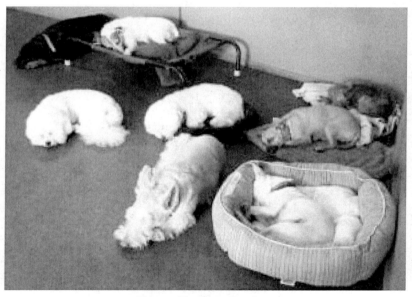

Happy Sleeping Pooches

PARK PET RESORT
ONLINE REGISTRATION FORM

BOARDING: Check in as early as 7 AM; check out by 12 noon.
Price shown covers period from 7 AM to 12 noon the next day.
1–4 days: One dog $37.50; two dogs $32.00 ea; additional dogs 10% ea.
5–9 days: One dog $35.50; two dogs $30.00 ea; additional dogs 10% ea.
10–15 days: One dog $32.50; two dogs $28.00 ea; additional dogs 10% ea.
16–30 days: One dog $30.00; two dogs $25.00 ea; additional dogs 10% ea.
12 hours overnight: Drop at 7:00 PM, pick up at 7:00 AM. $25.00 ea.
Day care fees for pickup after 12 noon: Noon–4 PM $12.00 ea; 4 PM–7 PM $17.00 ea; 7 PM–9 PM $22.00 ea.
Respite care for post-surgery or non-communicable illness:
7 AM–7 PM $25.00; Overnight $42.00.

For comparison, Motel Six, within one mile of the Park Pet Resort, charges $43.19 per night for a double room. Of course, this does not include a "ranger" to tuck you into bed.

In the late '40s and early '50s Dad charged $2.00 a day to board a small dog, $3.00 for a large dog and $1.00 for a cat. He charged $5.00 for a trim and bath for most dogs. Considering the inflation over 60 years, multiply these fees by 10 and you'll see that not much has changed. The services today, however, are more in tune with today's idea of the pet as family. Many owners would not dream of leaving their four legged "child" in a cage.

Vets generally agree that 99% of their complaints come from people unhappy with their boarding and grooming services. If the non-professional part of practice is first class and separate from the clinical area, these headaches can be avoided.

Seminars: Greyhounds, Cardio, and Behavior

Jan Wolf was a wonderful veterinarian who died too young. We became friends after he bought my storefront practice on the north side of Kenosha. Managing a full-size animal hospital and a clinic eight miles away turned out to be more than I wanted to handle. Within a year Jan had outgrown the clinic and purchased and remodeled a machine shop on the main drag in town. Fortunately for him, within two years, Wal-Mart opened their first superstore in the area across the street from Jan's animal hospital. His practice took off, and Jan never looked back.

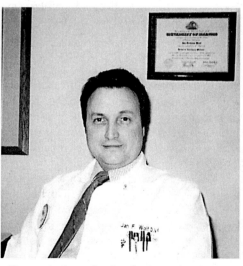

Jan and his wife, Terry, were from Riverside, Illinois. They were classmates in high school, just as my wife, Carol, and I were 20 years earlier in La Grange, next door to Riverside. Over the years we talked about combining our practices, but we could never figure a way to dispose of the duplicate equipment and property. Sadly, 20 years later, Jan died of a coronary at the age of 50. I was in the process of selling my practice. Dr. Scott Petereit bought both practices, combined them, and fulfilled our dream. Today, Wolf-Merrick is a cutting-edge facility.

Soon after Dr. Wolf came to town, Kenosha went to the dogs—literally. Five Greyhound tracks were to be built in Wisconsin, including one in Kenosha. Three syndicates were competing for the rights to build and operate the local track. Visions of Vegas danced in their heads. With threats from state humane societies

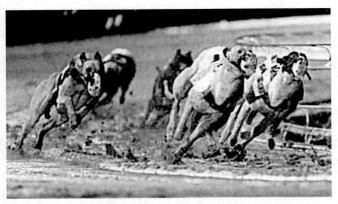
Greyhounds rounding the turn after the "rabbit"

about the Wisconsin weather, one of the groups hired me to research the effects of cold on Greyhounds. My research of all available information on the effect of cold weather on Greyhounds proved the fears to be groundless. Dogs spend only a very minimal amount of time out in the cold, and it has no effect on their health or running ability.

Dr. Wolf and I were inexperienced treating Greyhounds, as were most other vets in the area. We thought organizing a Greyhound seminar would be appropriate. Since I had been in contact with experts in Florida to write my report, I called on them again to obtain speakers for our proposed meeting. In the spring of 1990, shortly before the Dairyland Greyhound Track opened, we sponsored a Greyhound seminar that attracted over 150 vets from the surrounding area.

Local veterinarians began to see greyhound patients, both from private clients and kennel operators. We learned soon enough that racing dogs are not pets. Every decision made by the kennel owner is based on economics—is it worth spending the dollars against the possible return. In other words, how much bang for the buck? The life span of a racing dog is short.

On November 10, 2009, the Milwaukee Journal/Sentinel reported, "In 1989, state regulators with dollar signs in their eyes approved five operating licenses for pari-mutuel greyhound racing in Wisconsin. For a time, race fans and bettors flocked to the tracks in Geneva Lakes, Kaukauna, Lake Delton, Hudson, and Kenosha, generating millions for the state and the developers. But once the door opened for Indian casinos, attendance and revenue began to drop. One by one, the tracks went out of business." Efforts by the local Menominee Indian tribe to combine the track with a casino failed to pass the state legislature.

The sport reached its peak in 1992, when attendance approached 3.5 million, and nearly $3.5 billion was bet on 16,827 races at more than 50 tracks in the United States. Since then, revenue has dropped by nearly 50 percent and 13 tracks have closed.

Wikipedia states:

> After the dogs are no longer able to race (generally, a greyhound's career will end between the ages of four and six), or possibly when they no longer consistently place in the top four, the dog's race career ends. The best dogs are kept for breeding purposes. There are both industry-associated adoption groups and rescue groups that work to obtain retired racing greyhounds and place them as pets. In the United States, prior to the formation of adoption groups, over 20,000 retired greyhounds a year were euthanized; recent estimates still number in the thousands, with about 90% of National Greyhound Association–registered animals either being adopted or returned for breeding purposes (according to the industry numbers, upwards of 2000 dogs are still euthanized annually in the U.S., while anti-racing groups estimating the figure at closer to 12,000.)

Cardiology and preoperative blood testing was becoming common in small animal practice in the early '90s. With help from Vetronics, a company offering online cardiology diagnostics, Dr. Wolf and I sponsored a cardiology seminar. Preop electrocardiograms (ECGs) could be sent over the phone to a specialist for screening. It proved to be a hit with the 75 vets who attended. Their clients appreciated the up-to-date services available for their four-legged companions. It was now possible to do preop heart screening. The tracings were transmitted to specialist, analyzed, and a reply sent immediately. Preop blood analysis was also available due to the advent of high-quality blood analyzing machines. When offered these preop diagnostic services, 30% of clients—especially those with older animals—said, "Yes."

Our most successful meeting was the "Super Puppy Seminar." Nearly 200 veterinarians, clients, humane society–types, and interested parties attended.

Animal behavior training was just catching on in the vet world. Peter Vollmer was a popular author whose book, *Super Puppy,* sold over 500,000 copies. The best advice I ever received from Peter was the secret of the Hollywood dog trainers—Liver Treats. Peter reported most of the handlers training animals for television or movies used freeze-dried Liver Treats as a motivator. The dog in the movie knew, "Perform your task successfully, and you get a yummy." To this day I have a bag of Liver Treats in my car to reward any dog that approaches. When I carried them in my lab coat in practice, animals would often run into the exam room. They knew a treat was waiting.

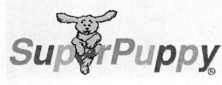

The canine nose is twenty thousand times as sensitive as humans. Dogs are routinely used to sniff out drugs and explosive materials in airports. There is evidence they can be trained to detect certain types of bladder cancer in humans. Notice how happy dogs seem when hanging their heads out of moving cars. Think of all those smells out there to enjoy.

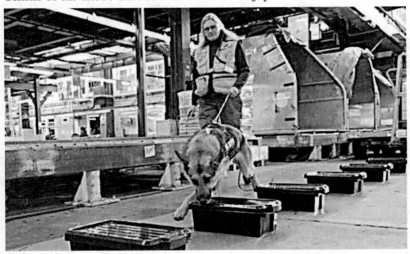

Norm Abplanalp

"With a name like Smuckers, it has to be good." Likewise, with a name like Norm Abplanalp, he's got to be Swiss. As it happens, Norm is of Swiss descent. I first met Norm over 50 years ago, when our families took a ski trip to Boyne Mountain, Michigan, along with Norm's brother-in-law, Dr. Bob Sternloff, a good friend and client. I learned that Norm had attended the University of Illinois School of Architecture at the same time I attended vet school. Our buildings were directly across the street from each other, but we never met. Over time, and after many hours spent on the slopes or at his cottage at Lake Tichigan, 20 miles from my home in Kenosha, we became good friends. He designed my first house and redesigned my animal hospital while I cared for his Beagles.

Norm was in private practice in suburban Chicago until 1966, when he became the head architect for Montgomery Ward, the large catalog/department store with headquarters in downtown Chicago. The concept of regional storage facilities was just taking hold with the national chains. These could supply next-day delivery to all stores in their region and avoid each store stocking a large inventory.

Norm and his associate architect thought this would be a good time to explore solar power to heat the facilities. Can you believe it? They were seriously considering solar 40 years ago! At that time, Dr. Franklin Swanson at the University of Wisconsin was America's leading authority on solar power. Norm decided it would be worth a trip to visit Dr. Swanson and pick his brain for ideas he could use in designing the new storage facility. Dr. Swanson was happy to oblige.

Back in Chicago, Norm designed a building with solar cells on the roof and set about to figure the energy savings. Alas, with the price of oil then at $2.10 per barrel, the building would need 35 years to break even. Norm came up with a radical idea.... What if the price of oil increased to the unheard of price of $9.00 per barrel? Eureka! The building would pay for the solar panels in less than 4 years!

With the evidence in hand, Norm proudly went to the Board of Directors with his new design and energy-saving plans. Alas, it was not to be. The board scoffed at Norm. Who could ever imagine that oil prices would ever approach $9.00 per barrel in our lifetime!

Four years later, in 1973, the Arab/OPEC oil embargo sent oil prices through the roof to $27 per barrel. They haven't approached $27 per barrel—let alone $3 per barrel—since then, and they likely never will. The moral of the story is, "Never make small plans or dream small dreams."

Serendipity strikes again. After composing this story in late 2010, I received the following email from Norm on New Year's eve:
Hi John,

> Yesterday's Tribune featured the ten hot spots in Chicago. One of them, a trendy Asian restaurant, Japonais, is a favorite of movie stars and big-time pro athletes. Japonais is located on the lower level of the old Montgomery Ward catalog building, complete with a terrace on the river. When I first came to work on Chicago Avenue I was warned about that basement—critters lived down there!
>
> You have, no doubt, heard of Google's buy-out offer of Groupon for a paltry $5+ billion. Groupon is the major tenant housed in the catalog building. Some person is sitting in my old location, making millions. Times change.
>
> Happy New Year,
> Norm

For the benefit of any uninformed, I quote the following from the Groupon Web site:

> Groupon is a Web company with 5 million members, offering them discounts to hundreds of companies. Launched in November, 2008, Groupon features a daily deal on the best stuff to do, see, eat, and buy in more than 300 markets and 35 countries, and soon beyond. We have about 1,000 people working in our Chicago headquarters, a growing office in Palo Alto, California, as well as regional offices in Europe and Latin America and local account executives in many cities.

Norm eventually retired from Montgomery Ward in 2001, a year before the company filed for bankruptcy and nine years too soon to share in the Groupon billions. He and Lois were then able to travel.

Norm's older brother, Charles, had been a pilot in the Second World War. During a mission to bomb southern German cities, Charles was shot down over Muswangen, Switzerland, while returning to his base in England. A long day flight over and back from Munich leaving them vulnerable for many hours. With his plane critically damaged, Charles was just hoping for a place to land outside of Germany. Unfortunately, he was killed in the crash – all of his crew survived. Norm was only 14 years old at that time and had always idolized his older sibling. Norm decided to explore the area where the incident took place on his next trip abroad. Norm kindly wrote of his miraculous trip to Switzerland. His account follows...

I was doing some business in Salt Lake City and preceding my next scheduled visit, I called Harold (my brother's co-pilot) and Bonnie (his wife), making arrangements to meet with them. On the appointed day, I finished my business early and spent a few hours in the LDS Genealogy center and toured Temple Square. It was a wonderful experience. Returning to the hotel, there was a message from Clinton Norby's flight engineer, stating he would pick me up and drive me down to Provo. We had quite an evening together.

After some conversation and a delicious piece of chocolate cake with ice cream, Harold said, "Well, Norm, are you ready to see my war room?" It was a chilling experience for me. After all those years, he had devoted a part of their home to store keepsakes from that fateful day in 1945. Pictures of my brother, remnants of the airplane, the silk escape map, on and on. He described how he spoke to the high school students every year, explaining WWII and the high cost of freedom. He said that he always held up a large photo of Charles, in full uniform, that was taken in front of the farmhouse in Michigan. I am the little kid sitting on the stoop. I was touched beyond words.

Norby brought along a book he'd purchased in a local military base store. The book contained pictures of the crashed airplane and documented the event in Switzerland. I regret that I've never been able to find a copy of the book, nor did I photograph the gathering of everyone that evening.

My wife, Lois, and I visited the crash site in Muswangen a few years after receiving Norby's report of events leading up to the crash. After reading his detailed account, seeing the actual crash site became an uppermost thought in my mind. Not being sure of my emotions,

POLEBROOK POST

351st Bomb Group Association 8th AIR FORCE

508th   509th   351st   510th   511th

POLEBROOK, NORTHAMPTONSHIRE, ENGLAND

VOL. XXIX NO. 2   351st Bombardment Group H Association Inc., W3058 Greiner Rd., Appleton, WI 54913   SPRING 2009

> Dear Rick,
> The following is a condensed version of what happened to the Torchy Tess and crew on February 25, 1945. I have enclosed photographs of the crashed Torchy Tess, and of the flight jacket that I am looking for. Thank you for your interest. I appreciate all you do to preserve the legacy of these heroes of WWII. You are a hero as well.
> Charles Vance Gividen

Torchy Tess
Told by Clint Norby

On February 25, 1945, a B-17G, #43-37854, named *Torchy Tess*, piloted by 2nd Lt. Charles Abplanalp from Chicago, Illinois, and co-piloted by 2nd Lt. Harold Gividen, from Mapleton, Utah, took off from Polebrook, England to bomb the railroad marshalling yards at Munich, Germany. As the crew of the *Torchy Tess* neared their target there was an explosion which quickly filled the plane with black smoke. The *Torchy Tess* had been hit by flak, causing extensive damage on the left front side of the plane. Two of the crew were injured in the blast. The pilot's windshield, both front and side, was damaged so that he could not see out. However, the pilot was not injured. The pilot's rudder controls were shot away, so the co-pilot had to do the flying. By this time the *Torchy Tess* had dropped out of formation and the crew was all alone, so Cpl. Paul Livingston, the radio operator, was asked to call for fighter support; however, the radio was shot up and not working. Our No. 3 engine had stopped and our No. 2 engine was running away, so the co-pilot feathered it. We had an oil leak going into the engine, which meant it was not getting proper lubrication, so eventually both Nos. 1 and 4 would freeze up on us and then we would have no power to fly.

Because of the damage to the flight controls and engines, the plane was not too stable, so during the time after we were hit, the plane was gradually losing altitude. Many of the flight instruments were damaged, so all the co-pilot could do was set a heading of what he could determine was west toward Switzerland.

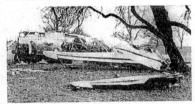
B-17 #43-37854 *Torchy Tess* crash landing in Switzerland.

The pilot asked if we still had bombs in the bomb bay. The bomb bay doors were only one-third open and all the bombs were still there, so I cranked the doors open. As soon as they were open the pilot hit the salvo switch, but only the bombs on the right

cover story continued on page 4

I decided that it would be best if I visited without any advanced notice. It seemed to be a simple trip. After all, the town is only made up of a couple hundred people, and the crash was in an orchard.

Driving up from Lucerne, we turned onto the approach road, and there was Muswangen atop a small hill, completely surrounded by orchards. Approaching the first orchard on the right, we noticed a monument, stopped the car, and walked in to check it out. As we explored, we noticed a man at the edge of town; he was intently watching our every move. After a while, I walked up to him and announced, "My name is Abplanalp." His instant reply was, "pilot, bomber." Then in German and

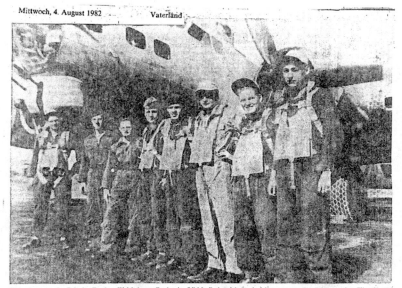

Mittwoch, 4. August 1982 — Vaterland

Dokument aus der Zeit des Zweiten Weltkrieges: Rechts im Bild befindet sich der in Müswangen verstorbene Bomber-Pilot Charles Abplanalp, zweiter von rechts ist der damals 20jährige Co-Pilot Harold V. Gividen, der nun Müswangen nochmals besucht.

Harold V. Gividen, Co-Pilot beim Absturz bei Müswangen:

«Drei der vier Motoren setzten aus»

«Wir hatten den Auftrag, den Güterbahnhof von München zu bombardieren.» Harold V. Gividen, der Co-Pilot auf dem amerikanischen B-17-Bomber, der am 25. Februar 1945 bei Müswangen eine Bruchlandung machte, erinnerte sich in einem Gespräch mit dem «Vaterland» zwar nicht mehr an die Bruchlandung, aber an verschiedene andere, interessante Einzelheiten aus der Kriegszeit 1945. Er war damals 20 Jahre jung.

Von Antoinette Spichtig

Der damals 20jährige Co-Pilot aus Utah, Harold V. Gividen, kann sich leider bis heute nicht mehr erinnern, was sich damals vor 37 Jahren, am 25. Februar 1945, auf dem Feld bei Müswangen zugetragen hat, weil er bei der Bruchlandung schwere Kopfverletzungen erlitt, die eine völlige Amnesie über die Ereignisse dieses Tages brachten («Vaterland» von gestern). Er konnte sich aber erinnern, dass sie an jenem Tag den Auftrag erhielten, den Güterbahnhof von München zu bombardieren.

Zusammen mit «vielen» andern Flugzeugen seien sie früh morgens vom englischen Stützpunkt 110, bekannt als Polebrook, in der Nähe von Peterboro, zu ihrer zweiten Mission gestartet. Ueber Süddeutschland sei ihr Flugzeug aber ins Feuer der deutschen Flugabwehr geraten und stark beschädigt worden. Der grösste Teil der Instrumente, und was unmittelbar danach geschah, kann sich Gividen nicht erinnern. Nur dank Fotos und Berichten, die er sich im Laufe der Jahre gesammelt hat, weiss er, wie das Flugzeug nach der Bruchlandung ausgesehen hat (vgl. «Vaterland» von gestern), und angesichts dieser Bilder ist es für ihn heute noch ein Wunder, dass er und seine Kollegen überhaupt noch aus diesem Wrack entsteigen konnten. Von den acht Besatzungsmitgliedern erlitten nur drei Verletzungen. Der Pilot überlebte die Bruchlandung allerdings nicht.

Einer dieser drei verletzten Besatzungsmitglieder war Co-Pilot Gividen. Er wurde, angesichts seiner Verletzungen, ins heutige Kantonsspital übergeführt, wo er während eines Monats von einer Schwester Zimmermann liebevoll gepflegt worden sei. Sie habe zwar kein Wort Englisch gesprochen und er kein Wort Deutsch, erinnert sich Gividen, aber sie seien trotzdem sehr enge Freunde geworden.

ziehe er es vor, mit einem seiner beiden Pferde tagelange Ausritte in die «Wildnis» zu unternehmen.

Beruflich ist Gividen aber nicht etwa Pilot, sondern arbeitet schon seit rund 30 Jahren bei US-Steel in der Produktions- und Planungsabteilung. Während zweier Jahre wirkte er als Mormonen-Missionar in Texas und engagierte sich auch sehr für die Pfadfinder.

Seine Frau Bonnie und er haben sieben Kinder zwischen 16 und 31 Jahren. Eines seiner Kinder starb allerdings kurz nach der Geburt. Zudem ist er stolzer Grossvater von elf Enkelkindern.

Frau Jung: «Ich salutierte»

ES. «Plötzlich ist ein Nachbar gekommen und hat gesagt, ein Bomber sei abgestürzt.» Marie Jung-Käppeli war die erste Person, die zum in Müswangen notgelandeten amerikanischen Bomber kam. «Die Flieger sind langsam aus dem zerschlagenen Bomber herausgekommen und ich habe salutiert», erklärte sie dem «Vaterland». Die Flieger hätten immer wieder auf den Boden gezeigt, offenbar um zu fragen, wo sie sich befinden. «Zu-

fractured English, he directed us to the local Gasthaus, excitingly saying, "photographic."

We then drove into town and to the Gasthaus. There was a sign announcing, "Home of the Muswangen Motorcycle Club." We went in anyway and sure enough, there over the little bar was a picture of my brother and his entire crew.

The man from the orchard entered the Gasthaus shortly afterward, along with an interpreter. He had gone home and gotten dressed in fine clothes so he could properly escort us to the crash site and represent the village. Standing there next to the big pine trees that the plane hit gliding in, he described in detail his memory of the events that fateful day. His account matched Norby's writings, as if the pages were talking to us. He related that he was home on leave from the Swiss army that day and personally witnessed the whole thing, saying they were thankful the town had not been wiped out by the terrible crash. The plane had hit overhead wires, all the electricity was out, and the clocks stopped at 1:00 PM—none of which was exactly as Norby had written. We all stood there in the orchard, knee deep in alfalfa, the bells on the grazing cattle softly chiming in the distance, listening to him tell his story. The moment was magical.

As an interesting sidelight to that trip, the very next day we traveled to the village of Innerkirchen. It was about a two-hour drive southeast of Muswangen, south of Luzern, situated behind the famous Eiger Mountain. It is in this area of Switzerland where the Abplanalp name originates. Ironically, Charles's life ended so very close to the roots of his family heritage.

Reflecting back, it is clear that his life interests had a great influence on my life; my interest in art and art appreciation, my career in architecture and original design, and a lifelong interest in downhill skiing. One of his letters contained a little brotherly advice, "Take all the math you can hold." Of course, engineering is a part of my profession and it required taking all of the math I could hold. The legacy of art now continues through the lives of my children and grandchildren.

One never knows what twists and turns await us. Tomorrow can bring an encounter that may change us forever.

Shant Harootunian

"Shant" can be translated into English as "lightning bolt." A person with "ian" at the end of his name is Armenian. Like "–son" in English names, "Mac–" in Scottish names, and "–sen" in Swedish names, it means "son of."

Shant Harootunian, in person, is an apt name for any attorney. Shant—quick to act, unpredictable, high energy, and loud. Harootunian—proud, honest, reliable, intelligent, and stubborn. One could not ask for a better friend.

Shant's father, Sarkis Harootunian, came to the United States in 1913 as a young man of 18 years. He was able to emigrate from Armenia only because his older brother, Shant's uncle, Sumpad, would accommodate him at his house. Sarkis had come to the U.S. hoping to attend college. Sarkis was fluent in Armenian, Arabic, French, and Turkish, but neither he nor his brother spoke English. Sumpad told Sarkis, "Your plan is laudable, but it lacks two key ingredients—language and money." Even with the then-modest tuition rates, Sarkis had no funds for his education. Sumpad had an answer to solve this dilemma. Sarkis would get a job at the Royal Weaving Company in Philadelphia, Pennsylvania (then, the largest silk mill in the U.S.). While working there Sarkis could not only learn English, but also earn enough money to pay for his tuition. Sarkis applied for the job, was accepted, and commenced speaking with his coworkers as planned.

A few weeks later, Sumpad invited Sarkis to come to dinner with family and friends. Sumpad proudly asked Sarkis to show how good his English was after only a few weeks in America. Sarkis said something like, *"Wszelki. Ja jestem bardzo szezsliwe jest w Ameryce."* ("Hello everybody. I'm very happy to be in America.")—all in perfect Polish! It seems that all of Sarkis' coworkers were immigrants from Poland who spoke only Polish and were as completely ignorant of English as Sarkis. Sarkis eventually learned the English language well enough to enjoy a confortable life and send his three sons to American universities, where they earned advanced degrees. He never forgot the Polish language, which he retained for the rest of his life.

Following two years of Latin in high school, Shant decided to take another language. Sarkis recommended that Shant study French, German, or Italian. Shant chose Spanish. "It seemed easier than the others," Shant recalled, "Especially after having Latin the previous two years." Following graduation, Shant began his college studies at nearby Temple University. In that day, Temple was the college where children of blue collar workers typically enrolled.

Walking to class one day, Shant noticed a sign in a local black YMCA, "Spanish Teacher Wanted." Shant's college professor who had been his counselor during his second year at Temple University, recommended Shant apply for the job. When the sign was still there two weeks later, Shant couldn't resist going inside to inquire. The office secretary directed him to the Personnel Director/Principal. He asked Shant, "Have you taught Spanish?" Shant replied, "No, I've only had two years of high school Spanish." Out of sheer desperation, Shant was hired on the spot. During his four years of undergrad studies, Shant taught conversational Spanish to a group of senior citizens. He was skilled enough to keep at least one lesson ahead of his students. Unknown at the time, Spanish was to play an important role in Shant's future.

Fast forward to a four-year hitch in the Navy, marriage to Louise (also fluent in Armenian), and law school. One of Shant's first civilian jobs was as an attorney for American Telephone and Telegraph Company. At that time "Ma Bell" was the only game in town. Shant was put to work with a dozen other young lawyers doing all the scut work experienced attorneys didn't want to do. Filing legal briefs, chasing deadbeats, etc. kept Shant busy 60 hours a week. All during this time, Shant remembered the words of his high school Spanish teacher, "It's nice to have a knowledge of Spanish, but you have to combine that knowledge with some other skill to make real money."

One morning, Shant's boss came into the large office room where the young attorneys worked and asked, "Who speaks Spanish?" Since many had been in the service, they knew not to volunteer for anything. After the third loud request, Shant meekly raised his hand. "Shant, come into my office," his supervisor said. Shant's life was about to change forever.

He was to be part of a team that dealt with telecommunications services to Latin America and the Caribbean. Shant spent the rest of his 20 years with AT&T handling legal matters involving primarily Spanish-speaking countries, including Mexico, Columbia, Venezuela, Spain, Puerto Rico, and the Dominican

Republic. Shant even went to Cuba in 1988, where he helped install the first modern submarine telephone cable from Florida to Havana. This system increased the telephone service between Cuba and the U.S. by tenfold, thereby allowing thousands of Cuban refugees in the U.S. to call their relatives back in their native country. Shant gained many friends during his time in foreign countries. He always felt his knowledge of their native tongue earned him respect and appreciation in their eyes, especially in business affairs. The words of his high school Spanish teacher turned out to be true!

Now happily retired from New Jersey to Georgia, to work on his golf game, Shant and I recently worked the long par five at our Kiwanis Golf Tournament. For a modest donation of $20 per foursome, the group was allowed a "Tiger Drive" of 325 yards. Most groups readily took advantage of the opportunity.

Shant often surprises the Spanish-speaking groundskeepers on the local course by bantering with them as we pass them on the fairway. I can only imagine their surprise. They usually give that look which says, "My God, a gringo who is fluent in Spanish. What were we talking about?"

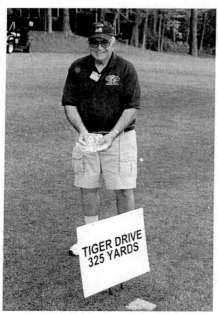

Shant Harootunian • 2009

Elective Surgery & Animal Cruelty

With the controversy about ear cropping and euthanasia raging in the veterinary press and lay publications such as *Dog Fancy*, it's no wonder the general public might rightly be confused.

I gave up ear cropping in the mid '70s. It was about the time the veterinary profession began to question the need or ethics of ear cropping and other cosmetic surgeries on animals. Most of my colleagues in Kenosha decided we would refrain from trimming ears. Clients we couldn't talk out of doing the surgery were referred to vets out of town, who gladly accepted the business.

It was about that time I was visited by Dr. Richard Crawford, a grade school classmate from suburban Illinois. Dr. Crawford had graduated from Kansas State Veterinary College, worked as a federal meat inspector and had recently opened an animal hospital in suburban Milwaukee. His practice was slow in attracting new clients. Since he knew I had learned how to do ear trims from my dad, Dr. A. C. Merrick, he wondered if I would show him how to master the art. I use the term "art" on purpose, because ear cropping is definitely an art form. There is much guess work on the part of the surgeon. Will this Boxer have a large head and need a more massive set of ears? Will this Schnauzer be dainty? Getting a look at the parents will help determine the end result the surgeon wants to achieve.

I told Dr. Crawford I would call him when I scheduled my next ear trim. He could observe and pick up the technique very easily. After the first few trials, he should have the technique down pat. I'd be available for consultation. When I decided to refrain from ear cropping, I sent all people who inquired to Dr. Crawford. Many of the local vets did likewise.

Many years later, in the mid '90s, I received a nice handwritten letter from Dr. Crawford thanking me for making his early retirement possible. He also included a thank you from his wife for the many travels they had enjoyed because of his expertise in ear cropping. Evidently, Dr. Crawford had become the ear crop expert of the Midwest. He frequently had two or three litters of pups to crop on the same day.

Ear crop surgery is an art. It's easy to botch the job so the dog will never look attractive. Beauty, of course, is in the eye of the beholder. I'm sure other dogs don't think it makes them any more handsome. In fact it may inhibit some of the "body signals" dogs send with their ears to other ani-

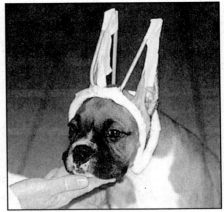

mals. I must admit, I had very mixed emotions while reading the letter. After reflection, I was at peace with my original decision.

I believe ear cropping will eventually go the way of firing in horses. This was a method of causing massive inflammation in the horses leg by inserting red hot needles into the affected tendons. The theory was this would stimulate better healing. Firing has been banned in many states and countries such as Great Britain. I can't really believe we were taught the firing techniques in vet school in the early '50s.

Declawing cats is another controversial subject. There are pros and cons, pluses and minuses. One side argues that cats should be left the way nature intended. This enables them to defend against attackers and rip expensive upholstery. I hardly ever removed all four claws, since cats do very little damage with their rear claws. About the time I started refusing to perform ear trims I also stopped doing declaws.

The surgery was crude and left the cat in considerable pain for a length of time. Sometime around the mid-eighties a new declaw technique was introduced, shown on the next page.

This involved removing the claw at a joint and closing the incision with medical Superglue. This technique has been modified by using a laser instead of a scalpel, with excellent results.

There are currently no federal laws concerning cruelty to animals. Each state and local governing body has their own set of statutes. This makes it easy for owners of "puppy mills" and others accused of animal abuse to simply move operations to another jurisdiction. Groups like the Humane Society and SPCA have long lobbied for action on a country-wide scale. Cases like the dog

New Declaw Operation for Your Pet

The conventional DECLAW procedure used nail clippers to cut off the claw at about the skin line. The incision was then closed with stitches. This method could cause extreme pain to the cat if the bone was shattered. Walking on sutures also caused discomfort. Regrowth of the nail was a possibility. It usually took a week for the cat to be walking normally again. For these reasons, Dr. Merrick refused to perform declaw surgery until the new Declaw method was introduced.

The new DECLAW operation (which we use at Merrick Animal Hospital) dissects the entire claw from the nailbed. Therefore, there is no shattered bone pain or possibility of regrowth. The incision is brought together with a new tissue adhesive (also used in human orthopedic surgery), that holds the skin together until healing takes place. This adhesive also has pain-killing and clotting effects on the tissue. The cat is usually back to normal within 24 hours after surgery.

DECLAW surgery is best performed at three months of age before the kitten has fully developed bone structure. It can also be done on older animals, especially when performing other surgeries such as castration or ovariohysterectomy.

DECLAW surgery is ususally done only on the front feet. By retaining the rear claws, the cat is able to climb a small tree or roll over an defend himself from attack by another animal.

fighting conviction of football star Michael Vick have highlighted the problem.

Modern "factory farming techniques" have magnified the scale of animal abuse. FactoryFarming.com describes factory farming as an attitude that regards animals and the natural world merely as commodities to be exploited for profit. Wikipedia states the following:

> Confinement at high stocking density requires antibiotics and pesticides to mitigate the spread of disease and pestilence exacerbated by these crowded living conditions. In addition, antibiotics are used to stimulate livestock growth by killing intestinal bacteria. There are differences in the way factory farming techniques are practiced around the world. There is a continuing debate over the benefits and risks of factory farming. The issues include the efficiency of food production; animal welfare; whether it is essential for feeding the growing global human population; the environmental impact and the health risks.

In animal agriculture, this attitude has led to institutionalized animal cruelty, massive environmental destruction, resource depletion, and human health risks. When most animals were raised on family farms, it was easier for the farmer to bond with his herd. I don't want to imply farm animals were treated like pets, but it was easier to identify with the individual in a herd of ten to twenty animals—be it chickens, pigs, horses or cattle. Factory farms often contain 30 to 50 thousand chickens, hundreds of con-

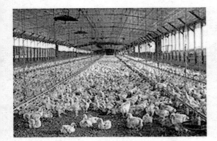 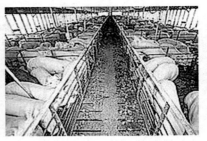

A commercial chicken house.   A gestational sow barn.

fined pigs, dozens of young male calves and hundreds of cattle. Downwind from a factory farm is often unbelievably nauseating.

Euthanasia is defined as "painless, easy death" or "painless death to avoid suffering." The practice in human medicine has come to the forefront in recent times. It has been practiced in animals since the advent of recorded history. I recall on the farm in the late thirties, my uncle killing our beloved farm collie with a rifle. Shep had developed a large growth on his front leg. When he could no longer move normally, there was no thought of taking him to the vet. Shep was an outside dog. He could hardly make it in and out of his doghouse, so Uncle Wendell decided to end his suffering and that was that. Sadness all around but no guilt.

In the mid '40s, I was employed as a kennel boy in Dad's animal hospital. Dad had read about electrocution as an alternative to the concentrated anesthetic we were using at the time. A client dropped off a young emaciated puppy suffering from distemper. Dad said he would take care of the euthanasia and disposal. He decided this pup would be a good subject to test his electrocution method. Dad and his assistant attached metal clips to each of the wires of a commercial extension cord. They proceeded to secure one clip to the anal area and the other to the nose of the semicomatose pup. Upon plugging the cord into the wall outlet, the pup gave a mighty yell and bounded off the table, seemingly no worse for the shock. In fact, it seemed to brighten his spirits. Dad concluded it was a sign that this little guy might survive. Thoughts of euthanasia were abandoned; therapy was in order. "Shocker" as he was named, was given to a new owner two weeks later, almost cured of his respiratory problems.

Our usual method of euthanasia was an overdose of Nembutal (sodium pentobarbital) anesthesia. One could buy a commercial bottle, but Dad made up his own. This was a throwback to his days as a farm vet where most vets made up many of their medicines. The powder was dissolved in saline to a strength ten times the normal anesthetic. This was then administered intravenously to the subject. Sleep was quick—within a matter of seconds—death was within a minute or two. This was easily done with most dogs. Cats were another matter. Dad found that a cat wrapped in a blanket was very calm. Injecting the drug through the blanket, directly into the heart, took only seconds and was easier on the animal and restrainer alike.

On one especially busy day, a cat was dropped off for euthanasia. He was placed in a cage in the cat ward. Hours passed and there was never a time when two people were available to perform the task. I decided, "Who needs two when I can do it myself?" The cat was an old calm male. After wrapping him in a blanket, I quickly injected the lethal dose into his chest. He immediately gave a loud cry and ejected himself into the air from the blanket restraint, turning and biting at the first thing he found. Unfortunately he chomped down on my right hand, causing a large laceration between my thumb and forefinger. Since that time, I've relayed the story, to clients who ask, of "My worst injury in practice was caused by a dead cat."

Euthanasia today is much more animal and people friendly. Most vets recommend counseling the whole family prior to the procedure. Many encourage family, including children, to witness the event. Usually a mild sedative is administered prior to the actual lethal injection. Struggles are rare, and death is indeed peaceful. There is still a lingering doubt in some quarters about the disposal of the body. A vet in a suburb north of Milwaukee was found to have used gravel from his parking lot to fill the urns returned to clients, instead of the actual cremains of deceased animals. He was fined and subsequently lost his license to practice for a time. Occasional stories in the paper like that and about bodies illegally given to universities for research attract attention. This has led most research groups to post the places they acquire cadavers.

Specialists & Pet Insurance

Be prepared to pay twice what you would in Kenosha, but I assure you, if Dr. Vainisi doesn't know how to cure Buffy's eye problem, no one in America does. Sam Vainisi was one of the first veterinary ophthalmologists in the country. Each week he traveled from his home in Denmark, Wisconsin, outside of Green Bay, to the Berwyn Animal Hospital in suburban Chicago, Illinois, and to the Milwaukee and Lincoln Park Chicago zoos. Dr. Vainisi regularly made the newspapers with photos of him treating an eye problem in a 9,000 pound elephant, Siberian tiger, or horned owl, but he mostly treated pets. Just as human medicine has produced ever-increasing numbers of specialties, veterinary medicine responded likewise to client demand for better services.

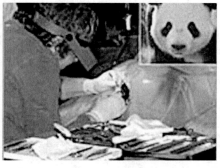

When the animal care staff at the Smithsonian Institution's National Zoo first noticed that Tian Tian (tee-YEN tee-YEN), the 10-year-old male giant panda, was suffering from an inflamed third eyelid in his right eye, the initial treatment was with a topical medication. When they realized that this did not resolve the inflammation, doctors performed an examination under anesthesia.

Dr. Nancy Bromberg, a veterinary ophthalmologist from SouthPaws Veterinary Specialist & Emergency Center in Fairfax, Virginia, removed the affected tissue. Veterinarians are now treating Tian Tian with antibiotic eye drops, and he is responding well.

As of 2010, the American Veterinary Medical Association (AVMA) lists 21 AVMA-recognized veterinary specialty organizations comprising 40 distinct specialties. More than 9,800 veterinarians have been awarded diplomate status in one or more of these 21 recognized veterinary specialty organizations by completing rigorous postgraduate training, education, and examination requirements. These board-certified specialists are ready to serve the public, its animals, and the veterinary profession by providing high quality service in disciplines as varied as internal medicine, surgery, preventive medicine, toxicology, dentistry, behavior, and pathology." Of the 90,000 veterinarians in the USA, more than 10% have advanced degrees.

Graduate veterinarians are trained to recognize and treat diseases in many species—horses, cattle, swine, sheep, dogs, cats, birds, and all manner of wild animals. No one can learn all there is to know about every animal, hence the need for limiting one's practice. Just as MDs undergo advanced training, vets are required to obtain advanced degrees and pass "boards" to qualify for certification as a specialist.

One of my great joys after 20 years of solo practice was having the ability to recommend a difficult case to a specialist in orthopedic surgery, ophthalmology, cardiology, or dermatology. Most professionals agree it's the wise doctor who knows his/her limitations.

For many years I would refer pets to specialists in Chicago, Milwaukee, or the vet school in Madison. There are now traveling surgeons who do their work in the local vet's hospital. This arrangement increases the chances of my patient being treated, because of the convenience for the client. Internal medicine specialists now routinely visit local practices and bring advanced portable ultrasound and other equipment to aid in the diagnosis of difficult cases. I sent patients with orthopedic problems to Chicago or the vet school in Madison. Each demanded a day of the client's time. Follow-ups could also be time consuming.

Meet Dr. Ianakov - OCSS

Most of our clients are aware of the excellent surgical procedures and facilities that we have here at Merrick Animal Hospital. We now have the services of "On Call Surgical Service." Dr. Lubomir S. Ianakov operates OCSS (On Call Surgical Service) out of Highland Park, Illinois and serves 60 veterinary practices in northeastern Illinois and southeastern Wisconsin. In the past 24 months, more than 1300 surgical cases were referred to OCSS.

On Call Surgical Service performs over 120 different surgical procedures and specializes in fracture pinning and plating, knee and hip problems, neurosurgeries, as well as soft tissue surgeries.

Dr. Ianakov's practice brings the surgical specialist to the patient rather than vice versa. This saves the owner the inconvenience of distant traveling, and allows the patient to be supervised by the veterinarian who is aware of the patient's clinical case history from the beginning to the end. Naturally the hospital is in a position to provide necessary recovery services, and most of all a "Completeness" in handling a surgical patient.

During the last ten years of practice, Dr. Lubomir S. Ianakov, an orthopedic and soft tissue veterinary surgeon had an "on-call surgical referral." He came to my hospital, bringing all the equipment he needed. I had only to provide the patient and a surgical suite. This eliminated the need for extensive out-of-town aftercare trips and enabled me to do the immediate after-care to my patient. I announced his availability in my newsletter.

There are many emergency clinics (ECs) around the country, usually open from 6 PM to 8 AM the following day. A number of these ECs have specialists in various fields who use the facility during daytime hours. This makes the specialists' services available to the local population and spreads the clinic expenses over a wider base, which in turn enables the clinic owners to keep fees as low as possible.

Some of the ECs in major cities are open 24 hours a day and are staffed by numerous specialists. These facilities treat pets following surgery at area vet clinics where all-night care is not available. They also provide care for cases that are beyond the capability of local vets.

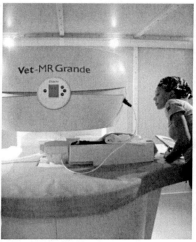

As a boarded orthopedic surgeon, Dr. Raymond Rudd saw complicated cases from the surrounding area. He recently expanded his animal hospital in my hometown of Peachtree City, Georgia to include a MRI and dental suite. He sold his practice to Veterinary Corporation of America (VCA) so he could spend a year in Afghanistan treating war dogs.

The demand for and ability to pay for diagnostic tests and state-of-the-art treatment has made the need for veterinary insurance greater than ever before. Jack L. Stevens, DVM, president and founder of Pet's Best Insurance stated in a recent article:

> The landscape for pet insurance has improved, primarily because of the basic principal necessary for all insurance—"risk transfer." There must be sufficient risk of not being able to afford to replace an item or restore health without insurance for the concept to be a viable option. As pet care costs continue to escalate, I predict not having pet insurance will be a greater risk than people are willing to accept or can comfortably afford.

When veterinary care was usually only a few hundred dollars for a serious illness or injury, there was little need for pet insurance. However, the environment for pet care has changed regarding the value of pets. In the past two decades pets are no longer disposable or simply replaced by a majority of pet owners. Today's pet owners increasingly view their pets as children or at least as important members of the family.

Treating the pet based on symptoms and experience (empirical care) is no longer the norm. Sophisticated diagnostics and treatments are expected and accepted by a greater number of pet owners. Euthanasia is becoming less of an option for bonded pet owners when health can be restored.

So far, the veterinary profession has avoided the quagmire involved in "managed care" human insurance. All popular vet insurance plans have the pet owner pay for the services in advance. The bills are then submitted, examined, and a reimbursement is made to the owner. Most plans return approximately 90% of the fees.

The Jan. 2, 2012, issue of *USA Today* reports, under the headline "Quirky perks for workers: Pet Insurance, Massages":

> Firms such as S. C. Johnson, TD Bank, and Travelocity provide discounted health coverage for workers' pets through Petplan Pet Insurance. "Petplan has seen tremendous growth in this area of voluntary benefits," co-CEO Chris Ashton says, "In this struggling economy, employers are increasingly looking for low-cost options to keep their employees happy."

The cost for an individual owner depends upon the age and breed of the pet, zip code, and deductible of $50, $100, or $200. The cost is typically between $1 and $2 per day. In 2011, my two-year-old lab/shep mix, Fritz, was quoted $49.92 per month—approximately $600 per year. This was the Gold Plan with no deductible—100% coverage for 100-pound Fritz.

Itch, Itch, Lick, and Scratch

Labor Day in Kenosha meant the school year was about to start, the annual Labor Day picnic would be held in Union Park, and the allergy season was upon us.

Duchess, our 100-plus-pound Lab/Shepherd alternated sleeping in bedrooms—Carol's and mine or one of the kids. As the fall progressed, her itching and licking increased and she was no longer a welcome sleeping companion. Flea powders and cortisone controlled her symptoms, but they were no cure. I determined to learn how to do allergy skin testing to enable me to control her dermatitis. The time was 1982.

John Kunzi, a friend and colleague, practiced in suburban Milwaukee, Wisconsin. He mentioned he had purchased the new allergy test kit and would be willing to test Duchess so I could learn the technique. The animal cannot be given steroids for two weeks prior to testing.

An area 6"×8" is shaved on the dog's chest, then 50 or 60 dots were applied with a mark stick, like stars on a flag. A bleb of prescribed injections was injected at each site, beginning with sterile water. The second injection is histamine. There should be an immediate reaction to histamine—reddening and swelling—but none to the sterile water. If there is no reaction to histamine, it indicates the animal has recently received steroids, and the rest of the test must be postponed until the steroid clears the system.

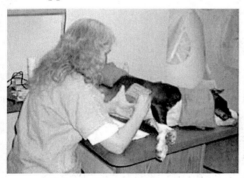

Skin testing for diagnosing environmental allergies

Next, a standardized group of allergens are injected—different ones for different areas of the country. Northern climate trees, grasses, weeds, kapok, and wool are used in the Midwest. In addition, extract injections of house dust mites and fleas are given.

Reactions of inflammation and swelling indicate the animal is allergic to the allergens injected. A vaccine is compounded of extracts of all the offending substances. Starting with minute quantities, the patient is given injections of ever increasing quantities over a two-month period. This allows the animal's body to build up an immunity to the various allergens. If the results are promising, the therapy is continued for two years. Positive clinical results are seen in approximately 80% of the cases.

Skin testing revealed Duchess was allergic to eight substances including weeds, fleas, and house dust mites. These mites are microscopic bugs that live in house dust by the millions.

I was encouraged by the beneficial results Duchess was showing her allergy treatment. I was determined to learn all I could, short of going back to school, about animal dermatology. While attending a dermatology seminar given by Dr. Kevin Schultz, I learned he was seeing patients twice a month at the Berwyn Animal Hospital (BAH).

BAH is a large small animal hospital in west suburban Chicago. At the time BAH had seven veterinarians and a staff of 32. BAH had six referral specialists flying in from around the country every month to treat area patients. Now, in 2011, there are 14 veterinarians on staff, many with advanced degrees in a dozen veterinary specialties. The staff has grown to 60, including 25 technicians.

Dr. Les Fisher sold the BAH to Dr. Herb Lederer in 1970 when Dr. Fisher became Director of the Lincoln Park Zoo in Chicago. The practice was growing and needed to expand or find a new building. About that time a suspicious fire gutted a large supper club a block south of BAH. The person or persons who torched the building were never found. Rumor had it the owners forgot to pay their "mob dues." In any event, Dr. Lederer was able to purchase the burned-out building, remodel it, and move his practice down the street into a state-of-the-art facility. He kept the old building and remodeled it into a pet store.

Dr. Schultz readily agreed to my request to shadow him for a couple of days. This turned into a bimonthly ritual which lasted over a year.

Dr. Schultz saw as many as 25 to 30 patients a day, rotating among three of the eight BAH exam rooms. While one dog was resting following his skin test, another owner was being grilled to elicit a full, specific history, and the third was in the process of receiving discharge instructions. I assisted wherever I could and

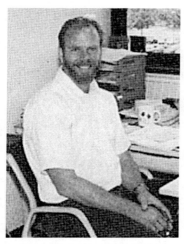

Kevin Schultz, DVM, PhD

took copious notes. I felt I was in a "master class" similar to one Socrates could have taught 2,000 years ago. Dr. Schultz later used his many talents to guide research at Merial, Ltd., where he served as Chief Scientific Officer and Global Head of Research and Development until his retirement in 2008. He is currently the Chief Scientific Officer of Tyra Tech.

As I developed a reputation as a "skin" specialist" in Kenosha, my records revealed fully 20% of the animals I treated had symptoms of skin disease. I stressed to any referred clients that I had an "interest" in dermatology, but I was not a board-certified specialist.

About that time I went with Carol to see our human dermatologist, Dr. Sydney Kaplan. When Dr. Kaplan started his specialty practice in 1960, he had office hours in Racine and Kenosha, Wisconsin, and Waukegan, Illinois. He would spend one or two days a week in each city. There were not enough referrals to support a single location. Twenty years later he could afford to spend all of his time in Waukegan, since patients were then willing and able to travel.

I mentioned to Sydney, whom Carol and I now considered a friend, my growing interest in veterinary dermatology. Dr. Kaplan replied, "John, you must go back to medical school and get your specialty in dermatology. Believe me, I've got the best job in the world. My patients never have middle-of-the-night emergencies, they never die, and when they're unhappy with me—no blame—they just go see my colleague Harry Schwartz. How can you beat that?" I had to admit, it sounded tempting, but I had too many mouths to feed and couldn't afford to take an extended sabbatical.

Some of the things I've learned about animal dermatology are:
1. Contact allergy causes the most intense itching. Many animals are very sensitive to ScotchGard. If people didn't wear clothes, no one would use it. I recommended clients provide a cotton throw to allow their animal to avoid the product.
2. Food allergies are difficult to diagnose. It is recommended to start with one product—cooked rice. After two weeks, add one

food weekly. If the allergy returns, eliminate the offending item. Then add another item, slowly working up to a balanced diet the patient can tolerate.
3. Common signs of allergy are "face rubbing" and "paw licking."
4. Skin infections commonly follow allergy. They need vigorous, long-term treatment.
5. Poor treatment results are often due to thyroid deficiency in dogs. Low thyroid levels subject the animal to more skin infections.

My advice is the same now as ten years ago. When in doubt, consult a specialist. Both you and your pet will appreciate their services. When I sent clients' difficult cases to Dr. Schultz, or any other specialist, I counseled them as follows, "Expect to pay twice what you do in Kenosha, but if Dr. Schultz can't solve Buffy's skin problem, no one in the country can. You can be satisfied you've done everything you can for your baby."

Allergy Testing Available

Most of us know someone who has allergies and the symptoms of sneezing, wheezing, and itching that can be so miserable. But more and more people are surprised to find out that another kind of friend can have allergies, too. Our pets! Although it usually affects dogs, cats can have allergies, too.

Pets with allergies usually do not wheeze and cough, but they do a lot of itching. They will scratch, lick, and bite at themselves to relieve the itching and this in turn can lead to open sores with secondary bacterial infection. It can become and unending cycle.

There are three types of pet allergies. Flea Allergy Dermatitis, caused by the saliva from fleas; Allergic Inhalant Dermatitis, caused by airborne irritants such as pollens, mold spores, house dust, etc., and food allergies, caused by any number of things that pets eat.

Food allergies can usually be cleared up by putting your pet on a special restricted, hypoallergenic diet. About three weeks away from the food allergen will give the skin time to heal and confirm the diagnosis of a food allergy.

Flea and skin allergies can best be determined by skin testing. Dr. Merrick has been skin testing for allergies during the past year. Experience has shown that winter is the best time to test as the animal's body has had a chance to recover from its reaction to whatever weed or grass or tree caused the allergy.

The testing procedure only takes about one hour. Antihistamines or cortisones given to prevent symp-

Mary, and a cooperative "Cricket", await results from an allergy test.

This appeared in my 1985 newsletter

Petco & Animal Hospital of Oshkosh

Welcome to Pet Food Warehouse Stadium in beautiful San Diego to watch the Chargers NFL team play. That would have been a mouthful if the PFW hadn't changed their name to Petco in 1997.

My practice was growing, but too slowly for me. I wanted to hire a full-time associate but couldn't afford one. I read an article in *DVM Magazine,* a monthly trade journal, about a new concept—vaccination clinics in Pet Food Warehouse stores located in shopping centers across the country. Calling the company produced the name of the veterinarian in charge of clinics in the Midwest. Carol and I soon visited Dr. Joel Locketz at his clinic in Minneapolis, Minnesota. In exchange for using the PFW stores as vaccination clinics, I would pay Dr. Locketz a small percentage of my gross. He in turn paid half of his fee to PFW.

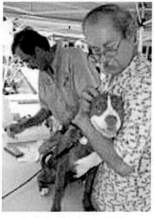
Petco Vaccination Clinic

Visiting one of the seven clinics Dr. Locketz operated around the Twin Cities convinced us this was a "no-brainer." The clinic was scheduled to run from 7 to 9 PM. We arrived at 6:30 to set up and found 12 people, pets in hand, already in line. Joel and his assistants would see 32 pets that evening.

Over the next few years my association with PFW—now Petco—proved to be the best practice builder I'd ever had. New potential clients moving into town would make Petco one their first stops. My handouts were on every checkout counter. Posters advertised the next vaccination clinic. We also drew blood for heartworm testing. Heartworms had recently become a major health problem in the northern Illinois/southern Wisconsin area. This also provided a service to clients who couldn't come to the animal hospital during daytime business hours. Only cursory examinations were done. If a problem was noted, we recommended they take their pet to their own vet for diagnosis and treatment. Naturally, many of these pets became long-time patients of mine.

Soon after I began my vaccination clinic in Kenosha, Dr. Locketz called for advice. Petco had recently opened stores in Oshkosh and Appleton, in the Fox Valley, 75 miles north of Milwaukee. He was getting very negative feedback from local vets about operating a vaccination clinic. In fact, he reported the local vet association had voted to "blackball" anyone who operated in the Petcos. I called a couple of vet friends and received the same news. No one was willing to break ranks.

My experience in establishing clinics in Petco stores in Kenosha had been very positive. It seemed to be a plus for my clients and my bottom line. My business grew by 22% the first year I was with Petco. Such business expansion is unheard-of in an established practice. The vaccination clinics provided a service to clients who were unable to bring in their pets during normal 8-to-5 office hours and appealed to clients who were unwilling or unable to afford full-service veterinary care. The hours were Tuesday evening from 7 to 9 PM and Saturday from 1 to 3 PM. Tracking the source of new clients is an established good business practice. The Yellow Pages advertising and my own clients always topped my new client referral list, until Petco became our leading client referral, by far.

With these facts in mind, I was sure I could easily convince one the local Oshkosh–Appleton veterinarians to establish a vaccination clinic. I was wrong. After talking to a couple of veterinary acquaintances in the area, I was surprised at the animosity and anger expressed by the idea of offering something that might limit their practice.

This confrontation reminded me of a somewhat similar incident which took place in the same general area some twenty years earlier. A client in the Green Bay area called up his veterinarian to inquire about prices to euthanize his aging spaniel. When informed by the receptionist of the fee of $25.00, he remarked, "Wow, that seems awfully high, I'll call around to get other prices." "Don't bother," the receptionist stated, "everyone has the same price." "You must be mistaken," the man replied. "No, that's everyone's price," she stated, "all the vets got together and set the price a couple of years ago." Bad mistake! The client happened to be in charge of the regional IRS office. Legal action ensued, with the IRS threatening to suspend all the veterinarians' licenses. Eventually, the individuals were put on probation for a time and fined a few thousand dollars each. The government was sending a message: "We will not tolerate price fixing, whether it concerns airline tickets, drug prices, or professional services."

Dr. Neil Rechsteiner of Green Bay purchased Dr. Bill Horne's practice. He related the following.

> The interesting story about the Green Bay veterinarians is true. I think the story happened in the early 1970s before my time, but Bill Horne told me the same story many years ago. Bill said the same thing about the receptionist quoting an euthanasia fee and the stating that every veterinarian in town was the same price. I think Bill said it was a State investigation and all the veterinarians were called together for a meeting with the investigators. Most of the veterinarians were not very concerned, except Bill. Bill hired an attorney to come to the meeting with him. At the meeting, all the veterinarians realized how severe the problem was, and they all hired Bill's attorney right after the meeting. I do not know about the fines or penalties that resulted. I think they were minor and the State required that every veterinarian agree to never discuss fees with each other again. This was unfortunate, because prior to this problem, everyone in town were close friends and talked together frequently. After the problem, they broke off their close communications and the friendships weakened. Interesting!
>
> — Best Wishes, Neil

In relating the story to an MD friend, he asked, "How do oil companies get away with the same thing? Every gas station in town raises and lowers prices within minutes of each other." "Good question," I replied, "I don't have an answer. I imagine they must do it in a way which bypasses government regulations."

My son, David, worked at the time for a veterinary distributor, selling drugs over the entire state. He volunteered to talk to a couple of friends who owned vet practices

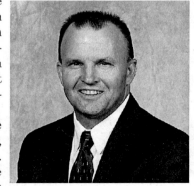

David Merrick • 1999

in the Oshkosh-Appleton area. He was surprised at the hostility they expressed.

David called me shortly afterward with the news that a young, experienced vet was looking to move from her present position as an associate vet in a town near Oshkosh. Dave arranged a luncheon meeting with Dr. Diane Grede. She immediately dispelled any doubts as to her ability or desire to have her own practice. She also lived just a few miles from Oshkosh. We decided she would keep her day job while I lined up a building, equipment, and most importantly, financing. I had started an outpatient clinic on the other side of Kenosha 20 years before, so I knew what it would take to build a full-time practice.

Building a stand-alone animal hospital was beyond my means. I did not have any desire to build something I could not control from 120 miles away. The local realtor I hired proved to be experienced and well connected to money supplies. The bank he recommended agreed to lend me $50,000 after the three-year business plan I presented showed a break-even point after 24 months. In short order, I was able to lease 2,000 square feet in a new mini strip mall, across the interstate highway from the Oshkosh airport. Oshkosh is famous for the world's largest Fly-In Convention.

EAA Air Venture Oshkosh (the new name for the Fly-In Convention, as of 1998) now serves as one of the world's premier aviation events, attracting top government officials, corporate leaders, and hundreds of thousands of aviation enthusiasts. It spans the entire spectrum of aviation and attracts 10,000 airplanes each year. The more than 500,000 aviation enthusiasts who attend the event annually supply the local and state economies with more than a $110 million boost during the week-long summer event. The air show is seven days long and typically begins on the last Monday in July. The Wittman Regional Airport control tower is the busiest control tower in the world during the gathering.

The site I intended to lease and remodel was not zoned for an animal hospital. My application for a zoning variance was approved by the Oshkosh Planning Commission.

The Oshkosh Northwestern newspaper reported on November 8, 1997, "Kenosha Man Hopes to Get Paws on Washburn Site." The article stated the need for a veterinary clinic in the area and had the backing of the Oshkosh Development Corp. I was quoted as saying, "It's hard to start out on your own right after vet school because of the high costs involved. This is a wonderful opportunity for this person." The article continues, "Merrick intends to hire a vet to run the new animal hospital and sell it to them in three or four years." This timetable proved to be accurate. The Animal Hospital of Oshkosh opened in the spring of 1998 and was sold to Dr. Diane Grede in July, 2001.

The executive director of the Oshkosh Commercial Development Corp. said the animal clinic adds a dynamic to the west side. The zoning change passed unanimously. With David's help, I was able to open the doors of the Animal Hospital of Oshkosh in the spring of 1998, just short of one year from start to finish. Dr. Grede had begun the vaccination clinic hours at the local Petco two months earlier, so she had a small client base before actually opening the practice.

As with most new businesses, I had underestimated the capital required to get the Animal Hospital of Oshkosh (AHO) into a positive cash flow. Each month, however, showed a steady growth. In our initial conversations, I told Dr. Grede that I had no intention of keeping the practice more than three or four years. I hoped to get a return on my initial investment and maybe a little extra profit.

After two and a half years, AHO was profitable. Dr. Grede reminded me of my "promise." My recollection was of a "goal," not a promise. Nevertheless, I began to figure exactly what the practice was worth. As usually occurs, Dr. Grede thought my asking price was much too high and in turn, I couldn't believe how little she valued the practice. David counseled both of us. "In twenty years of dealing with owners and associate vet buying practices," he said, "every associate thought they paid too much and every owner thought they received too little." We managed to settle in the middle range, with neither of us too happy or sad.

Because of her dedication and hard-working associates and staff, Dr. Grede was able to purchase the lot next door and build an ultramodern 5,000 square foot animal hospital.

In 2006 the Oshkosh Chamber of Commerce presented the Animal Hospital of Oshkosh with its Small Business of the Year award during its 99th annual meeting. The Oshkosh Northwestern newspaper reported the event as follows: "In the midst of flat panel monitors and high-tech equipment, Dr. Grede and the staff of 18 continue to mix old-fashioned, patient-centered care with the latest advances in veterinary medicine."

By 2011, AHO's staff had grown from Dr. Grede and three lay staff members to four associate veterinarians and 22 lay staff members. Again, good guys finish first.

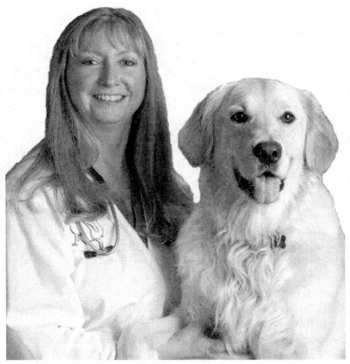

Diane K. Grede, DVM, and Hazel • 2011

Noah's Ark—Lion, Tiger, and Bear

"Lions, and tigers, and bears—oh my!" No Dorothy, this isn't Kansas. This lion, tiger, and bear are living in Noah's Ark, an animal rehab center in Locust Grove, Georgia, 20 miles south of Atlanta. Rescued eight years ago during a police drug raid in Atlanta, the three furry friends were only two-month-old cubs at the time. They had been obtained as "status symbol pets" by the drug lords. Attempts to separate the youngsters led to crying, wailing, and hunger strikes, so the staff decided to see if these three large carnivores could be raised together. Eight years later, Baloo, a 1000-pound bear, Shere Khan, a 350-pound tiger, and Leo, a 400-pound lion, are still the best of friends. They eat, sleep, and play together in their two-acre yard with private "clubhouse." Their celebrity status has earned them spots on *The Today Show* and *National Geographic* TV.

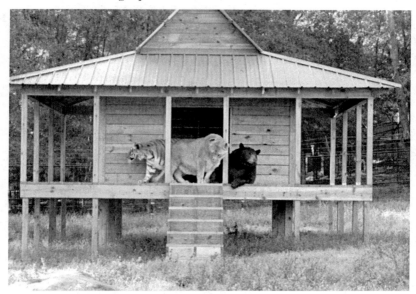

Shere Khan, Leo, and Baloo on their clubhouse porch

This unique facility, founded in 1978 by Jama Hedgecoth, also features a children's care home. As the name implies, the organization was founded to protect children and animals from abuse and neglect. It relies solely on donations; admission is free. As a result, the Ark is a favorite for school and church groups. Many bring picnic lunches to enjoy on the spacious grounds. An estimated 100,000 people tour the facility each year, learning about wildlife protection, preservation, and conservation. With over 200 acres, Noah's Ark provides a nurturing sanctuary for more than 1,000 animals. The cost to feed them is more than $10,000 per month. In 2008, the Ark turned away more than 1,200 animals due to lack of adequate funding to support and provide habitats for them.

Recently, three tigers were given a new home at Noah's Ark when a small traveling circus closed down. They are slowly adapting to their new environment outside of their previous cage confinement.

On a recent visit, Diane Smith, assistant to Director Jana Hedgecoth, made me aware of an unusual case. Goats can have from one to five kids. Twins are the most common birth rate. Four or five is somewhat rare. A goat had delivered four babies earlier in the month. One was still born, two were normal births, and one was dystocia (difficult, delayed birth). Circulation had been compromised to the rear quarters during delivery of the last kid. The baby goat was not able to use her rear legs, dragging herself by her forelegs. At first the mother ignored the infant. Animals seem to sense that a cripple will not survive, so they don't waste time or energy caring for them—preferring to care for those who have a better chance of survival. Eventually, as the baby continued to crawl around and attempt to nurse, the mother and staff became involved in its care.

After surgery to amputate both rear legs below the knee, the baby goat, now named Mollie Mae, continued her daily improvement. Her appetite and exercise, though limited by her condition, were excellent. The staff was surprised one morning to observe Mollie Mae attempting to walk upright on her front legs, like a gymnast running across the floor on her hands. Within a few days Mollie Mae was "running around" chasing her siblings and Mom.

Ms. Smith asked if I had access to some kind of device to assist Mollie Mae in getting around. My first thought was to construct a "rickshaw" similar to ones I made for dogs with paraplegia while in practice. By combining aluminum rods with wagon wheels from Ace Hardware, I could make a device which allowed the animal to pull itself around by their front feet. Ten years into retirement, I had no access to materials or the ability to construct something that would need to be expanded as Mollie Mae grew.

"Handicapped Pets" came to our rescue. Located in Nashua, New Hampshire, HP manufactures "Walkin' Wheels" for pets of all sizes. They will adjust without tools to fit animals (mostly dogs) from 20 to over 100 pounds. They even offered a courtesy discount because of the Ark's charity status.

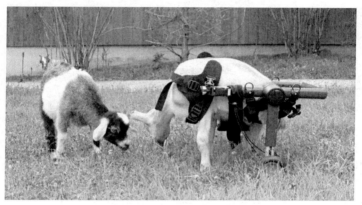

Maggie Mae with her new wheels

Approaching full growth at one year of age, Mollie Mae is an especial favorite of wheelchair-bound visitors. She typifies the dream of Noah's Ark founder, Jana Hedgecoth. As a four-year-old girl, Jana dreamed of taking care of animals and children that were unwanted, to provide them a "home" in every sense of the word, and to allow anyone to see them "for free." Her dream became reality.

St. Andrews and Mr. James Herriot

Honoring Mr. James A. Wight

While all Muslims must visit Mecca in their lifetime, veterinarians should visit Trisk, in North Yorkshire, England.

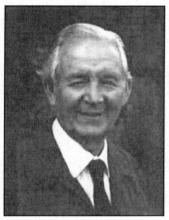

Mr. James A. Wight (James Herriot)

Veterinarians around the world can thank James Wight for the incalculable good he did for our profession with his stories about veterinary practice in pre–World War II northern England. Because of restrictions on advertising, Mr. James Wight chose a pen name (James Herriot) of a famous football (soccer) star when publishing his work. Only MDs and PhDs were allowed to use the title "Doctor." Other professionals were called "Mister." People with royal titles were addressed as "Sir."

In the United States, Wight's books were considered too short to be published separately, so several pairs of novels were spliced into larger volumes. The title, *All Creatures Great and Small,* was taken from the second line of the hymn, "All Things Bright and Beautiful," after a suggestion by Wight's daughter, who thought the book should be called *Ill Creatures Great and Small.* Stories abound from veterinarians visiting Dr. Herriot's Surgery (clinic) and being surprised to be given the grand tour by the man himself. No super ego here, just mutual respect for a colleague. Fortunately, his son, James Jr., joined him in practice and was able to relieve some of his professional burdens.

His is a story about pride, and honor, and respect, and dedication, and morality, and integrity, and veracity, and principle, and humility. Mr. Wight represented those qualities of character as well as anyone could have imagined. He described to an adoring world audience the demands and rewards of the average veterinarian. No superdoc, just your average guy with an extraordinary talent of dealing with the two and four legged animals that came his way.

I know very few veterinarians who also wouldn't be given very high marks on those qualities. Why is this? Physicians used to be held in that kind of esteem by the general public, but no more. The average MD now pays up to $20,000 per year in malpractice insurance. Veterinarians (except equine) pay less than $500. I believe it's the same quality of spirit that makes better people/clients out of individuals that care for creatures and share their homes and lives with them. This innate sense of compassion for another sets them apart. Veterinarians are fortunate to interact on a daily basis with these individuals.

I believe this helps account for the 70% acceptance rate of women in vet school applications over the last few years. Women are nurturers by nature. Men, in general, are drawn to professions where they can make more money. The need to be able to support a family surely enters into their decision. As more women live independently, the wage gap will close.

To Trisk and St. Andrews

Herriot's former Surgery at 23 Kirkgate, Thirsk is now the "World of James Herriot" tourist attraction.

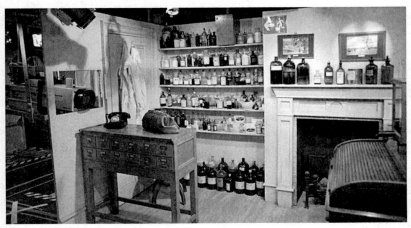

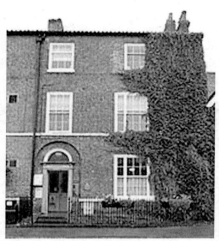

With the preceding as a prologue, my brother, Phil, and I drove our rental car the short two-hour drive from Birmingham to Trisk in April, 2009. Phil, a retired tour business operator, had made reservations at the The Gallery bed and breakfast next door to Herriot's Surgery. Phil had spent some of his 32-year Regular Army career in England, but he had not been to St. Andrews. Trisk, a typical north England town, is right on the way from Birmingham, England to St. Andrews, Scotland. Narrow streets are lined with adjacent homes and businesses. Herriot's Surgery was exactly as seen on the PBS Television production which ran for seven years. This was due to erecting an exact duplicate of Herriot's Surgery adjacent to the original, which incorporated lights and microphones to produce quality television. The original Surgery is now called The James Herriot Museum. Included in the museum are the actual primitive tools and instruments used by vets 60 to 70 years ago. Video clips are available showing what vet practice was like in pre-war England. I know of no better way to see what advancements have been made in medical practice in the last century. The visit to Trisk was a pleasant prologue to our golf at St. Andrews. The trip of a lifetime—a visit to my hero's home and the home of golf. Who could ask for more? Well... maybe a little better weather.

Phil and I arrived at the first tee of the "Old Course" at 10:00 AM for an eleven o'clock tee time. The early May day had started out cold and wet. For the uninitiated, no one is allowed in the St. Andrews club house except members. No one is permitted in the caddy quarters except caddies and employees. Guests and golfers are left out in the weather. We'd called ahead to inquire about the weather, thinking golfing might be cancelled due to the forecast. No such luck.

"This is St. Andrews," replied the starter, "We rarely cancel. It's a little misty today, ..." (translation: occasional heavy rain) "... a little chilly, ..." (45°F.) "... and a little windy" (20 to 30 miles per hour). Burrrrrr! When our tee time arrived, the group ahead consisted of four middle-aged local ladies. No buggies (motorized golf carts) are allowed at St. Andrews, so they each pulled a trolley (golf cart). One after another they drove their ball 150 yards down the middle of the first fairway. I said to Phil, " If those gals can do it, so can we." Phil replied, "This is St. Andrews." And off we went.

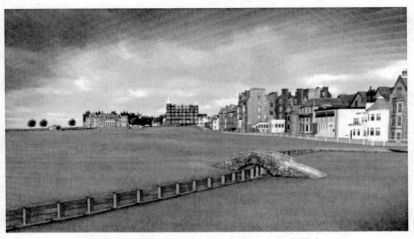

The Old Course is home to *The Road Hole,*
the 17th, one of the world's most famous golf holes.

Masters 2009–2011

Ginger's voice sounded concerned. "Dad, are you sitting down?" My first thought pictured one of my grandchildren in an auto accident. "Who's hurt and how bad?" I responded. "Nothing like that, Ginger replied, " I have two tickets to the Masters this Sunday." I could hardly believe my ears. Ginger sounded serious, and she rarely plays practical jokes. I told her, "Yes, I'm sitting down. Give me all the details."

Ginger, my second daughter, lives an hour north of me in suburban Atlanta. She is currently in charge of ReLo for Coca Cola Refreshment. As such, she moves hundreds of Coke employees around the world every year. It seems that one of the major national legal firms—who has Coke as one of their top clients—sponsors "A Week at the Masters" every year for 100 of their best friends. The executive who was to have received our two tickets had gotten an ultimatum from his wife. "If you desert me and the kids again this spring, be sure and pack well, because I'll throw everything you leave out on the street." He got the message and Ginger got the tickets.

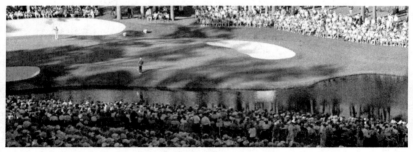

For non-golfers, Wikipedia describes the golf tournament:
The Masters Tournament, also known as "The Masters" (sometimes referred to as "The U.S. Masters "outside of the United States) is one of the four major championships in professional golf.

Scheduled for the first full week of April, it is the first of the majors to be played each year. Unlike the other major championships, the Masters is held each year at the same location, Augusta National Golf Club, a private golf club in the city of Augusta, Georgia, USA. The Masters was started by Clifford Roberts and Bobby Jones.

Jones designed Augusta National with course architect Alister MacKenzie. The tournament is an official money event on the PGA Tour, the PGA European Tour, and the Japan Golf Tour. The field of players is smaller than those of the other major championships because it is an invitational event, entry being controlled by the Augusta National Golf Club. The tournament has a number of traditions. A green jacket has been awarded to the winner since 1949, which must be returned to the clubhouse after a year.

The idea for Augusta National originated with Bobby Jones, who wanted to build a golf course after his retirement from the game. He sought advice from Clifford Roberts, who later became the chairman of the club. They came across a piece of land in Augusta, Georgia, of which Jones said: "Perfect! And to think this ground has been lying here all these years waiting for someone to come along and lay a golf course upon it." Jones hired Alister MacKenzie to design the course, and work began in 1931. The course formally opened in 1933, but MacKenzie died before the first Masters Tournament was played.

As with the other majors, winning the Masters gives a golfer several privileges which make his career more secure. Masters champions are automatically invited to play in the other three majors (the U.S. Open, the British Open, and the PGA Championship) for the next five years, and earn a lifetime invitation to the Masters. They also receive membership on the PGA Tour for the following five seasons and invitations to The Players Championship for five years.

Because the tournament was established by the amateur golfer Bobby Jones, the Masters has a tradition of honoring amateur golf. It invites winners of the most prestigious amateur tournaments in the world. Also, the current U.S. Amateur champion always plays in the same group as the defending Masters champion for the first two days of the tournament.

Although badges (tickets) for the Masters are not expensive, they are very difficult to come by. Even the practice rounds can be difficult to get into. Applications for practice round tickets have to be made nearly a year in advance and the successful applicants are chosen by random ballot. Tickets to the actual tournament are sold only to members of a patron's list, which is closed. A waiting list for the patron's list was opened in 1972 and closed in 1978. It was reopened in 2000 and subsequently closed once again. In 2008, the Masters also began allowing children between the ages of 8 and 16 to enter on tournament days free if they are accompanied by the patron who is the owner of his or her badge.

Every golfer I know would give anything, except his favorite putter, just to be able to attend a practice round. Masters tickets aren't impossible to find, but they are among the toughest tickets in all of sports to get. And if you are able to find Masters tickets, it will probably require a lot of money—perhaps even thousands of dollars—to purchase one.

But there is some good news: During tournament week at the 2011 Masters, Augusta National announced it was making a small number of tournament tickets available for the 2012 Masters, with a random drawing following online registration. The club also announced changes in how it handles practice-round ticket requests.

Unlike the other golf majors, the Masters has very tight restrictions on the number of Masters badges that are available. It is virtually impossible to buy Masters golf tickets directly from Augusta National, so it makes a lot of sense to get an all-inclusive Masters package from one of the many sports ticket agencies.

This was the back story to my surprise and shock when Ginger called. I could hardly believe my ears. Masters tickets! Not for practice rounds, but for the final day on Sunday. She had already made reservations for a motel room 20 miles west of Augusta. Everything closer was booked months in advance. We drove for three hours through the budding Georgia spring. Cherry trees and azaleas were in full throat, shouting, "Look at me. Aren't I the prettiest plant you've ever seen?" The grass was just beginning to lose its winter look of faded beige. The motel was our first—and only—disappointment. We learned firsthand why they had a few rooms available. A broken lock on the front door, torn curtains, faint odor of tobacco and other drugs were in the air. We were determined not to shower and slept in our clothes on top of the faded blankets. I wished I'd brought some insecticide to neutralize any possible bedbugs.

Shortly after dawn we were up and on our way to "Breakfast at the Masters." Our tickets (badges) were to include parking in the tennis court of an estate across from gate #9. The entrance was modest by modern mansion standards. We were greeted by multiple hosts and hostesses, our cameras and cell phones were requested (confiscated), and we were shown to the huge tent attached to the sunroom. Tuxedoed waiters served whatever one's heart desired. The Waldorf couldn't have put on a better spread. We were told to make ourselves at home whenever we felt the need for food or refreshment all day long. Within an hour we were on the course, passing row upon row of cars parked inside the fence, 400 yards from fairways. Upon leaving the parking area, we went through a security check similar to airport screening. We were informed that cell phones, cameras, and recording devices were not allowed inside the grounds. Anyone found with recording devices would immediately be expelled and his badge confiscated. The patron who sold us his badge would also lose it permanently.

I wanted to be on the second fairway by 9 AM. John Merrick was to tee off at 8:50, and I wanted to see my namesake in person.

Both John and his playing partner hit drives of 300 yards, approach shots of 170 yards and two-putted for pars. The pros make it look so easy—smooth swing, perfect follow through, and a touch of the cap to polite applause. Actually, it's a wonderful coincidence that a golfer of the same name was in contention for the Master's crown in 2009.

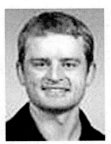

John S. Merrick
Age 29 • Long Beach, Calif.

I tell my friends I wish the golf genes worked in reverse so I could inherit some of the young man's talent. John was two under par at the time, about 16th place.

Ginger and I made it our mission to find a weed on the Masters grounds. After looking on and off all day, there was not one to be found—zippo, nada. The Masters has a weed patrol that's beyond anything I've ever witnessed. Most people have seen parts of the Masters tournament telecast for the last 30 years on CBS. The pristine nature of the surroundings has been wonderfully described many times. Believe me, Augusta National Golf Course is more spectacular in person. After three hours of tramping around to see as many of the pros as possible, we headed back for lunch. Again, all you could eat and more. Our table companions were two gentlemen from Calgary, Canada. They were oil people who were clients of the legal team that supplied our tickets. I inquired about their opinion of the Canadian Health

System. They both heartily endorsed it. "Of course, you need to get private supplemental insurance," one said.

Back on the course, we sat in the large bleachers adjacent to the 11th green and 12th tee. To our astonishment, my name was at the top of the huge "leader board." John Merrick, leading the Masters at 8 under par. John had managed to shoot 66, the low round of the day, and finished tied for sixth place. What mixed emotions I felt—happy to see "my" name on the leader board, and sad, because I was unable to get a picture for posterity. We left as the three-way playoff began.

The crowds were 30 to 40 deep. I'm sure the people at home watching on TV got a better view than 99% of the spectators.

The Masters came into my life again this year—2011.

Doctor Bill Walker had passed after a six month battle recovering from surgery to remove a cyst on his lower spine. Bill was 91 and had served in the Air Force, making 65 Atlantic crossings ferrying planes to the war zone and wounded troops back home in WWII. After the war, the GI Bill allowed him to become the first in his family from Huntsville, Alabama to graduate from college. Bill practiced dentistry in suburban Atlanta for 35 years, retiring to traveling and golf in 1985.

Bill first purchased Masters tickets in 1955. At the time badges were easy to buy and cost $15.00 per day. Every year Bill would receive a fresh batch of tickets. On the days he and his wife, Billie (Elizabeth), couldn't attend, friends or family were happy to go. Bill had a house (cottage) in the northeast Georgia mountains, 150 miles from Atlanta. His wife had recently died following two years of fighting lung cancer. Afterward Bill spent the bulk of his time in the home of my good friends, Dr. Richard and Judith Moore. Richard recently retired from his OB/GYN practice, leaving it the hands of two of their three MD daughters. Judith had worked as a financial and legal analyst for the FHLB (Federal Home

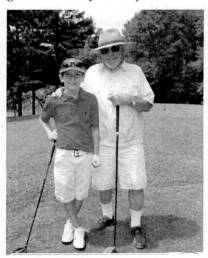

Bill Walker with his great grandson, Eli Presberg

Loan Bank) and the FSLIC (Federal Savings and Loan Insurance Corporation in the late 1980s.

Prior to his illness, Bill played nine holes of golf three or four times a week. I'm sure he was an excellent golfer in his younger days. He scored near 50 every nine holes we played. Bill's death occurred one month prior to the Masters of 2011. This would be the last time the family could attend, as there is no longer any "legacy" plan to pass on tickets from deceased badge holders. Judith called me to see if I would house/farm-sit their animals. Included on their 69 acres are four horses, one pony, one goat, 20 free-range chickens, one house dog (Wendy), one house cat (Grey Socks) and three barn cats (No Name One, Two, and Three). Richard and Judith don't count the deer, foxes, coyotes or raccoons as part of their menagerie. I was to live in their house and feed and care for the dog, cats, and chickens while the family was in Augusta. A next door neighbor, Keith Varnado, was in charge of the remaining large farm animals.

Richard informed me that he and Judith were taking two of their horses with them so they could ride while other family enjoyed the golf. They were renting the "guest house" on an estate a short distance north of Augusta. Their horses were stabled in a friend's barn. The remaining horses were all little shy until they discovered the carrots I brought every AM and PM. Then they followed wherever I went, except in the henhouse to gather eggs.

The first day was uneventful until I was awakened by a violent thunderstorm after midnight. All electricity was off. I called Richard to get directions for a flashlight. Their mixed Lab, Wendy, was a little too heavy to jump up on the bed, so she settled for hiding underneath. Morning revealed the damage: three large pine trees brought down. One massive tree fell across the fence gate leading to the barn, ending up within three feet of the structure. Even the fence was spared by the huge lower limbs preventing the trunk from falling completely to the ground. Chopping the three downed trees into logs created a pile of sawdust 35′ long, 10′ wide and 12′ high. Richard plans to use it to fill in low spots all over the farm. The horses and goat were in their stalls during the storm, since there was no bed handy for them to crawl under.

The remaining days were quiet except for the rooster, who threatened to attack every time I came near any of his harem. The hens were unconcerned and continued to lay a dozen eggs every day. I gave farm-fresh eggs to all my neighbors that week. They were sorry to see an end to my adventure "back on the farm."

New Zealand—Animals and Gardens Down Under

Saturday morning, 6 to 10 AM in Atlanta. It's time to wake up and listen to Walter Reeves, "The Georgia Gardner" on the radio. Walter dispenses advice to amateur and master gardeners alike with good humor and knowledge gained from a lifetime of gardening experience, beginning with his growing up on the family farm near Atlanta, Georgia. Since I'm an early riser and a recent master gardener, I listen to Walter as often as possible. In the spring of 2010, Walter announced he was planning a trip to New Zealand. The first 40 people who signed up would be invited to go along. I jumped at the chance. Individuals interested in fashion head for Paris or Milan; gardeners flock to New Zealand. Soon after New Year's Day, 2011, we headed for two weeks in NZ with a three-day side trip to Sydney, Australia.

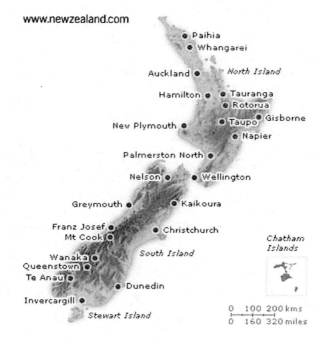

Some New Zealand Quick Facts —
Population: 4 Million
Capital City: Wellington, pop. 400,000
Auckland, pop. 1,400,000
Christchurch, pop. 400,000
Sheep, total head 45,000,000
National emblem: Kiwi, a flightless bird with hair like feathers and
   long beak. New Zealanders often refer to themselves as "Kiwi."
Demographics: The majority of people are of British descent; 14% of
   the total population are of indigenous Maori descent. Maroi is
   the official language, but English is most commonly spoken.

By geological standards, New Zealand, located some 1,200 miles southeast of Australia, is the youngest country on earth. It consists of two large and many small islands. During its long isolation, New Zealand developed a distinctive fauna dominated by birds. Until the "civilized" people from Europe arrived in 1770, there were no mammals on the islands, except for one species of bat. There are still no large predators or snakes; no lions, tigers or bears. There are, however, around 70 million possum. More about that later.

Our NZ tour guide , Julianne Drew, was half Maroi (pronounced "MARI")—the native people of NZ—and half Scottish. As a youngster she was forbidden to speak Maori, her native tongue, because she looked "White" and could pass. Fortunately, she was allowed to speak Maori as a teenager and is fluent in it today. At 52, she has been a tour guide for 25 years. Maroi are Polynesian, like Samoans. They were the first humans on the two islands around 1,400 AD. At that time there was only *one* mammal—a bat—on the islands.

From the outset, the country has been in the forefront of social welfare legislation. New Zealand was the world's first country to give women the right to vote (1893). It adopted old-age pensions (1898); a national child welfare program (1907); social security for the elderly, widows, and orphans, along with family benefit payments; minimum wages; a 40-hour workweek and unemployment and health insurance (1938); and socialized medicine (1941).

Despite having the most expensive health care system, the United States ranks last overall compared to six other industrialized countries—Australia, Canada, Germany, the Netherlands, New Zealand, and the United Kingdom—on measures of health system performance in five areas: quality, efficiency, access to care, equity, and the ability to lead long, healthy, productive lives, according to a new Commonwealth Fund report. While there is room for improvement in every country, the U.S. stands out for not getting good value for its health care dollars, ranking last despite spending $7,290 per capita on health care in 2007 compared to the $3,837 spent per capita in the Netherlands, which ranked first overall.

An OECD report in 2001 described the New Zealand tax system as one of the most neutral and efficient within its membership. New Zealand changed to the decimal system in 1965, then dropped the penny and nickel—rounding up or down to the nearest dime. A really good idea.

New Zealand fought with the Allies in both world wars as well as in Korea. In 1999, it became part of the UN peacekeeping force sent to East Timor.

Atlanta to Frisco, then a three-hour layover, then an 11-hour nonstop flight to Auckland. We crossed the international dateline and lost a day, which we gained back on the way home.

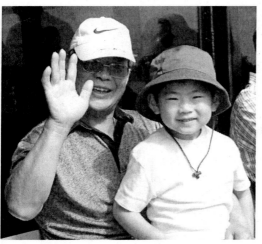

When boarding a harbor tour of Auckland on our first day, I missed a step, slipped and scraped my shin—blood all over. A Chinese man and his grandson gave me two Band-Aids. The six-year-old was very fluent in English, using words suitable for a teenager.

On to Longlands Dairy for a tour of their dairy farm followed by a delicious home cooked lunch. Dairy farming is one of the major industries in NZ. As the price of wool dropped over the years, dairy and tourism along with wool dominate the economy.

We then traveled to the Agrodome, where we saw performing sheep, sheep shearing, and a sheep dog exhibition. After the sheep parade to their stations, sheep dogs run across their backs and pose. There are ten kinds of sheep raised in NZ. All but the Marino are raised for mutton. I asked the sheep trainer/shearer how he

Rotorua • New Zealand

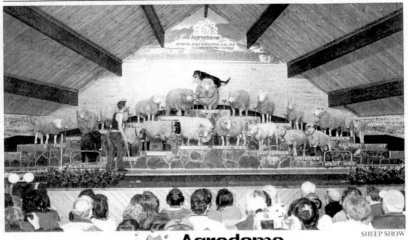

SHEEP SHOW

got the animals to stand so calmly while dogs ran across their backs. He replied, "We don't feed them in the morning. There's a cup of food at each station. They're happy to be fed breakfast."

NZ had upwards of 100 million sheep. The number is now down to 35 to 40 million. Even so, there are still ten sheep for every person in NZ. When England joined the Common Market, NZ stopped shipping whole individual cuts instead of carcasses. In 2008, sheep meat exports (mostly lamb) brought in more than half of the country's NZ$ 4.5 billion (US$ 3.5 billion) meat export revenues.

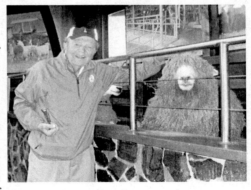

John with a future sweater

Saving New Zealand's Environment

The possum fiber in PossumSilk comes from the New Zealand Brushtail Possum, which is an introduced species that causes enor-

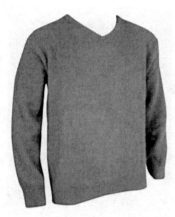

PossumSilk sweater

mous ecological damage to New Zealand's native forests and wildlife. Brushtail Possums reproduce prolifically in New Zealand's lush environment, which means they are not only eating the native plants and trees at a tremendous rate, but are also in direct competition for food with the native wildlife. At present there are approximately 80 million Brushtail Possums in New Zealand.

I bought a PossumSilk sweater in Rotorua, the nicest and warmest I've ever worn. PossumSilk™ is a blend of 50% marino lamb's wool, 40% possum fiber and 10% silk which is extremely warm, soft and lightweight to wear. PossumSilk also has superior anti-pill properties. The reason PossumSilk is so warm and lightweight is because of the possum fiber's unique hollow structure, which gives it excellent thermal properties.

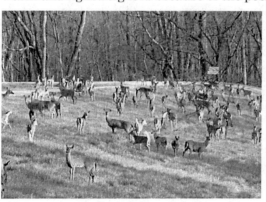

Herds of tame deer can be seen grazing along the highway. Juliann tells us NZ now raises thousands of deer for venison, which is exported for sausage, mainly to Germany.

The same 3- to 4-foot fence is used for deer, sheep and cattle. We asked, "Won't the deer jump that short fence?" Juliann replied, "No, why would they? They have all they want to eat, plentiful breeding partners and no arrows or gunshots to dodge."

We made a potty stop on the way to Wellington. Resting under an outside table of a bar (7-11–type store) was an Australian sheep dog. I got out to say hello. He immediately jumped up for attention and petting. I apologized that I had no Liver Treats, but maybe I could get some inside.

Inquiries to the bartender about dog treats were negative, but the lady/owner pointed to the dog's owner sitting at the bar drinking a beer. I introduced myself and complimented him on how good his dog looked. I guessed his age at 4 or 5, but James replied, "Actually Bob's 8 years old. He's a Huntaway." Bob had short hair and was about the size of a large Fox Terrier. James related, 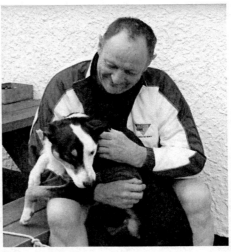 "Bob's a barker, not a herder, like regular sheep dogs. When I give the command, he barks—loud and long. That stops the sheep in their tracks. Then the herders can drive them where I want them to go." Commands may be indicated by a hand movement, whistle, or voice:

- Come-bye or just bye: Go to the left of the stock, or clockwise around them.
- Away or 'way: Go to the right of the stock, or counterclockwise around them.
- Stand: Stop; although when said gently, it may also mean just to slow down.
- Wait, (lie) down, or sit: Stop.
- Steady or take time: Slow down.
- Cast: Gather the stock into a group. Good working dogs will cast over a large area.
- Find: Search for stock. A good dog will hold the stock until the shepherd arrives. Some will bark when the stock have been located.
- Get out or get back: Move away from the stock. Used when the dog is working too close to the stock, potentially causing the stock stress. Occasionally used as a reprimand.
- Hold: Keep stock where they are.
- Bark or speak up: Bark at stock. Useful when more force is needed, and usually essential for working cattle and sheep.
- Look back: Return for a missed animal.

- In here: Go through a gap in the flock. Used when separating stock.
- Walk up, walk on, or just walk: Move in closer to the stock.
- That'll do: Stop working and return to handler.

I asked, "Is Bob an outside dog at home?" "Oh, no," James replied. "Bob sleeps with me. If I don't get in bed first, I have to push him off my pillow." Seems just like home in America

Continuing on our bus ride to Wellington, one of our group pointed to a shrub similar to Scottish Heather and asked the guide, Julianne, "What is that plant we often see along the road?" Julianne replied, "I'm not sure, I call it, 'New Zealand roadsideius.' " Walter chimed in that in the USA, he calls plants he can't identify, " 'ell if I know americus."

Through the Rimutaka mountain range to Upper Hutt, we visited the Efil Doog Garden—a magical delight, starting with

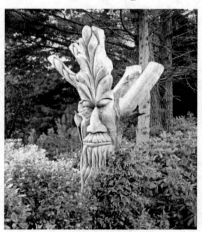 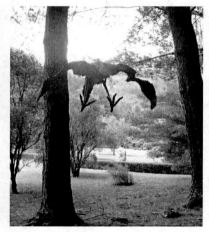

the name, "good life" backward. We enjoyed a box lunch while strolling the exotic forests with a large collection of sculptures and the art gallery of early NZ paintings. This is a *must see* on any New Zealand trip.

Outside of Wellington we again passed many herds of sheep and deer, both inside a typical three-foot high fence

A short ferry ride took us from Wellington to Nelson, then a Superior train ride along the west coast to Christchurch. We took a bus tour of the unique magical locations showcased in the *Lord of the Rings* movies, journeying to the remote and beautiful Mt. Potts's high country station. We saw how this peaceful mountain had been transformed into Edoras, the capital city of the Rohan

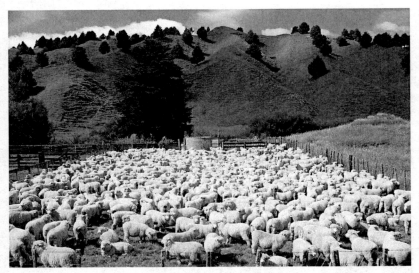

A herd of sheep near Wellington

people in the L.O.T. R. trilogy. I may be the only one of our group that has no idea what *Lord of the Rings* is about.

Then back home for a surprise—a dinner/theatre show at the Octagon Restaurant—an elegant way to end our stay in NZ.

The Octagon began as an Anglican church in 1873. The present owner, Harry Slade and his wife, the singer Natalie Slade,

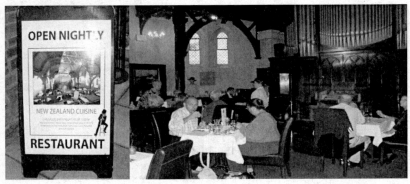

purchased the building in 1993. After extensive remodeling, it served as one of Christchurch's premier restaurants. The organ, purchased in 1933, was completely overhauled and blends well with the wonderful acoustics of the church/theatre. We were entertained by Natalie singing popular hits from the '40s to the '90s and a blind musician who played both piano and organ with his ever-present Labrador Retriever sleeping beneath his feet.

I was awakened by a minor earthquake (5.1) the day before we left Christchurch—just enough to shake the bed and cause some buildings to sway a little. What followed ten days later would devastate the city of Christchurch.

Christchurch, New Zealand's second largest city, is reeling after a devastating, 6.3-magnitude earthquake struck on

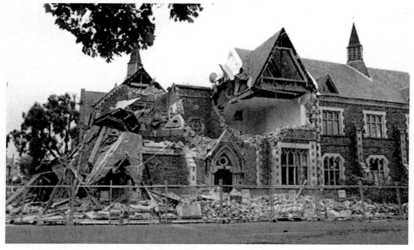

Christchurch Cathedral in Christchurch, New Zealand, stands in rubble after the 6.3-magnitude earthquake of 2011.

February 21, 2011. Many buildings, including the community's eponymous, signature cathedral, crumbled. The Octagon suffered extensive damage in the earthquake.

A poll taken two days after the quake shows that 40% of Kiwis support paying an earthquake levy to help pay for the rebuilding of Christchurch; 22% prefer more borrowing; 29% want spending cuts. When asked just whether they supported or opposed a levy, 57% supported it. Yet the politicians are choosing spending cuts instead. The death toll is now over 150.

Cardiac Surgery—Dogs, Pigs, and daVinci

Routine open-heart surgery was decades away in 1951. The heart-lung machine was only a figment of scientific fiction. That didn't stop pioneers from trying to work out new techniques to treat heart problems surgically. There are literally dozens of congenital heart problems.

A congenital heart defect (CHD) is a defect, present at birth, in the structure of the heart and great vessels. Heart defects are among the most common birth defects and are the leading cause of birth defect–related deaths. Approximately 9 people in 1,000 are born with a congenital heart defect. Many defects don't need treatment, but some complex congenital heart defects require medication or surgery.

This was the background to a cooperative effort between surgeons the University of Illinois Veterinary School and a surgical unit headed by a full colonel at the nearby Chanute Air Force Base in Rantoul, Illinois. They wanted to find out how long an animal could have blood shut off to and from the heart which would allow time for surgical repairs of cardiac defects. As you can imagine, it is almost impossible to do surgery inside a heart with blood gushing from every direction. The goal was to see if the animal would survive without any secondary side effects after 120, 180 or 240 seconds of blood stoppage.

Pigs and dogs weighting around 100 pounds were anesthetized and intubated to provide oxygen and ether during surgery. After opening the chest, closing sutures were preplaced in the area of the heart to be opened. When all was ready, the vessels to and from the heart were clamped, the heart was opened between the preplaced sutures, and the surgeons went through the motions of repairing "a hole in the heart."

As I recall, the team achieved their goal of over 200 seconds of heart stoppage without the patients showing any adverse side-effects. My problem was getting positive verification. There are only nine living members from the first two classes of '48 who might have been involved in helping with the surgery. Only WWII vets were accepted in 1948 and 1949, and all would be approaching 90 or beyond. After emailing and writing to all, I heard from Keith Etheridge and George Scott. Both remember the incidents very well. George was involved in making up all the packs, and Keith in the cleanup. Neither remember any exact particulars. Keith wrote:

> Hi John. I remember the incident. Dolloway, Linker, and I were the only singles our junior and senior years and lived in the loft in the old cattle barn converted to vet clinic. We received lodging for cleaning instruments from LA and SA surgery. Dragutin Maksic also lived with us as he was getting accredited. The farthest east part was kennel, next LA surgery, then a SA surgery with two tables. I remember the incident but didn't participate unless I cleaned up afterwards. Witter would be the clinician either year and Brasmer the junior year and Schilling our senior. I know Witter is deceased, but I don't remember seeing obit's for Brasmer or Schilling. Another lead might be Dolloway who lives in Washington. — Keith

Upon further research, I discovered that Drs. Witter, Brasmer and Schilling are all deceased.

One of the many changes in veterinary curriculum is in the teaching of surgery. In my junior year we were divided into teams of three, alternating one surgeon and two assistants. The assistants prepared the animal, giving anesthetics, intubating to provide oxygen and continued anesthetic, and preparing the belly, leg, etc. for surgery. Animals were obtained from the local shelter or pound. The younger patients were castrated or spayed (ovariohysterectomy) and adopted. Older animals were routinely euthanized after sometimes performing 3 or 4 surgeries on the same patient.

Sometime after the influx of female students and the rise of the animal rights groups, stricter rules on practice surgery were instituted. In July, 2010, a communication from

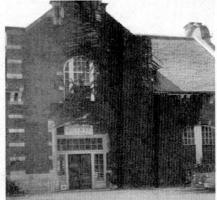

U. of I. Veterinary Clinic • 1948-60
Converted from an old stable

the Michigan State University Veterinary School stated:

> MSU no longer will use live animals to teach veterinary students surgical techniques, a spokesperson for the College of Veterinary Medicine said Thursday. Linda Chadderdon, spokeswoman for the college, said the university will switch from live animals to alternative methods of animal surgery education, such as animal cadavers, beginning in the fall. An official announcement is expected Friday.
>
> Currently, MSU purchases animals, mostly dogs, that are bred for scientific purposes. The animals are put under anesthesia during the process, called terminal surgery, then are euthanized. Chadderdon said the college slowly has been parting from this method for a number of years while it searched for alternative ways to teach surgery to veterinary.
>
> Bryden Stanley, an assistant professor of small animal clinical practices, said the college spent the past several years testing alternative methods of teaching students animal surgery techniques. Starting in the fall, the college will use animal cadavers and models to teach students. Stanley, who helps organize the courses that teach terminal surgery, said the alternative teaching methods will be as effective, if not more, than surgery on live animals. "It will be skill-based, and they will have practiced so many times, when they do come to the live animal, they will be better prepared," Stanley said.
>
> Animal science freshman Lauren Follmer said she does not think switching from live subjects to cadavers and models will hinder the learning process, although she said it depends on what surgical techniques are being taught. "It depends on what they're trying to learn," Follmer said, "There are some things that it's better if it's live, but for some of the more basic things, I guess it'd be perfectly fine (otherwise)."

When my clients would marvel at the advances being made in human surgery, I reminded them that all these wonderful techniques were perfected on animals long before being approved for people. This was verified by a visit in 1990 to the Pewaukee Veterinary Service, owned by brothers Randy and Jeff Schuett in Pewaukee, Wisconsin, a Milwaukee suburb. At the time they were involved with teaching human surgeons laparoscopic techniques.

They would provide the patients (pigs weighting around 150 pounds) and do the preop and anesthesia. Board certified surgeons actually did the instruction. This was done many times a year at a facility in Naperville, Illinois. Randy emailed me recently,

> John, nice to hear from you. I have had the opportunity to help with a number of research-type projects that have been a little different. We first did some heart transplants with a surgeon from St. Luke's in Milwaukee. After that we did a lot of laparoscopic training using pigs as models, that lasted for many years, and occasionally I still do one of those labs. One of the most unique things that I did was to help develop a technique to perform embryo transfer in black bears so that some day we could use the technique in pandas. Even though that hasn't happened yet, that project started a lot of other projects with black bears that are still ongoing. You should give me a call some time or come and visit and I could fill you in all the details. Take care. — Randy

Fast forward 20 years to 21st century. Heart/lung machines allow surgeons to routinely bypass the blood to and from the heart, allowing adequate time to perform many cardiac procedures hitherto impossible.

I had the thought of never retiring. Maybe I'd sell my practice to a younger vet and work a lot less and travel a lot more. Developing macular degeneration, dry type, in my left eye in the fall of 1998 shot down that idea. I mentioned the possibility to my optometrist, Dr Joe Romanak, that he had given me a bum pair of glasses. He assured me it was much worse than that. Subsequent visits to an ophthalmologist confirmed Dr. Joe's diagnosis. My left eye slowly developed a blind spot in the middle of my field of vision. Fortunately my perimeter sight was still clear as a bell. As I have aged the blind spot has gradually reduced in size.

I had recently diagnosed a congenital heart problem in Dr. Romanak's, Toy Poodle, Packer. Ultrasound studies by Dr. Wolf confirmed the diagnosis. Packer had a patent ductus arteriosus (PDA), a condition in which the ductus arteriosus does not close. (The word "patent" means open.) The ductus arteriosus is a blood vessel that

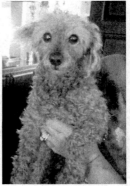

Packer

allows blood to go around the baby's lungs before birth. Soon after the infant is born and the lungs fill with air, the ductus arteriosus is no longer needed. It usually closes in a couple of days after birth. PDA leads to abnormal blood flow between the aorta and pulmonary artery, two major blood vessels that carry blood from the heart.

I referred Packer to Dr. Walt Weirich, a cardiology specialist at Purdue University, who performed surgery the following week. In the summer of 2012 Dr. Romanek informed me that Packer will be celebrating his 16th birthday this fall.

I had bypass surgery in 1992 to replace five blocked heart vessels. By 2003 I had two stents placed to open up closed arteries. They plugged in six months. Two more stents placed in 2005 plugged in six months. I was on a number of heart meds and had a cholesterol level well below 200, but it was no help.

Enter Dr. Averal Snyder and his assistant "da Vinci." Not Leonardo, but a robotic surgical assistant that is allowing surgeons to perform wonders. Dr. Snyder performed my da Vinci cardiac surgery in February, 2009.

This is where a machine is used to perform surgery while being controlled by the heart surgeon. The main advantage to this is the size of the incision made in the patient. Instead of an incision being at least big enough for the surgeon to put his hands inside, it does not have to be bigger than three small holes the diameter of lead pencils, for the robot's much smaller "hands" to get through.

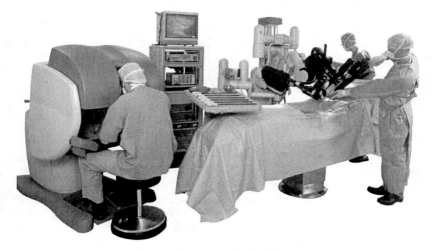

Surgical team with da Vinci.

Risks

The development of cardiac surgery and cardiopulmonary bypass techniques has reduced the mortality rates of these surgeries to relatively low ranks. For instance, repairs of congenital heart defects are currently estimated to have 4–6% mortality rates. A major concern with cardiac surgery is the incidence of neurological damage. Stroke occurs in 2–3% of all people undergoing cardiac surgery and is higher in patients at risk for stroke. A more subtle constellation of neurocognitive deficits attributed to cardiopulmonary bypass is known as postperfusion syndrome, sometimes called "pumphead." The symptoms of postperfusion syndrome were initially felt to be permanent, but were shown to be transient, with no permanent neurological impairment.

Transmyocardial Laser Revascularization

Transmyocardial revascularization (TMR) is a surgical procedure for inoperable coronary artery disease patients with angina (chest pain). Patients with coronary artery disease are treated with interventional procedures (angioplasty and stenting), coronary artery bypass grafting (surgery) and medications to improve blood flow to the heart muscle. If these procedures do not eliminate the symptoms of chest pain (also called angina), transmyocardial laser revascularization or TMR is another treatment option physicians can offer to patients.

How does TMR work? TMR is a treatment aimed at improving blood flow to areas of the heart that were not treated by angioplasty or surgery. A special carbon dioxide (CO_2) laser is used to create small channels in the heart muscle, improving blood flow in the heart. TMR is a surgical procedure. The procedure is performed through a small left chest incision or through a midline incision. Frequently, it is performed with coronary artery bypass surgery, but occasionally it is performed independently.

Once the incision is made, the surgeon exposes the heart muscle. A laser handpiece is then positioned on the area of the heart to be treated. A special high-energy, computerized carbon dioxide (CO_2) laser, called the CO2 Heart Laser 2, is used to create between 20 to 40 one-millimeter-wide channels (about the width of the head of a pin) in the oxygen-poor left ventricle (left lower pumping chamber) of the heart. The doctor determines how many channels to create during the procedure. The outer areas of the channels close, but the inside of the channels remain open inside the heart to improve blood flow.

The CO2 Heart Laser 2 uses a computer to direct laser beams to the appropriate area of the heart in between heartbeats, when the ventricle is filled with blood and the heart is relatively still. This helps to prevent electrical disturbances in the heart. Clinical evidence suggests blood flow is improved in two ways:

1. The channels act as bloodlines. When the ventricle pumps or squeezes oxygen-rich blood out of the heart, it sends blood through the channels, restoring blood flow to the heart muscle.

2. The procedure may promote angiogenesis, or growth of new capillaries (small blood vessels) that help supply blood to the heart muscle.

TMR usually takes one to two hours. The procedure may last longer if it is combined with other heart procedures. Another benefit is the postop reduced recovery time. I was home the day after surgery and playing golf two weeks later.

Dr. Snyder related that 40 of the 41 patients he had performed TMR experienced very good results, less angina and more energy. I did not seem to get the same improvement—no better, no worse. When Dr. Snyder explained the TMR procedure to me, I asked where was he located in the operating room. "I'm across the room from you at the di Vinci console." "Do you sew up the cuts in the heart or the holes made by the inserted rods?" "No, the laser immediately seals the heart muscle and the holes in the chest close by themselves." "If da Vinci is doing all the work," I asked facetiously, "then why am I paying you the big bucks?" Dr. Snyder replied, " Just like the pilot in a 747, I know which buttons to push, which levers to pull, and when to do it." Even though da Vinci costs a million dollars, it is not able to perform without someone at the controls.

It's been 60 years since that experimental open heart surgery on pigs at the vet school in Champaign. Already medical scientists are growing bladders and tracheas from the patient's own stem cells. These can replace worn out or diseased organs without the need of long term drugs to avoid rejection. Just as the computers get smaller and faster year by year, medical science explores new frontiers at a ever-expanding rate. I only hope and pray the politicians and governments keep up with the progress.

Five-Finger Discount

Amy Whitehouse (not her real name) responded to my ad in the Kehosha News for a receptionist/lab tech. She seemed perfect—five years experience working at another local animal hospital, mature (probably not going to have more kids), and a pleasant phone voice. What could go wrong? I found out soon enough after talking to my colleague and good friend, Dr. Jim Nordstrom. As a partner/owner of Kenosha Animal Hospital, Jim could fill me in on the reasons Amy was available. He responded they had to let her go but was reluctant to explain why. After some prodding, he related the following tale of woe.

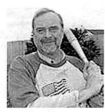

Dr. James Nordstrom

Over the past few months Dr. Nordstrom and his partner, Dr. Jim Watts, noticed an increase in business but a decline in profits. An audit of the books revealed startling evidence that someone was stealing from the front desk. Further investigation documented supplies were also slipping out the back door. Two employees, Ms. Whitehouse and a maintenance worker were methodically helping themselves to cash and supplies. Estimates range from $10,000 to $20,000 that was pilfered over a two-year period.

I asked what action was taken. Jim responded, "We called the police after we confirmed our suspicions. They investigated and came up with evidence which we used for dismissal. You need to be careful, for employees are quick to sue if you don't have very solid proof of wrongdoing. In the end, we decided not to prosecute. The bad publicity would do more harm than good."

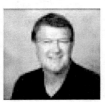

Dr. Frank Pisarik

A recent conversation with Dr. Frank Pisarik, at that time a new associate in the practice, added more flesh to the story. A long-time receptionist mentioned to Dr. Pisarik that she suspected one of the staff was stealing.

Very few, if any, theft controls were in place at the time. Auditing the books revealed a major loss of income over the previous few months or longer. The police advised them to have all staff take lie detector exams. After the announcement, three employees quit. No charges were filed, but the thefts stopped.

I have mixed emotions about their decision. The publicity may be temporarily detrimental to the practice, but it would quickly pass. I believe the better action is to expose the criminals for what they are. This will alert other businesses in and around thr community to be careful when hiring these individuals. I admit this can be a problem for the practice, as theft is difficult to prove in court, and people can sue for false arrest.

About that same time, my animal hospital experienced a couple of break-ins. Someone—police suspected teenagers—broke windows on the unlighted side of the building to gain entrance. They proceeded to take cash and a few selective drugs. I had been advised to always leave a few singles and $10 to $15 in change in the open register. Most thieves will take the cash instead of the entire register. The police advised installing a motion detector and recommended an ex-cop to do the job.

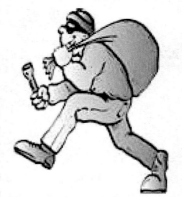

Steve Clancy knew his business. He installed motion detectors in the front office and pharmacy. He then applied silver tape to all the outside windows. Next he placed conspicuous red signs in the windows, advising anyone that the windows and interior are wired to the police station. Actually, there was no electronic hookup to the "cop shop," but Steve assured me thieves would not be willing to take a chance. Most would sooner look for an easier target. Sure enough—we never experienced another break-in.

Wikipedia reports, "Retailers report that shoplifting has a significant effect on their bottom line, stating that about 0.6% of all inventory disappears to shoplifters. In 2001, it was claimed that shoplifting cost U.S. retailers $25 million a day. Observers believe that over half of shoplifting is from employee theft or fraud and the rest by patrons.

On a personal note, I recall one of our three boys being caught stealing something at the local grocery. An email to all five kids brought immediate responses from the three boys. The youngest—about 7 or 8 at the time—wrote, "As I recall, it was at a grocery store (Sentry?). I was the culprit. I think I was "learning the ropes" from my older brothers. The item was a box of candy cigarettes, and as I walked through the doors to leave, someone ran up behind me and caught me, upon which I immediately spilled the beans on the others. I had to write a letter of apology to both the manager and checkout lady. The two older boys deny, then and now, any involvement in the crime.

One of my daughters responded, "The only thing I ever stole was a '$100,000' candy bar. I walked out of the store—it was next to Sears—then I freaked out and walked back in and threw it into a shelf. I could not handle the guilt. I did not even make it 50 feet from the store. My friends made fun of me for months." Maybe it's in the genes.

I was in an incident that took place 30 years earlier. One afternoon, after 7th grade school at St. Francis Xavier was over, a number of the "guys" would head to the bowling alley or downtown La Grange. We had a passion for Yo-Yos. They cost 25 cents at the local 5 and 10 store. We had a better idea. Two or three of us would distract the clerk, providing cover for the loner to swipe a Yo-Yo. After a time, two of our group, Bill Duffy and Bob Sheen, declared, "This is too easy. We are the best shoplifters in the city. We can even steal 'the kitchen sink'." To prove their boast, they marched down the street to Montgomery Ward. We followed at a discreet distance. Bill and Bob entered the front door and headed for the plumbing section in back. The rest of the group observed the caper from the hardware section. The boys picked up a kitchen sink, faucets and all, and proceeded to carry it out the side door and around the corner to the adjacent alley. We didn't do "high fives" at the time, but it would have been appropriate.

Veterinarians do not have the same problems as retailers because most of our inventory is behind a counter. Veterinary offices may be tempting for thieves. It might be easy to re-sell stolen goods, or you might have cash on hand. Management experts recommend making your business less attractive to criminals:
- Keep equipment and supplies locked up and out of plain sight.
- Deposit receipts at the bank daily.
- Keep delivery doors closed / locked even during business hours.
- Establish internal controls to cut employee theft.
- Use a safe and protect the key/combination.
- Make a standard opening and closing procedure for the office.
- If you have an alarm, arm it every time and change the pass code regularly.
- Keep your building(s) well lit, inside and out.

The FTC has announced that enforcement of a law covering "identity theft" began on April 1, 2010. Compliance with the rule means developing a written document that thoroughly details the measures your practice will take to protect the personal identifying information of its employees and clients. As always, a written plan is worthless unless all of the staff understand and implement the plan; therefore, all staff must be trained, and sign documents that confirm they've been trained. Last, but not least, all vendors and service providers who have physical or electronic access to sensitive information (e.g., insurance agents, accountants, copier companies, cleaning services, etc.) should be contacted and notified that you also expect them to comply with the rule and take all reasonable measures to protect the practice's information as well as those of the clients. Documentation in writing of your program is critical; not just the policy and its updates, but also the training and notifications.

The AVMA has developed a guide with examples, and the FTC has recently released a "Do-It-Yourself Program for Businesses at Low Risk for Identity Theft" document to provide guidance.

Many large practices offer retirement plans. "Sadly, this is an area of employer theft," Robert Powell reports in a recent issue of *MarketWatch*. "Most of the time, the money you contribute to your 401k ends up in your account. But there are times when it doesn't," according to the U.S. Labor Department's Employee Benefit Security Administration. Roughly once a week in July alone, some of the 150 million Americans covered by the more than 700,000 employer-sponsored retirement plans received notice that their hard-earned money ended up in the wrong pocket.

There are things you can do to protect your retirement savings long before your employers end up in a labor department press release for the wrong reason.

Participants need to monitor their account statements to ensure that their contributions are being timely deposited and invested in the right funds," said David Wray, the president of the Profit Sharing/401k Council of America. The experts recommend you monitor on a regular basis and leave no stone unturned. "Most firms provide account balance information via a variety of ways," said Tom Kmak, the chief executive officer of Fiduciary Benchmarks. Usually, you can get your account balance on the Internet, via an 800 number, and in hard copy once per quarter. "Check all three to make sure they are in sync," said Kmak, even if it means checking after every paycheck.

I mentioned this story about employee theft to Mary Kay Rudd, who was the long time office manager of a large practice. I inquired if she had had any similar incidents in her practice. Her response follows:

> Funny you should say this. We had an employee, over a 3-year period, steal over $50,000. She was our morning receptionist. She stole money out of the night bag every morning and reprinted the night report. Then she would delete the transaction out of the client's account. We caught her by accident and really don't know how much she stole. It included cash, fake returns, food and items off the shelf, and payment for her own pets. She denied it for a year until we finally got the case heard in court. She lied to her lawyer and the judge. Luckily, I had insurance and had actually switched companies during this time so I was reimbursed by both companies, and she is paying me some piddling amount every month. Eventually, she is suppose to pay the insurance companies back too. She is on probation for 20 years, and she's only about 27 years old! Her parents were jerks too, especially her father, who believed her lies. It was obvious she lived beyond her $12/hour means. You probably saw her, very short red, curly hair. I have not seen or spoken to her since our court date two years ago. It was very difficult to prove our case. I have been told by other vets that they just write it off or ask the offender to please repay the money. Yeah, right. I am sure I lost more money than I was able to prove in court. She got first offender status, so if she stays out of trouble, sees her probation officer, and pays everyone back, she has no criminal record at the end of the 20-year period. The judge structured it this way so that she had to make restitution. Otherwise she could have gone to jail for a few years and walked away with $50,000 plus. She also got unemployment of $3,000 from the State of Georgia, since she was innocent (lying) until proven guilty. It's too much trouble for the state to go back and try to collect this money back from her. I tried to get the State to look at her case, but no one cared.
>
> I believe VCA (Veterinary Corporation of America) has had trouble with theft, but I don't remember details about the one story I heard. They have a Code of Business Conduct Handbook that all employees must sign at hire.

They have a mechanism for whistle blowers to alert the company, should they feel the need, and remain anonymous. Violation of company policy may result in disciplinary action, including discharge. Serious violations can result in suspension without pay, and theft will result in termination. VCA states they may seek civil remedies from the employee, and they may seek reimbursement. Of course, it is difficult to catch and prove your case against an employee. I had an employee who changed the time on the computer so she wasn't clocking in late and I caught her on a fluke. There was another employee who was leaving early at night and pretending to forget to clock out. Both of these employees were fired.

When I was giving management seminars, I advised my audience to not lose any sleep over five-finger discounts, shrinkage, or bad checks. Do what is prudent and affordable to prevent loss, but be aware that you will lose 1% to 3% every year no matter how hard you work to prevent it. Just add 2% or 3% to your fee schedule. This is the rule of thumb for all major businesses. It's a form of insurance. The 99% of honest people pick up the tab for the 1% who aren't.

I'm reminded of the old saying, "When a pickpocket meets a saint, all he sees is his pockets."

Corporate Vets

"Shirt-tail relatives—that's what we are," I told Steve Avery. We were visiting my grandson, Adam Robinson, and his wife, Kristin, when they brought my first great granddaughter, Elle, home from the hospital. Steve, as Kristin's dad, is unrelated to me by blood, but we have common offspring. Steve is the CEO and CFO of a group of 30 or more anesthesia practices around the country. In the last 20 years professional corporate companies have grown exponentially.

Professional corporations (abbreviated as PC or P.C.) are those corporate entities for which many corporation statutes make special provision, regulating the use of the corporate form. The first laws that permitted the formation of professional corporations were intended to give licensed professionals such as attorneys, architects, engineers, public accountants, and doctors some of the tax advantages enjoyed by corporations without also giving them the benefit of limited liability. If a regular corporation—which is a distinct entity under the law—becomes insolvent, its creditors can only claim business assets for the repayment of debts, not the personal assets of its owners.

Over the last few years, Veterinary Corporation of America (VCA) grew to become the largest pet health care provider in the country. Under their new name, VCA Antech, they became a publicly-owned company in 2001. VCA Antech stock is traded on NASDAQ under the very appropriate symbol, "WOOF." VCA operates more than 540 animal hospitals in 41 states across the nation in the VCA network. These hospitals are staffed by more than 2,000 fully qualified veterinarians, over 200 of which are board-certified specialists. The growth of another large corporate practice, Banfield, the Pet Hospital, based in Portland, Ore., was fueled by its partnership with Petsmart. It employs more than 1,900 veterinarians at more than 720 hospitals nationwide. VCA treats more than 1.5 million animals annually, compared to Banfield's 4 million.

"VCA, Banfield, and smaller corporate practices make up about 5 percent of U.S. practices," says Dennis M. McCurnin, DVM, MS, Dipl. ACVS, professor of veterinary surgery and management at Louisiana State University's School of Veterinary Medicine. He is also a veterinary practice consultant. "Are they going to take over the practice of veterinary medicine? No, I don't foresee that," Dr. McCurnin says.

Today, we have some 80,000 veterinarians in the U.S. and about 60 percent of them are in companion animal practice. About five percent of the companion animal practices are corporate and 95 percent are private. The AVMA noted that the average number of veterinarians in private practives is two.

Quality of life has become an important issue for practitioners. In the past, many owners and associates worked 50 or more hours a week, in addition to being on emergency call. Today, new graduates want to work 40 hours a week or less, with no emergency duty.

There seems to be a disconnect between living a good lifestyle and repaying debt, however. The mean educational debt in 2008 was $119,803, as reported by the AVMA. The mean starting salary for small-animal exclusive practice in 2008 was $64,744 (*Journal of the AVMA;* Oct. 1, 2008). The ratio of debt-to-starting-salary is near 2-to-1. The increase in salaries, however, is lagging behind the increase in educational debt.

Another factor in the growing debt issue is the difference between today's graduates and those of 20 to 30 years ago. Newer graduates may not be as interested in ownership because of the increased hours usually required of owners. According to a *Veterinary Economics* survey, 59 percent of female and 48 percent of male associates don't ever plan to own a practice. This seems to cross the gender line, as both males and females seem to share this feeling.

Veterinary schools are about 80 percent female in current classes. The gender shift and generational differences seem to make today's graduate more likely to seek work with controlled hours, nights and weekends off, and mentoring and benefit programs. Since the larger corporate practices were introduced about 15 years ago, the opportunity to have a controlled work week, minimum management duties, retirement plan, and benefits has changed the employment picture for both new graduates and specialists. Many large practices are offering shared jobs and daycare for veterinarians with young children. Practices with one or two veterinarians often do not provide the schedule flexibility and benefits provided by larger private and corporate practices.

"Again," Dr. McCurnin says, "the question that comes up frequently deals with the future of private and corporate practices.

How will pet insurance affect the level of patient care? Will corporate practice eventually replace private practice as we know it today? Who will buy all the one- and two-person practices when the owners want to retire? Will a balance exist between corporate and private practice?

"Will we then have become dinosaurs that roam the earth and die off? I do not believe this will happen, but our profession is changing and individual veterinarians must change as well.

"Practices must become more efficient and produce more revenue per hour to allow us to hire new graduates. Efficiency must include multitasking, operating two to three examination rooms simultaneously, delegating to highly qualified staff, using improved communication skills, and managing our practices as a professional business.

"I believe there will always be a place for private practice and that it will continue as the dominate form of business in the foreseeable future; however, one-person practices will decrease and three-, four-, and five-person practices will increase. Some small practices will be lost and others will become consolidated."

When Corporate Practice Calls — By Bob Womack

When Brian Harpster, VMD, MS, owned a practice, his wife claimed he worked 90 hours a week, though he says it was actually 60 to 70. His West Shore Veterinary Hospital in New Cumberland, Pa., had a staff of 30 and grossed $1.7 million annually.

At 51, he wanted to reduce his hours and still practice, while eliminating "the headaches and hassles" of management. In a decision he says was "50 percent lifestyle and 50 percent financial," he and his two partners sold the practice to VCA Antech in December 2002. They sold for 11 times the hospital's original cost in 1984, retaining ownership of the building and land, with VCA agreeing to pay for future renovations. Carrying low debt, they could use VCA's rent payments to defray the mortgage, which will be paid off next January.

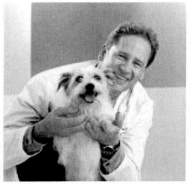

After the sale, Dr. Harpster's income was about the same, but his work week dropped to 40 to 45 hours. He now works 3½ days a week, 32 to 34 hours, at what is called VCA West Shore.

Independents Dominate

Todd Tams, DVM, Dipl. American College of Veterinary Internal Medicine (ACVIM), chief medical officer of VCA, says, "I talk to many veterinarians who express concern that large corporate groups are just trying to take over, but that's not the case. There will always be a role for veterinarians who want to operate their own practice."

The main reasons veterinarians sell to a corporate practice are "stress of ownership...and financial pressure. They'd like to get some money back out and cut back on their hours," Dr. Tams says. "A lot of veterinarians think they're burned out on veterinary medicine, but after six months, they often say, 'I realize now what I was actually burned out on was the stress of trying to run all aspects of hospital operations'."

For new veterinarians, a corporate practice's internship, mentorship and continuing education programs are draws, Tams says. The groups also can "put buying pressure on vendors in a lot of markets" to get better prices. "Corporate practice has probably been good for the profession as a whole." When a corporation buys a practice, it often aims to "upscale medical quality to the high end of the standard of care," Tams says. "We [at VCA] definitely want to practice a high level of care, and sometimes higher fees come with that.

I signed up for Groupon in Atlanta after reading an article in *Time* magazine. Excerpts follow:

> Groupon, the category leader, offers its subscribers—who number more than 50 million and are growing at a clip of 3 million a month—discounts on goods and services, but only if a critical mass of people agree to buy the deals that are e-mailed to them each day. The discount could be up to 90% off on a car wash, a restaurant meal, a cooking class, dental work, or just about any product or service available in the 500 cities and 35 countries where Groupon operates. Social commerce, the Web's next big honeypot, has a three-way payoff: you get a better price, the merchant gets a guaranteed slug of added business and potential new customers, and Groupon takes a cut.

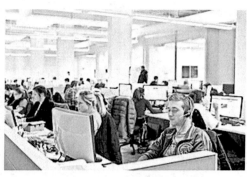

Groupon CEO Andrew Mason, in a room built for an imaginary employee. The company has been hiring more than 100 real employees each month.

"Groupon has cracked the code on a model for local advertising and local commerce," says James Slavet, a partner at Greylock Partners, a venture-capital firm in Silicon Valley and a Groupon investor. "Long term, this is a business that will do for retail what Google's done to search and search advertising."

By late 2008, Groupon launched. It worked—spectacularly, virally, to the point of overwhelming some merchants who were early participants: think of a flash mob that gets hungry for Greek food or decides to go bowling. Within a year, Groupon had 1 million adherents. Merchants across Chicago, and then in neighboring cities and states, lined up to get in.

A company with Google-like potential? No wonder Google felt compelled to buy Groupon, making an astonishing offer of $6 billion for it last December. Equally astonishing, Mason and his partners turned the Googleplexers down. "We have a lot of options," says Mason.

Veterinary Economics Magazine reported in May 27, 2011:

You may not run your veterinary practice like a trendy restaurant, but perhaps it's time to start marketing like one.

Surely you've seen the deals by now: $20 for $40 worth of food at a local bistro or $35 for a $70 massage at the downtown spa. Groupon is the big name, but there are plenty of other similar services, both local and national. And if you haven't already participated in one of the services, you may be missing out on a golden marketing opportunity.

Here's a look at how veterinary practices participated in Groupon promotions and emerged with a whole new group of clients—all at no initial cost to the practices.

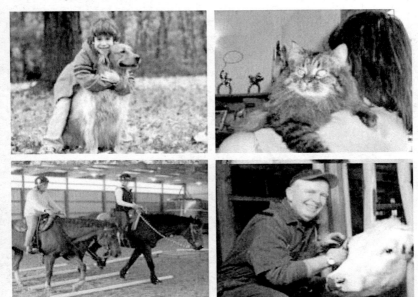

The practice: Country View Veterinary Service; Oregon, Wis. **The mastermind:** Dr. Emily Leuthner, practice manager **The deal:** $22 for one grooming session ($50 value), $40 for a six-week obedience class ($85 value), or $40 for five days of doggy daycare (up to $85 value)

The practice sold 171 packages during the promotion, which ended in February. Dr. Leuthner first gained inspiration after talking to her hairdresser, who sold 750 Groupons in a single day. She contacted the company, who worked with her to develop the specifics of the offer. The company's "city planners" then worked to schedule the listing and write promotional copy for the Web site. All in all, Dr. Leuthner says it was a pain-free process.

"I was pleased; it was a very positive experience." Dr. Leuthner says. "Our deal ran on Super Bowl weekend, and Groupon cut us a check within 48 hours." I was shocked when we had over 75,000 hits on our website on Super Bowl Saturday.

Dr. Leuthner says sites like Groupon are far superior to newspaper and phone book ads because they're simply a better bang for the buck. It costs nothing to offer a deal on Groupon, and businesses receive roughly half of the proceeds from each Groupon sold. But the real deal is in the new clients your practice can receive from the promotion, Dr. Leuthner says.

"We've definitely received new clients from it," she says. "Even if none of the deals had sold, it didn't cost us a penny to reach out to more than 30,000 potential clients. You just can't find that kind of exposure anywhere else. You definitely take a hit in terms of the revenue you'd normally receive from these services, but you're bringing in new clients." To offset that possible income loss, 171 Groupons generated 90 new clients and 20% were never redeemed—all profit to the clinic.

And depending on what kind of deal you offer, clients may end up investing in more. For example, they may need to update their pet's vaccines to take advantage of daycare or boarding services at your practice. That's extra revenue for your practice, and perhaps a lifelong client. In fact, 27% of those with Groupons utilized other services

Don't expect much of a direct profit from a deal-of-the-day type of service, Dr. Leuthner says, but think of it as a marketing tool that costs your practice nothing.

"Ultimately, you're not laying out any money for the advertising, and you're getting a lot of exposure." A veterinarian in Tennessee said it best. "The clients we've received from it have been great, so it's definitely been worthwhile. And even if you only get a few clients from it, they may end up coming to your clinic for years. That's several thousand dollars worth of revenue." This is true "target marketing" at its best.

Dr. Leuthner related the mixed animal practice has 6 full-time and 2 part-time veterinarians with 29 support staff—one lonely man in the midst of the harem of 36 females.

On October 22, 2011, the Associated Press reported, "Groupon, which had to delay its initial public offering (IPO) of stock this summer after regulators raised concerns about the way it counts revenue, is discounting its expectations for the IPO. In June, it was valued as high as $25 billion, but in a regulatory filing Friday, the company said it expects a value less than one half that at between $10.1 billion and $11.4 billion." To paraphrase former Illinois Senator Everett Dirksen: "A billion here or there—either way, you're talking about real money."

Braelinn Village Animal Hospital, Inc., in Peachtree City was a recent purchase of VCA. The owner, Ray Rudd, MS, Diplomat American College of Veterinary Surgeons (ACVS), is a boarded veterinary surgeon. Ray's wife, Mary K. Rudd, MPH (Masters of Public Health Nutrition) and PhD (nutrition), was the practice manager until her recent retirement. Having worked in hospital and public health settings made her familiar with running medical facilities.

As a member of the Army Reserve, Dr. Rudd is currently (August, 2011) serving in Afghanistan caring for the "war dogs." He frequently assists in surgery to repair wounds on humans, friend and foe alike.

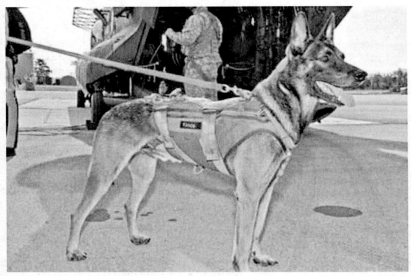

Conversations and personal communication with Mrs. Rudd revealed the following:

Braelinn Village Animal Hospital was a fit for VCA because:
- We had revenues approaching $3 million and employed 6 full time veterinarians, including my husband, Ray Rudd, MS, Diplomat ACVS.
- We were the largest and most successful hospital on the south side of Atlanta.
- Fayette County is an affluent area.
- We also had state-of-the-art equipment—the first and only private practice in Georgia with MRI.

VCA is following in Banfield's lead by branding products with a VCA label. So far this includes flea and tick products, heart worm preventatives, and shampoo products. They plan on adding prescription medications. They offer an online pharmacy and automatic shipments of products to combat the loss of sales to PetMeds and similar companies.

I would not recommend using a broker, because VCA will tell you exactly what information they want and need in order to make an offer. A lawyer will be necessary to advise the seller after a contract offer is made. The whole process took about six months, and we were paid in cash.

VCA recently bought VetStreet, a service that allows clients to view their pets medical records and request prescription refills and appointments via email. They are also attempting to form relationships with major humane societies, and in some cases local humane societies, to drive traffic to VCA hospitals.

VCA has continuing educational requirements for their doctors (30 hours/year) and offers a lots of continuing education in-house. They are very concerned with the quality of medicine practiced and also with appropriately charging for those services.

Even with the departure of two veterinarians and my husband, the rest of the hospital staff has remained stable. This was my main concern, because our hospital relies heavily on our technician staff, who are mainly RVT, highly trained and very dedicated.

There was constant corporate pressure to achieve a certain profit. I could not adapt going from an owner to an employee.

I can relate to Mrs. Rudd's assessment of corporate America. One of the joys of self-employment is being able to analyze a situation, assess what action to take, and pull the trigger. This is diametrically opposed to the bureaucracy of committee and the CYA culture. The old saying "If you can't stand the heat, get out of the kitchen" only partly applies here. Self employed entrepreneurs have a different kind of heat in our kitchen. At least we know who to blame when things go wrong. We see him/her every day in the bathroom mirror.

Lake Shore Animal Hospital

Lake Shore Animal Hospital was not even close to Lake Shore Drive in Chicago. The three-story, ultra-modern animal hospital was on a busy street, Chicago Avenue, but close to the notorious Cabrini-Green Housing Development. Built in 1965 by Dr. Lloyd Paschun and his wife Mary, the hospital rivaled any in the Midwest. Elevators carried patients from the first floor reception to exam rooms, treatment, surgeries and hospital cages above.

Rumor had it Mary was not only the business manager but also the source of financing the project. It always a puzzle why this magnificent structure was built on the edge of the highest crime area in Chicago.

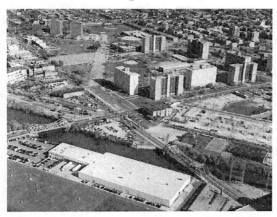

Cabrini-Green was a Chicago Housing Authority (CHA) public housing development on Chicago's Near North Side. It was bordered by Evergreen Avenue on the north, Orleans Street on the east, Chicago Avenue on the south, and Halsted Street on the west. At its peak, Cabrini-Green was home to 15,000 people who lived in mid- and high-rise apartment buildings totaling 3607 units.

Unlike many of the city's other public housing projects like Rockwell Gardens or Robert Taylor Homes, Cabrini-Green was situated in an affluent part of the city. The poverty-stricken projects were actually constructed at the meeting point of Chicago's two wealthiest neighborhoods, Lincoln Park and the Gold Coast. Less than a mile to the east sits Michigan Avenue with its high-end shopping and expensive housing.

Over the years, gang violence and neglect created terrible conditions for the residents, and the name "Cabrini-Green" became synonymous with the problems associated with public housing in the United States. Specific gangs "controlled" individual buildings, and residents felt pressure to ally with those gangs in order to protect themselves from escalating violence. Police were reluctant to enter the area without backup protection.

The last of the buildings in Cabrini-Green was demolished in March, 2011. The area has been undergoing a redevelopment since the late 1990s, into a combination of high-rise buildings and row houses, with the stated goal of creating a mixed-income neighborhood, with some units reserved for public housing tenants.

Enter Leonard Wilson, DVM (not his real name). Leonard had just graduated near the top of his class from Ohio State University in June, 1966. His proud parents presented him with a brand-new, shiny Chevrolet to mark the occasion. He had accepted an offer to start his working career at the LSAH. Leonard was a farm boy with an interest in small animal medicine. LSAH would provide an excellent education. Little did Dr. Wilson realize his education would begin earlier than he planned.

Dusk cast long shadows on the skyscrapers as Dr. Wilson arrived at LSAH around 8:30 PM. Finding the hospital closed, Leonard parked on the street in front of the building and registered at the small hotel across from LSAH. Imagine Dr. Wilson's shock the next morning when he awoke to find his beautiful Chevy parked where he'd left it, missing all four tires, the battery, radio, and typewriter. The thieves were not interested in his textbooks. I wish I knew what happened to Dr. Wilson. No one at LSAH has a clue. Maybe he'll read my story and fill in the blanks.

My friend, Norm Abplanalp, when asked about Cabrini-Green, wrote the following;

> When I started at Montgomery Ward's in 1978, my business life changed a lot.
>
> The Ward's office tower, located on Chicago Avenue, was directly across the street from a cluster of low-rise units that were a part of Cabrini-Green. The catalogue house stretched some 1200 feet along the side street to the north was diagonally across from the infamous high-rise units. It was the route I drove every day to work.
>
> Upon arrival at the Ward's complex I was instructed to be very careful of my exposure to the street and the parking ramp, which, along with all buildings, were heav-

ily guarded 24/7. Employees that used train service were escorted to the station by security guards, they moved in packs for safety. The place was an armed encampment—a long, long way from my quiet life working in suburban Park Ridge.

My first office was located on the 23rd floor of the office tower. One Monday morning when I arrived for work, there were bullet holes in the upper section of my window. Police were called, and they placed soda straws in the holes to track the trajectory. The shells were embedded in the ceiling tiles. They pointed to one of the units in Cabrini-Green.

A number of land parcels just east of the parking ramp were converted to play yards for the Green—basketball, toddler playgrounds, and similar facilities. At least one notorious bar was purchased and torn down to help reduce the troublemakers on the route to the train station. Slowly the area south and east of the Ward's complex changed into artist studios and galleries, along with some very trendy restaurants. The artists have now moved out, because it's just too expensive an area.

Cabrini is now totally gone, but the memory lingers on.

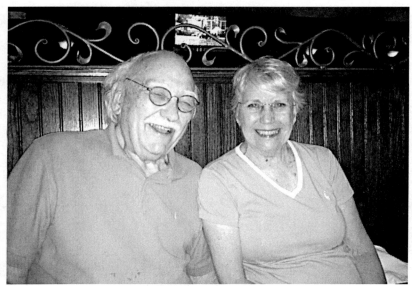

Norm and Lois Abplanalp

The Chef's Sons—Taste of Kenosha

My book is titled *The Veterinarian's Son,* so it seems natural to seek the stories of three of my favorite establishments in Kenosha, now run by sons or grandsons. Radigan's, Bartley House, and Andrea's.

Carol and I drove up to Kenosha, Wisconsin, to answer an ad in the JAVMA describing an animal hospital for sale. The fall colors were beginning to appear—hints of yellow, gold, brown, and red among the greenery. It was sixty miles, on the dot, from Brookfield, Illinois, up Highway 45—no interstate highway yet. The animal hospital was built within five acres of oak trees. It was the prettiest sight I'd ever seen. At least that was my first impression. Carol agreed, love at first sight. We met Mrs. Annette Fortmann, Dr. Abe's widow, on the circular drive in front of the establishment. Dr. Abe had died a year earlier of an undiagnosed brain tumor. He went from good health to migraines to death in a matter of a few months. The hospital was being leased to a young vet who was moving to Milwaukee. A call to my banker, Uncle Byron Merrick, assured me a loan for the down payment would be provided. All that was left was to sign a couple of papers, set a closing date, and find a good restaurant for dinner. Mrs. Fortmann recommended Ray Radigan's on Lake Michigan, just south of Kenosha. This was a very pleasant beginning to my 45 years in Kenosha.

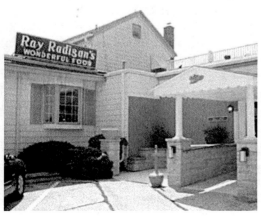

Ray Radigan's may have been founded in 1933, but the roadhouse location on Sheridan Road, just north of the Illinois-Wisconsin border, suggests it has been there much longer. A recent review stated, "While most restaurants promise wonderful food, most don't live up to the promise, though fortunately, Ray Radigan's does." Starched white tablecloths, a tasteful spray of flowers, and a formally set table set the mood. Rolls warm from the oven were accompanied by butter with the restaurant's name stamped on.

A wonderful meal—a martini, followed by small filets—ended our first day in our future home town. The drive back to Brookfield was uneventful. Carol snuggled and slept on the way.

Over the next 40 years I cared for many of Ray's dogs. After Ray retired, his son, Mike, continued the Radigan's tradition of excellence.

The story—told as "mostly true"—was that Bartley O'Mara's dad was a Kenosha bookie in the twenties and thirties. He started the restaurant/bar as a front for his bookmaking operation. It became more successful as time went on and prohibition ended. I

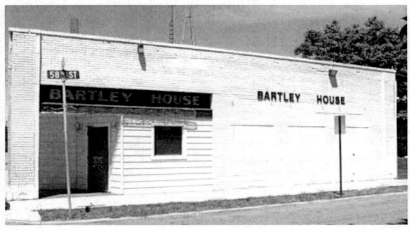

may get to hear the "real" story someday from one who would know how it all began. Bartley was a client for many years. His son, Bart Jr., and daughter, Maureen, now manage the establishment. It sits in the "old" part of town, right by the elevated Northwestern Railroad tracks which carry commuters from Milwaukee to Chicago. You would never find it without local knowledge or Google.

On a recent visit to Kenosha following my grandson Joe Vlahovic's marriage to Crystal Koba, I decided to invite the wedding party to an early supper at the Bartley House. Stopping by the establishment after lunch at Andrea's, I was greeted at the back door by the ever lovely Irish lass Maureen O'Mara, in her "work

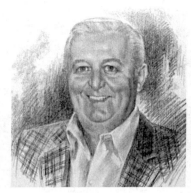

Bartley O'Mara, Sr.

clothes." When I inquired if she could accommodate 25 for dinner around 5 PM, she replied, "For you, Dr. Merrick, of course we can." When our party arrived, Maureen had ordered two extra waitresses and arraigned for Bart to show up a little early. Our hostess, Maureen, now stunning in her "evening work clothes," escorted us to our private tables. The meal was a five-star success. Nothing had changed in the ten years I'd been gone. "If it ain't broke, don't fix it."

My oldest son, Bill, bussed tables for The Bartley House when he was 16. Bart Jr. was also a busboy at the time. Bill recalled the best part of his job was being relieved from kennel cleaning duties. The worst was being stiffed by a crabby older waitress.

Andrea's has been a Kenosha fixture for 100 years. Started as a combination tobacco, candy and ice cream store, it has grown into one of those small town places where you can always find just the right, unique gift for anyone on your list. One can also get a delightful lunch before, during, or after shopping. It's still one of the few shops with a large selection of tobacco products. The third generation of Andrea's now manage the operation. Many of the seven Andrea kids went to school with my six. A page from Andrea's Web site follows.

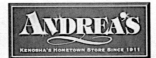

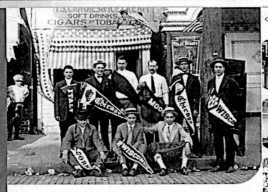

Original store 1912. Jack Andrea top row, second from left.

ANDREA'S HISTORY
THIS IS THE STORE THAT JACK BUILT

The year was 1911 and young Giacomo Andrea, who recently arrived from the Italian province of Calabria, set up shop in a piano crate on Holland Avenue (now called 22nd Avenue) He sold tobacco and candies to men and women who were on their way to and from work at the Vincent-Springs factory and the other area businesses.

Four years later, Jack, as he came to be known, moved his business to a store on 60th Street. Fans whirled above the Italian marble soda fountain counter where Jack dispensed ice cream extravaganzas that soon became Sunday afternoon traditions. The business grew, as did Jack's family. Jack moved to the current location at 2401 60th Street, filling the store with the sweet smells of confectionary and filling the apartment above with Jack's family, aunts and uncles. On cool summer evenings, friends would drop by to have sodas, smoke cigars, and talk into the early hours of the morning. During the day, children would rush in to buy penny candies and sugar cones filled with the rich ice cream that was now being made on the premises. In fact, it was at Andrea's that the rippling process was invented (fudge-ripple ice cream), as Antonio "Tony" Grassonio brought artistry to the manufacture of ice cream.

In the 1950's the second generation of Andreas took up where Jack left off ...still making "with love" old-fashioned sodas, sundaes, and thick malts and expanding the restaurant to serve complete meals. The tobacco shop also grew, offering custom-blended tobaccos and a larger selection of pipes and accessories.

In 1968 Andrea's closed for two weeks to remodel the building, which is now numbered three. The original entrance at the corner of 24th Avenue and 60th Street was bricked in to form the back wall of the humidor room. The Italian marble soda fountain counter was moved to its present home in the café. A bay window was installed to showcase the expanded gift collection. Where passers-by once looked in to the ice cream manufactory, they now saw gleaming table-top arrangements and cozy holiday gift displays.

It's been nearly a century since Jack opened his piano crate for business. And yet, Andrea's continues to value the friendships with the generations of Kenoshans who grew up with us. We hope that our commitment to service and quality will continue to foster the family traditions that were established so many years ago. In fact, we're dedicated to the proposition that the good old days are today at Andrea's.

CLICK ON PHOTOS BELOW FOR A DETAILED VIEW.

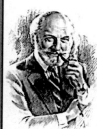

AL ANDREA

For three generations Andrea's has excelled in the premium cigar and tobacco industry. Second-generation Al Andrea (Jack's son) was a proponent of "all things in moderation." He worked tirelessly in the industry to emphasize quality over quantity in the enjoyment of fine tobaccos. In the 1960's, Al introduced his own custom blends of pipe tobacco, among them Andrea's Prime Time and Hunter's Moon. He also travelled throughout Europe, building relationships with the premier makers of handcrafted smoking pipes in Dublin, London, and Milan.

This same expertise resides in Andrea's today, where third-generation David Andrea, Scott Bruss, and staff are able to match the right product to your taste, temperament, and leisure time.

There will be no third generation of Merrick veterinarians unless my grandchildren choose to follow in the path of their forebearers. I was the only one of my father's children to take up the torch. My six kids are all following different paths. Who knows what roads the next generation will embark upon.

The Marvelous Mahones

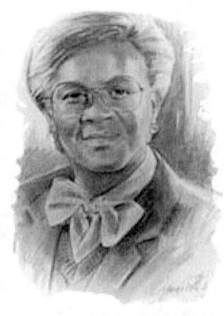

Malcolm X, the black civil rights activist assassinated in the mid-sixties, stated in a TV interview, "When I'm in a new town and looking for my people, I ask for the directions to the Lincoln school. Sure enough, it's located right in the black neighborhood." The same was true in Kenosha at that time. Imagine my surprise when Googling my black friend, Mary Lou Mahone, before beginning to write a story about her wonderful family. Google popped up loads of information about "The Mary Lou Mahone Middle School," which was located smack-dab in the center of an affluent middle-class neighborhood on the west side of town.

Kenosha, the city, is the county seat of Kenosha County in the State of Wisconsin in the United States. With an estimated population of 97,856 in 2009, Kenosha is the fourth-largest city in Wisconsin. Kenosha is also the fourth-largest city on the western shore of Lake Michigan, following Chicago, Milwaukee, and Green Bay. Kenosha lies on the southwestern shore of Lake Michigan, 32 miles (51 km) south of Milwaukee.

Historically, Kenosha was a very difficult place to be a person of color or other minority. In the 1950s, Kenosha had a population that was 5% black and 3% Hispanic. Racine, a city of similar size ten miles north of Kenosha, had double the number of minorities as Kenosha. This may have been due to the influence of Johnson's Wax, one of Racine's largest employers. The housing in Kenosha was "redlined," just as in most other northern cities.

Art and Mary Lou (Lou to friends) Mahone were pillars of Kenosha's minority community when I began practicing in Kenosha. They were one of the few black families to own their own home on the north side of town, miles away from Lincoln School. In the span of 20 years they would have nine children.

At the time, 1960, there were no blacks on the police or fire departments. There was not one black school teacher in the Kenosha public school system. My friend, Dr. Bob Sternloff, Director of the Kenosha Recreation Department, told me he had strongly recommended that the schools hire a black physical education instructor. Despite being much more qualified than the other candidates, he was informed his job would be in jeopardy if he pushed the issue.

Mary Lou worked in the catalog department of the downtown Sears store. She was the first African American PTA president in Kenosha and the first African American to run for the Kenosha Unified School District No. 1 Board of Education. She volunteered many hours working for equal rights and a good quality of life for all children. Mary Lou was also an original founder of the Boys and Girls Club of Kenosha.

Art, after working briefly at American Motors, was a welder at Allis Chalmers in Deerfield, Illinois. He joined the faculty at Gateway Technical College as a welding instructor and taught there for many years. He had been the Heavyweight Golden Gloves contender in Kenosha and had earned a brown belt in the Korean martial arts, Tae Kwon Do. Art died at home after a long illness in 2010.

To supplement his income, Art worked for me as an all-around assistant. Any job requiring "heavy lifting" was saved for Art. Art was very strong, but had a firm, gentle manner with animals. They sensed he

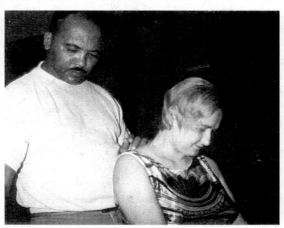

Carol Merrick having her hair styled by Art Mahone

was the leader of the pack. My guess the same applied at home. Art was also an excellent hair stylist. Carol used his services whenever she could.

Despite their many achievements and accolades, Mary Lou and Art were most proud of their offspring. Each was successful in their own right. Carrying on the Mahone torch is Ardis of Kenosha, WI; Bruce (Lisa) of Ft. Myers, FL; Malcolm of Chicago, IL; Cerci of Sioux Falls, SD; Sydne of Coralville, IA; Jonathan (Yvonne) of San Antonio, TX; Timothy of Kenosha, WI; Sean (Tamarah) of Troy, MI; and Jennifer of Kenosha, WI.

Mahone Middle School, built in 2002, was named after Mary Lou Mahone. The history page on the school Web site follows:

About Mary Lou Mahone

A woman of substance and elegance, Mary Lou Mahone played a big role in Kenosha. She was a dedicated leader and activist to her community achieving much in her life, from being the first black PTA president in Kenosha, to being a charter member of the Boys and Girls Club.

Mary Lou Mahone was also a strong guiding spirit, bounding people with love and prayer. In her private life she was a lover of literature and music, a gourmet cook, and a keeper of African American culture. Due to her life work, Kenosha has been made a better city for everyone. She died on June 8, 1999.

To honor their parents the Mahone children have established the Mary Lou and Art Mahone Fund in conjunction with the local Liberal Arts Carthage College.

The Mary Lou Mahone Endowment Fund was created in 1999 as an open Field of Interest Fund within the Foundation, to celebrate her life and legacy. The Fund's mission is to address the needs of disadvantaged individuals through the creation of opportunities in youth leadership activities, women's health initiatives, and senior citizen programs.

Through the community's generous response to the fund's ideals, and through such fundraising efforts as the annual "Reaching for Rainbows" Gospel Fest, the Mary Lou Mahone Golf Classic, and the Jazz & Blues Festival, the Endowment Fund has grown to more than $600,000.

What's in a Name?

Over 500 years ago Shakespeare had Juliet give voice to this classic verse:
>'Tis but thy name that is my enemy;
>Thou art thyself, though not a Montague.
>What's Montague? It is nor hand, nor foot,
>Nor arm, nor face, nor any other part
>Belonging to a man. O, be some other name!
>What's in a name? That which we call a rose.
>By any other name would smell as sweet

My friend, author and colleague, Dr. Jack Antyles wrote a story in one of our veterinary journals about what clients name their pets and how this might give vets a clue about the pet and clients nature. He made the point that most people give their pets positive, classic names, e.g., Prince, Duke, Lady; or descriptive names, e.g., Blackie, Dusty, Spot. No one names their pet, "Welfare Recipient." I once had a client who named their overactive Boxer puppy "Damnit." You only had to spend five minutes with Damnit to see how appropriate his name was.

At one time in the 1960s I had three clients whose names presented a problem. Each of the men had divorced and remarried. Each had acquired a pet of the same breed and name as in their previous union. When Mrs. Weber called for an appointment for her Siamese cat, Snookie, was she Dr. Weber's first or second spouse? When Mrs. Grinder called about her Basset, Droopy, was she Mrs. Grinder two, or the first Mrs. Grinder ("Miss Charlotte"), our kids ballet teacher? Each woman would be asking for an appointment for an animal with the same name. The receptionists would pull both animals' records and identify which was which when the owner showed up. The third duplication was made moot when the second Mr. and Mrs. Henry Sampson and their Toy Collie, Lady, moved to Colorado.

My dentist, Dr. Warren Johnson related this story during an office visit around 1960, treating his Cocker Spaniel, Blackie. It seemed he was contacted by a repo guy looking to take back a Cadillac that he had stopped paying for. Only problem was Dr. Johnson didn't own, and had never owned, a Cadillac. Another

Warren Johnson had used his name and address to buy the car in Milwaukee six months previously. That's a good story, but unfortunately, in the 60 years of passing time, memories can conjure up "facts" that are unrelated to the truth. A call to the real Dr. Warren Johnson produced the actual story, with the computer help of his granddaughter, Hannah Johnson.

Every dental practice has a history of a chain of events. In 1950 my office was above the Lincoln Drug Store with other doctors and a dentist. Some of them were moving to other areas and it looked like they were being replaced with apartments for families—not a good mix with professional offices. I began to look for a new place to practice. Two empty lots on 38th Avenue and 75th Street were owned by the city, and I bought them. Shortly after that the Lincoln Food Store's owner died and that was a block away from the lots I had purchased. At that time it was large enough for two dental offices and since it was one large room, it could easily be divided into two separate offices that would be adequate for two dentists. I asked Dr. Evo Sentiere if he would be interested in being a partner in this project and he said yes. We would then have ground floor offices.

I sold the two lots to a building contractor to get money to buy, convert, and equip the new office. That was the last that I thought I had to do with the lots. That was not true. About a year later the contractor called one evening and wanted to know what kind of lots I had sold him. I asked him why? He said some lawyer had stopped his construction on them. I told him his trouble must be coming from before I owned them.

Then, it occurred to me that some friends of ours who lived next door to a couple whose name was the same as mine and who was going through bankruptcy, may cause me some complications. That is exactly what it was! The court thought that my lots were land he had owned and was selling them.

This was all cleared up with my going to the court and proving that I was not him and that the lots were mine and not his.

From time to time after that, every now and then, an attorney would call and try to collect from me some bill that the other Warren Johnson owed. But, by then I was aware of this issue and would tell them they had the wrong person and that would end it.

All of these calls finally ended when the other Warren Johnson died.

                    Sincerely,
                    Warren Johnson, with the
                    help of Hannah Johnson

Animals' names haven't changed much in the last fifty years. Compare that to the ten most common girls and boys names of 1960 and today.

Most Popular Children's Names			
Girls, 1960	**Girls, 2010**	**Boys, 1960**	**Boys, 2010**
Lisa	Isabella	**Michael**	Jacob
Mary	Emma	David	Ethan
Karen	Olivia	John	**Michael**
Susan	Sophia	James	Alexander
Kimberly	Ava	Robert	**William**
Patricia	Emily	Mark	Joshua
Linda	Madison	**William**	Daniel
Donna	Abigail	Richard	Jayden
Michelle	Chloe	Thomas	Noah
Cynthia	Mia	Jeffery	Anthony

Not one of the top ten girls' names of the '60s are popular today. Two of the boys' names still make the list. My guess is the popular names fifty years in the future will include many more Hispanic names: Pedro, Pablo, Manuel, Carlos, Maria, Conchita.

Most Popular AKC Dog Names, 2010	
Male	**Female**
Bear	Lady
Blue	Belle/Bell/Bella
Max/Maximus/Maxwell	Princess
Duke	Mae/May
Buddy	Rose
Jack	Daisy
Prince	Grace/Gracie
King	Baby
Bailey	Molly
Rocky	Maggie
Harley	Sadie
Jake	Ann/Annie
Shadow	Star
Lucky	Lily/Lilly
Hunter	Angel
Dakota	Coco/Cocoa
Lou	Sophie/Sophia
Midnight	Lucy
Cooper	Abby/Abigail

For the last several years running, Max had been the most popular name of all. Why? Because it is easy to understand, short (one-syllable) and it suits both large and small dogs, as well as cute and tough ones alike! This year Bear topped the AKC list.

Remembering Jesse Payne

Jesse was a southern boy—about as far south as you could get and still be in Illinois— from Cairo (pronounced like Karo syrup, not like the city in Egypt). Our affable anatomy teacher, Dr. Sinclair, loved to fire trick questions at the class. "What muscle squeezes the last drop of urine out of the penis?" I'm thinking, bladder muscle? stomach muscle? Without hesitation, Jesse answered, "deep digital flexor." "Damn," Sinclair said, "you're right."

Jesse had a philosophy that I adopted early on. It applied to baseball—Jesse was a great second baseman—and to life in general. "Take two and hit to right." Translated, it means, "Don't be in a hurry to make decisions. Wait for your pitch, and give the runner a chance to advance on his own three different ways—a wild pitch, balk, or stolen base." Helping your teammate is your objective. Hitting to right field allows the runner to reach third base on a single.

Jesse played fiddle in a country-western band. Whenever they had a gig at a local bar, Carol and I, accompanied by a number of classmates, attended to dance and cheer.

Jesse and I shared a taxicab job one winter during our junior year in vet school. The hours were 5 PM to midnight, seven days a week. With that schedule, I had no doubt they had a hard time filling the position. I mentioned the job to Jesse. Jesse said it sounded like just the job for us together. Jesse said, "We could work from 5 to 9 and study from 9 to 12 every other day." And so we did. It worked out even better than Jesse had foreseen. It was an ideal job. Start work around 3 or 4 PM and work until 10 or 11 PM, depending on the day and business. We paid our own gas, split the fares with the owner, and kept all of our tips. Paying 25 cents a gallon for gas in the '50s, we could clear $10.00 on a good night.

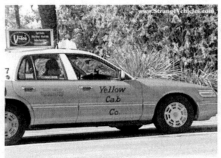

One afternoon, I took a soldier from the train station to a little town in Indiana, ten miles east of Danville. Illinois. About 40 miles each way. Total including tip was $25.00. Pretty good for the two-hour trip. We were usually busy from 4 until around 8 PM Most of the commuter trains or buses were in by then. Afterward, I'd park by the bus or train station to wait for a pickup or radio fare. It was a perfect time to do two or three hours of reading or cramming for tomorrow's quiz.

No one knows a city like a cabbie. Even today, I instinctually drive down alleys and look for short cuts, which used to drive Carol wild. You think she would have gotten used to it after 50 years. I was surprised to discover that most fares don't consider the driver is in the cab. Anything one can imagine goes on in the back seat—yelling, screaming, gossip, passionate lovemaking—the whole nine yards.

Jesse and I discovered we were both better than average ping-pong players. We noticed an announcement of an intramural table tennis tournament and decided to enter. Most of the matches took place in fraternity houses or the college union. We won better than half our games but were eliminated before the quarterfinals.

In 1997 my youngest daughter, Peggy, and her husband, Don Auxier, embarked on a delayed honeymoon, which included Tupelo on the way. I mentioned I had visited with Jesse and his wife, Loretta, at a reunion gathering and determined that they had retired to Tupelo. I called Jesse and inquired if they would be available for a visit from the newlyweds. "Of course," was his reply, "the sooner the better."

Arriving on their motorcycles a few weeks later, Peg and Don were greeted like long-lost relatives. After seeing Don's bright crimson cycle, Jesse remarked, "For another dime, you could have gotten a *red* one!" Within hours both couples were off to a cat-

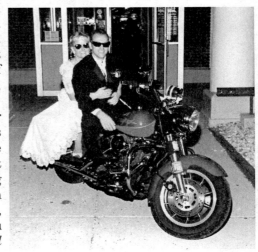

Peggy and Don Auxier

fish dinner at Jesse's expense. "I'll feel offended if you don't bunk with us tonight," Loretta said.

On the way home from supper Jesse stopped by his store to show off his establishment. While staring at the countless rows of bottles, Jesse said, "If I'd known how much money I could make selling booze, I'd have retired a lot earlier." He then showed Don the "peacemaker" he had hidden under the checkout counter. "I don't hesitate to show this magnum to customers," he said. Thankfully, Jesse never had occasion to use the weapon.

Jesse passed after a sudden illness within 8 months after Peg and Don's visit. I received the following obit. from the U. of I. veterinary school: "Dr. Jesse Payne, Jr. (54), of Tupelo, Mississippi, died August 17, 1998. His 40-year career with the Meat and Poultry Inspection Program of the U.S. Department of Agriculture was devoted to national policies for food safety and public health. During his career he held every elected and appointed position in the National Association of Federal Veterinarians."

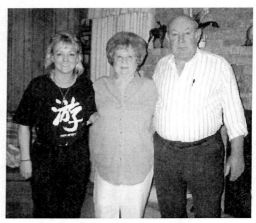

Peggy Merrick Auxier, Loretta & Jesse Payne

Jerry Banicki

Jerry Banicki was not your typical farm boy applicant to vet school after World War II. He had been accepted in the new school's second class (I was in the third), starting vet school in 1949 and graduating in 1953. His farming experience amounted to herding drunks out his dad's Chicago bar after a late night of carousing. He learned different languages by working in the family laundromat and bar, and Polish at home. There were always people from different countries he was interacting with, so he picked up a little bit here and there. Jerry had enlisted shortly after the bombing of Pearl Harbor and flew missions to bomb southern Germany.

Jerry's granddaughter, Mariah Moeser, wrote the following letter after consulting Jerry:

>Jerry entered the service in 1942, went through school at Kirtland AFB, then on to Barksdale. As he was pulling up to Barksdale for the first time, he saw a plume of smoke. The cab driver told him that it was a daily sight; once a day a B-26 went into the ground. He went from Barksdale to Eglin Field to Ascension Island to the Coast of Africa (the French Riviera, he thinks) and that's where they started flying missions. On his first mission, they returned and counted 300 bullet holes in the plane.
>
>The first time he went down was north of Rome, Italy. He was picked up by the British in a small one-seater. He doesn't remember much about the flight back, but he does remember people sitting on the tail of the plane to help it get in the air. He was in a hospital in Sicily for two months. The second time he went down was also in Italy, but he was captured by the Germans. He spent just under two years in a camp and was in isolation for 2 weeks. He has many stories from his time there.
>
>In one he mentioned was how he kept trying to dig escape tunnels—he says 100—and 100 times the Germans caught him. He had a ring from Kirtland or Barksdale that one of the Germans wanted. He told them that he couldn't get it off his finger, so they couldn't have it.

The German said he knew a way, and pulled out a knife to cut off his finger. Jerome soon found a way to get the ring off. He spoke 3 or 4 languages—Russian, Polish, German and English, I think—and so was called on to help translate at times. On Jan. 17, 1946, he separated from active duty, as a captain. Thank you, Mariah.

In a later communication from Mariah, she states:

> He was shot down a the second time in Italy. Once on the ground, he was shot in the back by the Italians and then captured by the Germans and sent to a POW camp in Germany. He lost 90 lbs while he was a POW. The camp was located north of Berlin on the Baltic-Stalag Luft or Luftwaffe-Stammlager (Luftwaffe base camp). These POW camps were administered by the German Air Force for Allied aircrews. Despite his capture, Jerry managed to smile for the camera.
>
> After his release, he walked two days to a British camp and, after retrieving the rest of the POWs from the camp, he left and was sent to Camp Lucky Strike for recovery before going home. At Lucky Strike they had them on a diet for a few days to ease them back into a regular diet of more and richer foods. He says that after those few days he was back to three meals a day, but it took him years to gain that weight back.

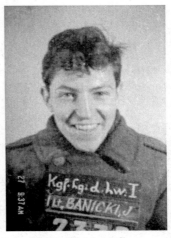

Jerry Banicki in a German POW camp.

Jerry was a survivor—in war and vet school. Jerry finished as one of the top students in his class. When asked about his motivation/drive, Jerry usually answered facetiously, "Greed." When pressed, he admits it was his life-long ambition to become a veterinarian. He remembers in grade school how he use to go to the animal shelter and visit. He always wanted to be a veterinarian. Jerry said sometimes he wished he had gone to med school, but then he wonders/thinks he may not have lived as long. Being a people doctor is too much stress, and he enjoyed working with animals.

After finishing vet school came the tough part.

The Veterinarian's Son — Jerry Banicki

As one could imagine, veterinarians were in short supply in a state without a vet school. Illinois was no exception. Jerry and wife, Bernice, determined Decatur would be an ideal place to start a small animal practice. Located some 80 miles west of Champaign and 150 miles south of Chicago, Decatur was a fast-growing city of 40,000. There were only three veterinarians in town—none focusing exclusively on small animals.

Bankers had not yet learned that veterinarians are the best credit risks among all professionals; their default rate is near zero. No one was eager to risk loaning money to a young, inexperienced veterinarian. He never asked a bank for money to start his business, but he did write 100 letters to friends and family asking for $100 to get started. He did not promise to repay the money, it was accepted as a gift. Jerry stated that he received approx $4000 but did not repay anyone. He even asked the dean of his vet school for money.

After surveying Decatur, Jerry and Bernice bought a house on a main street which could serve as both clinic and residence. Just as they were settling in and starting to get clients, disaster struck. The city closed the road in front of his building to widen the street. The only way to his practice was by a back alley. Naturally, drive-by traffic slowed to a trickle. Bernice stated at the time, "Business is so bad, we would love to see salesmen come in so we could have somebody to talk to." With a wife and two young children to support, Jerry would do it all and help anyone who asked, from inspecting stock yards and making house calls to taking care of smaller house pets.

The street was out for a year. During that time, since he was not able to keep the business going without additional income, he taught at a Milliken College nursing school for that year until the street reopened. Jerry dug out a basement under the hospital. Once they moved out, it was turned into the dog kennels. It was as large as the building itself. Jerry reports he would board or have 100 dogs in there. He said he would put them anywhere he could fit them—$2/day for cats and $3/day for dogs.

I guess the lesson is "survivors survive." The road finally reopened, business picked up, and Jerry's practice prospered. He retired in 1995, at that time four other vets were working at the hospital. He said that during his time there he tried to hire anyone who came along looking for a job, and he would have, at some points, five or six vets working for him.

Jerry's granddaughter, Mariah Moeser, reports that Bernice passed on November 29, 2011. Jerry died exactly two months later, on January 29, 2012. Their spirit lives on with the countless friends, clients and family they influenced.

War Stories

Gordon Becker's bio in our local Kiwanis directory is as follows:
War Veteran—WWII, India/Burma/China—85 missions. Served in U.S. Army & Air Force for 6 years (active) and 17 years (reserve). Colonel. At age 19 he was the youngest pilot and flight instructor in Baltimore area. He was fired for setting a "bad example" flying through a tree while leading a three-ship formation with British cadets! Retired: Chief, Flight Standards Division, Southern Region, Federal Aviation Agency.

Tom Brokow's bestselling book, *The Greatest Generation,* details the lives of many men and women who served in World War II and beyond.

In 2008, a New Orleans newspaper reported the following:
They were a swashbuckling lot—parachuting behind enemy lines, charging onto sandy beaches as bullets whizzed by, liberating countries from a totalitarian grip.

They jitterbugged the nights away, sang about faraway sweethearts, and painted the noses of their B-17 bombers with bawdy pinups. "They're overpaid, oversexed, and over here," the British groused about their American allies.

And now they're dying off, and with them the memories that defined what has been called the Greatest Generation. Once 16 million strong, U.S. veterans of World War II are dying at a rate of more than 1,200 a day. As their ranks shrink, the National World War II Museum is one of several organizations rushing to preserve the personal accounts of veterans. Other such efforts are sponsored by the Library of Congress and the U.S. Latino and Latina WWII Oral History Project.

In May, 2011, the Department of Veterans Affairs estimated that approximately 2,079,000 American veterans are still living. By 2020, most will be gone. There are 2,079,000 stories yet to tell.

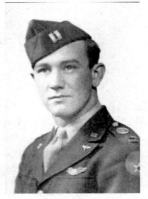
Capt. Gordon Becker
Age 22 • 1942

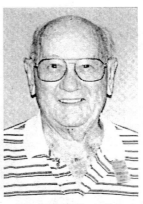
Colonel Becker, Ret.
Age 91 • 2011

Most who served their country 60 years ago are reluctant to recount the details of their service.

I play golf twice a week with one of those guys. Nine holes are all Gordon's aging knees will allow. He played to a 10 handicap in his prime. Now he's happy to hit the ball straight.

My guess is Gordon forgot to list his Baltimore "flying through a tree" escapade on his resume for the FAA job.

Gordon began flying lessons while still in high school, as a senior at the age of 16. He recalled the price was $5.00 per hour—$2.00 for gas and $3.00 for the instructor. By the age of 18 he had accumulated 180 hours of solo flying. He was 20 hours short of the requirements for a commercial pilot's license. His instructor offered Gordon a deal: We'll grant your commercial pilot's license, and you can pay us at the rate of $4.00/hour out of your earnings.

Gordon became a flight instructor.

My brother-in-law, Edward Scheffelin, served in the Pa-

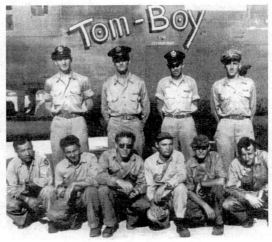

cific as a bombardier on a B-24. Scheff flew 44 missions and received the Distinguished Flying Cross.

In this 1943 photo (opposite page) Scheff is standing in the back right with a flying friend on his left shoulder. He is 23.

He retired in 1970 after 30 years of service.

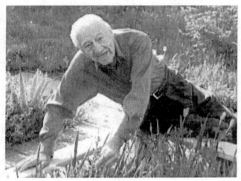

Scheff's pride and joy is his flower garden, encompassing both front and back yards of his home in Carmichael, California. He is pictured on his 90th birthday, in August, 2010, pulling weeds. What else makes a Master Gardener happy?

Scheff started the Visual Tutor Company, designing and producing mathematical instructional materials for children and youth with learning problems. The Quebec Association for Children with Learning Disabilities called Visual Tutor "A Good Aid for the Right Child."

In the early 1990s, the magazine published by the Reserve Officers Association asked World War II veterans to send in their experiences, and selected stories were published in the issue that coincided with the 50th anniversary of their experiences. Selected contributions, including Scheff's, were published in a 1996 book, *World War II Reminiscences,* edited by John H. Roush:

"Landing with an Angel"

First Lieutenant Edward J. Scheffelin joined the 72nd Squadron as a bombardier in B-24s in November, 1943, about four months after the Coral Sea battle. He was part of the 5th Bomber Group, 13th Air Force. At the time of this story he was stationed on Munda [in the Solomon Islands].

On the return from one mission against Rabaul, the weather was particularly stormy. It was pitch black except when thunderclouds 60,000 feet high were lit up like Christmas trees from lightning. They were too high to fly over, and it was too dangerous to try to fly under them. Too often those clouds blended with the ocean. Visibility was zero, and the area was dotted with tiny islands and tall mountains. Flying at about 20,000 feet, the pilot, Captain Tom Shearin, had to lace the plane around the menacing clouds. Because they could only use dead reckoning, those maneuvers caused their navigator to lose his position; they were lost.

With only a half hour's worth of fuel left, the crew began to get concerned. All had craned necks at windows, looking for something in the soup. Finally, First Lieutenant Scheffelin saw some anti-aircraft shells exploding in front of them. The navigator determined that the shells had to be coming from Rendova Island, where the United States had a small fighter base. Radio silence forbade any contact, but it gave them a position, and the plane made a beeline for Munda—home—about a half hour away. Captain Shearin had all four engines leaned out as much as he dared.

They entered the Munda traffic pattern. On downwind, one engine sputtered and quit. On final, a second engine fizzled out. A B-24 lands very heavily on normal landings, due to the short chord length of their Davis wings. Good landings required a touchdown speed of 90–100 mph, which also dictates that all four engines are operating. Somehow Shearin made it down in one piece on only two engines. As the plane taxied to the revetment area, a third engine gave up. Shearin parked it with only one engine running, and it had less than five minutes' worth of fuel left.

Had it not been for the anti-aircraft fired at them, the crew would not have known where they were in time. They would have gone down. Maybe on an island, maybe on the ocean. Unfriendly land, and unforgiving water. The angel that flew with that crew did not relinquish her duty.

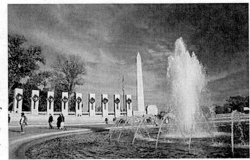

The World War II Memorial honors the 16 million who served in the armed forces of the U.S., the more than 400,000 who died, and all who supported the war effort from home. Symbolic of the defining event of the 20th century, the memorial is a monument to the spirit, sacrifice, and commitment of the American people.

The Second World War is the only 20th century event commemorated on the National Mall's central axis. The memorial opened to the public on April 29, 2004, and was dedicated one month later, on May 29.

Volunteers started Honor Flight Network, a nonprofit organization founded in 2006 to fly veterans at no cost to Washington to see the World War II Memorial and other monuments. Top priority is given to the senior veterans, World War II survivors, along with other veterans who may be terminally ill. Of all of the wars in recent memory, it was World War II that truly threatened our very existence as a nation—and as a culturally diverse, free society.

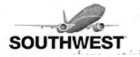

Official Honor Flight Airline

Lt. Dan Berschinski, a 25-year-old from Peachtree City, Ga. is part of the 5th Brigade, 2nd Infantry Division, which has been deployed with eight-wheeled vehicles, called "Strykers," to southern Afghanistan, a stronghold of Taliban forces. Since arriving in the summer, the brigade has lost more than two dozen soldiers.

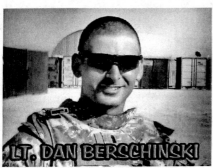

Dan graduated from McIntosh High School in Peachtree City, in a class between my grandchildren, Adam and Cc Robinson.

An excerpt of a column posted on Dan Berschinski's Web site by Hal Bernton on December 1, 2009:

> In 2007, Dan Berschinski graduated from West Point. He headed off to Fort Lewis, Washington, where, in July of that year, he led an infantry platoon to Afghanistan.
>
> Berschinski had both legs mangled and one arm badly injured by a land mine in August, and was sent for treatment to Walter Reed Army Medical Center in Washington, D.C.
>
> As for Berschinski, his homecoming has been a marathon of surgeries and rehabilitation. In recent weeks, he has walked on an initial pair of artificial legs. In the fall

of 2011, he expects to check out of Walter Reed Army Medical Center and begin outpatient therapy. In an interview on CNN aired in September of 2010, Dan expressed "No Regrets." One of the nurses appraised Dan as her most determined patient. The interviewer described Dan as both mentally and physically tough.

In the summer of 2011 I contacted Dan's parents to get an update on Dan's progress. They reported Dan was progressing beyond their wildest hopes. He reports to Walter Reed Hospital daily for physical therapy. Dan plans to return to school to get his MBA next year.

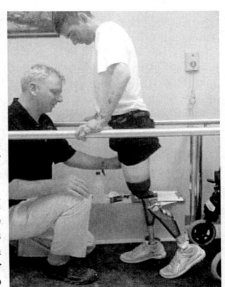

Learning to walk again • 2009
Photo courtesy of website maintained by Friends of Dan Berschinski.

Dan also encouraged everyone who had been supporting his recovery to think about supporting the Wounded Warrior Project instead.

Wounded Warrior Project (WWP) began when several veterans and friends, moved by stories of the first wounded service members returning home from Afghanistan and Iraq, took action to help others in need. What started as a program to provide comfort items to wounded service members has grown into a complete rehabilitative effort to assist warriors as they recover and transition back to civilian life.

The Army Wounded Warrior Program (AW2) is the official U.S. Army program that assists and advocates for severely wounded, ill, and injured soldiers, veterans, and their families, wherever they are located, regardless of military status. Warriors in Transition (WTs) who qualify for AW2 are assigned to the program as soon as possible after arriving at the WT. AW2 supports these soldiers and their families throughout their recovery and transition, even into veteran status. This program, through the local support of AW2 advocates, strives to foster the WT's independence.

I have written about five men who served their country in much different times. Sadly, Charles Abplanalp, killed in action in 1944, is no longer with us. Three others, Jerry Banicki, Gordon Becker and Edward Scheffelin are still "alive and kicking." Well, at least alive and moving. Daniel Breschinski at 28, is in his prime. The former three are all 90 years old. They were involved in wars fought 70 years ago. Given the current longevity figures, Dan could easily live until 2090 or 2100. In World War II, Dan would have come home in a body bag. I can't envision what "miracles" of technology and medicine await. Dan fully expects to have "new legs" grown from his own stem cells by the end of the next decade. I don't doubt it will happen. It should be a national priority to ensure that there is always government money available to provide the care these honored soldiers have earned.

Wikipedia reports:

> The dissolution of the Soviet Union was the disintegration of the federal political structures and central government of the Union of Soviet Socialist Republics (USSR), resulting in the independence of all 15 republics of the Soviet Union between March 11, 1990, and December 25, 1991. The broader result of the dissolution was the fall of communism as a global ideology between 1989 and 1991, and the end of the Cold War.
>
> Multi-ethnic communist federal states proved particularly vulnerable to disintegration during this time. The Soviet Union was but one example of three such states that collapsed in Europe as a result of the fall of communism, the others being the Socialist Republic of Yugoslavia, which broke up in a series of wars in 1991–1992, and Czechoslovak Socialist Republic, which had its peaceful velvet divorce in 1993.

The Soviet Union did not collapse because of a "Hot War" between East and West, but because of a "Cold War" based on ideas and market forces. The world began to see similar such events evolve in 2011 with the "Arab Spring" in the middle east.

I hope I live to see the day when America spends our treasure on spreading ideas by peaceful means. Changing hearts and minds should be our goal.

Second Time Around

Separation from a cherished pet has been equated to the loss of a loved family member—a child or spouse. I'm sure most veterinarians have heard clients remark—tongue in cheek—"My (dog, cat) means more to me than my (husband, kids)." It's seems natural to seek companionship after the loss of a spouse. As the population ages, the opportunities for "second time around" relationships increase. Chance often plays a role in facilitating these encounters.

Helen Skewes, who was the original motivator for my book, had been widowed for five years when she attended her 60th high school reunion in Ames, Iowa. She met her high school sweetheart, Dick Palmer, at the event. One thing lead to another and their relationship rapidly progress from dating to Helen moving to Dick's 400-acre farm near Tipton, Iowa. I received the following letter from Helen, which I will quote in part:

> I just did something I thought I would never do. I ran off with my high-school boyfriend. We have not been in touch with one another for 60 years, but our paths crossed last August and it's like I'm 17 again. The story is romantic but too long to share here. His wife of 50 years died last year after suffering with Alzheimer's for nine years. Together we have ten children, and were caregivers for 16 years. We decided life was too short not to have fun together, so although he sits on a 400-acre farm in Iowa, we took off on a two week odyssey. It was a trip he had been longing to take for ten years, and I loved every minute of it. I worried that my "good" reputation would be ruined, but I thought, "Oh, what the hell?" Conditions are different now, and I am so happy to be back in my life. Both our families are cheering us on, and who cares what the little old ladies at Tudor Manor [Retirement Center] think.

Helen's letter of July, 21, 2010 said in part, "We married a year and a half ago—January 13, 2009—but our ten children have not met. So we set up a big 80th birthday bash on July 20th in Iowa City, and made it mandatory that they all attend." The local newspaper carried the announcement that ten children, 15 grandchildren, and four great-grandchildren attended.

My brother Phil's wife of 43 years, Francine, died in 1996 after a five-month battle against cervical cancer. Retiring to Williamsburg, Virginia, after 30 years in the army, Phil managed various hotel/motels in Williamsburg-Hampton area for ten years. In 1990 he started a guided tour company, Colonial Connections, which gave group tours around the east coast.

Attending a friend's daughter's wedding, he encountered Phyllis Green, who had taken the Amtrack train from New York City to Williamsburg to attend the event. They reminisced about the time Phyllis was living in Williamsburg and the mutual friends they shared. Phil's travel business frequently took him to New York, where Phyllis was a sales manager for Pyle Coleman, arranging meeting space for Fortune 500 companies. He found many excuses to visit the empire city after that chance meeting. Phyllis lived in Battery Park, directly across from the World Trade Center. Phil had come to New York on Thursday, September 6, 2001 to look for a suitable restaurant for a senior tour to dine before attending the theater later that month. Phyllis worked in midtown near the theater district, so it was a natural that the two should meet and discuss the upcoming bus tour. Phil returned to Williamsburg on Saturday, September 9, 2001.

It was a beautiful fall weekend, not portending the events of Tuesday, September 11, 2001. Phyllis was an early riser and liked to get to work early. After taking the subway from Tower One to midtown, her friend in Wall Street called to tell of the first plane crashing into the building. Phyllis ran to the lobby to watch the TV and saw the second plane crash into the Tower Two. Life from that moment on would never be the same on the West Side Highway.

It took Phyllis ten hours to walk from midtown, criss-crossing the city and being stopped at every checkpoint for proof of residency. Fireman had run hoses through the lobby of her building for additional water to battle the blazes and keep them from spreading. Walking up to her 8th-floor apartment, Phyllis discovered everything covered in dust. Calls from Phyllis assured Phil she was shaken and exhausted, but surviving. On Thursday, September 13th, the residents were allowed 15 minutes in their buildings to gather personal items. Gathering some clothes, Phyllis slept on a girlfriend's couch for two months.

Two weeks after 9/11, Phil's tour group of seniors arrived in New York City after a tour of fall color in New England. They attempted to visit the site of the disaster but were unable to get closer than two blocks.

A Bell for Crabapple Elementary School

Tradition! Webster defines it as "The passing down of culture from generation to generation, especially by oral means." Wikipedia explains it this way:

> In the Broadway play, *Fiddler on the Roof,* the main character, Tevye, explains the roles of each social class (fathers, mothers, sons, and daughters) in the village of Anatevka, and how the traditional roles of people like the matchmaker and the rabbi contribute to the village. The song also sets the major theme of the show—the villagers trying to continue their traditions and keep their society running as the world around them changes. "Tradition!"

There was no tradition to pass on when Crabapple Lane Elementary School was built in 2003 in our adopted home town, Peachtree City, Ga.

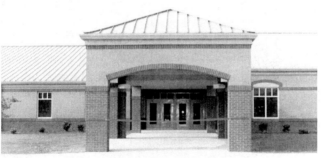

I had already donated receipts from a local Pike's Nursery, which allowed the school to receive "free" garden supplies. These were used to plant and maintain the school courtyard. Carol and I decided to donate our antique school bell. The provenance declared the bell had been cast by the C. S. Bell Company in Hillsboro, Ohio, around 1885. It had been in our family since 1963. The bell was a front-page feature on the September 11, 2006, edition of the Atlanta Journal Constitution commemorating the five-year anniversary of 9/11.

In 1995, the C. S. Bell Company was purchased by Prindle Station of Washogual, Washington, who promised to keep the original patterns.

460 A Bell for Crabapple Elementary

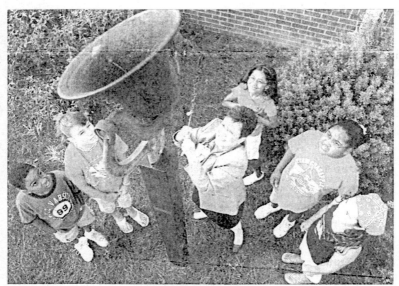

METRO ATLANTA: Every year on the anniversary of Sept. 11, Crabapple Lane Elementary School in Peachtree City rings its historic bell to honor those who died. Principal **Doe Evans** does the ringing Monday, surrounded by fifth-graders (from left) **Alex Saulsbury, Maddie Plant, Alyssa Mendez, Rhegan Mitchell** and **Lauren Phillips**. The century-old bell, donated when the school opened, is rung only one other time every year — on Veterans Day in November.

Atlanta Journal Constitution • September 11, 2006

Purchased as a "call to dinner" bell, it hung near our back door in Kenosha for nearly forty years. We couldn't bear to part with it, so we brought it along to Georgia. Without any kids to call or a place to hang, the bell remained silent for two years. At our annual neighborhood garage sale, we considered selling the bell. What price to ask? Google said old school bells sold for anywhere from $50 to $200. Then we came up with the idea to return the bell to its original purpose—calling school kids to class. Crabapple Lane Elementary school was just about ready for its first class in the early summer of 2003. Carol and I drove the mile to the school and entered to find the principal, Doe Evans, and the architect, Richard Powell, going over final plans. Both were enthusiastic about receiving the bell. The architect mentioned he could make the bell the focal point of the nearly finished courtyard. And so he did.

At a ceremony on December 12, 2003, Carol and I were honored guests at the dedication of the bell. The school presented us

BELLS ARE OUR BUSINESS

The C. S. Bell Company was founded over one hundred years ago by the grandfather of the present owners. During all that time, the Company has been owned by the family of the original founder, the name of the Company has been BELL, and one of the chief products has always been Bells.

During these one hundred years our Bells have been sold in every part of the world and they have become a standard of quality by those familiar with Bells. Our purpose, since we began manufacturing Bells in 1858, has been to furnish real Bell value. If you will consider the fact that there are more Bells of our make in use in the entire world than of all other makes combined, we believe you will come to the conclusion that purchasers of our Bells have been given that value.

Steel Alloy Bells are made of a mixture known only to ourselves. When

STORY OF THE BELLS

Throughout all ages, in all countries and among all peoples, bells have been the subject of veneration, symbolism, superstition, emotion and influence. They have been used for every sort of occasion, in times of great calamity or stress, in times of general thanksgiving, or public festivities, for private joys or sorrows.

There is no question but what it was a marvelous discovery to have found, in one stroke of an iron clapper against metal, the means of awakening the same feelings at the same moment in thousands of hearts and to have enlisted the winds and clouds as bearers of thoughts of men.

So personal are the feelings about bells that people often write to us about our bells as if they had lives of their own. One time, three of our bells in Pennsylvania spent a riotuous election night riding on a truck, but on the way home the truck overturned and the rollicking bells "died together." The next day, they were properly buried with all the school children in sorrowful attendance.

At Ellington Field, Texas, one of our bells became an enlisted man with the rank of Private First Class, a name — Oscar — and an official serial number!

Many of our Church Bells have been blessed and one of them listed among the "Bells that Changed the World." This bell, in the famous collection at the Mission Inn, Riverside, Calif., is the Father Damien Bell. It tells a story of true devotion and unselfish ministration to stricken brothers. It is the bell from the Church of St. Francis at the leper settlement on the Island of Molokai, one of the Hawaiian group.

But, of course, it has not only been the ca-

Above: Part of the C. S. Bell story. • Below: Commemorative photo.

"That a man is successful who has lived well, laughed often, and loved much, who has gained the respect of the intelligent men and the love of children; who has filled his niche and accomplished his task; who leaves the world better than he found it, whether by an improved poppy, a perfect poem, or a rescued soul; who never lacked appreciation of earth's beauty or failed to express it; who looked for the best in others and gave the best he had."

Robert Louis Stevenson

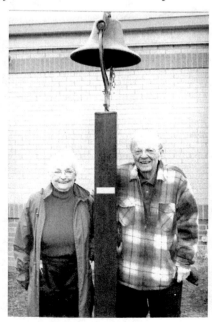

with a commemorative scrapbook with every class pictured, including a photo of Carol and me with the newly mounted bell.

Principal Doe Evans stated the bell will only be rung twice a year, on September 11th and November 11th. It will be used as a teaching moment to keep the tradition of honoring those individuals killed in the Twin Towers attack and the victims of all wars, past and present.

Crabapple Lane Elementary opened its doors on August 11, 2003. Sixty-six faculty and staff welcomed over 400 students for the start of our charter year.

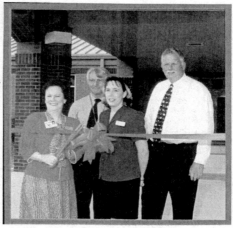

Mrs. Evans Klaus Darnall, Mrs. Walters, Mike Satterfield

Principal Evans, City Public Works Chief Darnell,
Assistant Principal Walters, and City Planner Satterfield

250 and Counting

I can picture it in my mind's eye: a Neolithic woman tending to an injured wolf cub (future dog), not aware she is the first animal doctor on the planet. The profession has come a long way in the succeeding eons.

Acupuncture has been used on animals for over 4000 years. Legend has it that veterinary acupuncture was discovered when lame horses used in battle were found to become sound after being hit by arrows at distinct points. In any event, there is evidence that Chinese "horse priests," the caretakers of the army's horses, practiced acupuncture during the Zang and Chow Dynasties around 2000–3000 B.C. Similarly, the International Veterinary Acupuncture Society (IVAS) website claims:

> Acupuncture may be defined as the insertion of needles into specific points on the body to cause a desired healing effect. This technique has been used in veterinary practice in China for at least 3000 years to treat many ailments. The Chinese also use acupuncture as preventive medicine against such problems as founder and colic in horse.

The Egyptian Papyrus of Kahun (1900 B.C.) and Vedic literature in ancient India offer one of the first written records of veterinary medicine. (See also Shalihotra) One of the edicts of Ashoka reads:

> Everywhere King Piyadasi (Asoka) erected two kinds of hospitals—hospitals for people and hospitals for animals. Where there were no healing herbs for people and animals, he ordered that they be bought and planted."
> The Talmud does state that no mares were exported from Egypt in Roman times without being subjected to a hysterectomy, which tend to prove that successful surgery was implemented in such an early period.

John M. Hicks, Jr., DVM, MPH, in a paper published in 2007, described the veterinarian's role in public health by citing the long history of veterinary accomplishments during the past centuries:

Veterinary Medicine in Ancient Civilizations

INDIA
- Hindu Vedas, well over a thousand years before Christ, set forth treatises on human and veterinary medicine.
- First writings on medicine of man and animals.
- Vedic veterinary medicine interprets that man learned the art of medicine from observing animals and birds.
- Later Greek and Roman veterinarians owe much to Hindu veterinary medicine.

EGYPT
- Veterinary Papyrus of Kahun (1900 B.C.), oldest veterinary medical writings yet discovered.
- Considered the "birthplace" of the great animal plagues of the Middle East (most likely anthrax).

BABYLONIA
- Babylonians emphasized preventive medicine (Judaic sanitary practices are considered to be of Babylonian origin).
- Code of Hammurabi (2200 B.C.), regulated both human and veterinary practice by laws.

GREECE
- Classic period of human medicine (470–146 B.C.)
- Age of the philosopher physician.
- Hippocrates of Cos (460–377 B.C.)
- Hippocratic System emphasized high standards of ethics, accurate observations, clarity and honesty in recording case histories, and rational treatment.
- Greek veterinarians were called *hippiatroi* (horse doctors, or *equarius medicus*) Also referred to as *medicus veternarius*, probably the origin of the word "veterinarian."
- During the first century, Greek *hippiatroi* attached to the Roman armies made contributions through writings on problems of animal disease observed in the army's horses.

Hippiatrika
- Likely the first comprehensive work on animal diseases that dealt with specific treatment for various diseases.
- Animal and human medicine were about parallel at this point.
- Veterinary medicine was considered to be superior to human medicine during this period by some historians.

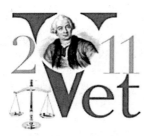

Claude Bourgelat
1712–1779

2011 is significant for the veterinary profession because it marks the 250th world anniversary of veterinary education. The world's first veterinary school was founded in Lyon, France, in 1761; and the initiative of French veterinarian, Claude Bourgelat

By the age of 49, Bourgelat was considered one of the finest horseman in Europe. He had 25 years of management experience at the King's Academy. On August 4, 1761, he obtained a grant of 50,000 livers (540 ounces of gold; worth around $750,000 in 2011).

The only requirements for admission to the new school was the ability to read and write. There was no age limit, only to present evidence of baptism and a certificate of good conduct.

Beginning in 1763, major epizootics, especially *Rinderpest,* raged in France. Bourgelat taught the students everything they needed to know in one year to send as many as possible to combat the prevailing cattle diseases. A veterinary historian, Dr. Vincent Krogmann, wrote, "The plague was stayed and the health of stock restored, through the assistance rendered to agriculture by veterinary science and art."

This convinced the king to decree in 1764 that Lyon be given the title "Royal Veterinary School," qualifying it for support by the state.

The American Veterinary Medical Association (AVMA) was founded in 1863, when 40 delegates representing seven states met for a convention in New York. Originally named the United States Veterinary Medical Association, the USVMA was renamed the AVMA in 1889.

By 1913, the AVMA consisted of 1,650 members, with membership open only to graduates of accredited veterinary schools. Today, the AVMA has more than 81,500 members engaged in a wide variety of work. In addition to treating pets, veterinarians work in a number of fields such as public health, agriculture, food safety, academics, and the military. The 21 recognized specialties range from Anesthesiology to Zoological Medicine.

A friend of mine was one of the featured speakers at the annual meeting of the Michigan Vet Med Society held in Lansing, Michigan, in the early 1980s. He was seated at the head table for lunch and asked me to join him. As luck would have it, I was ensconced next to the Dean of the School of Vet Med. I recalled the words of my friend, Dr. Erv Small, long-time Director of Clinical Veterinary Medicine at the University of Illinois, "Those of you who are not familiar with the protocol of academia, remember this: Around these hallow halls, Deans only answer to God—and then only occasionally." Dean Bradley monopolized much of our conversation, bemoaning his inability to keep any promising grad students in embryo transfer research. Texas A&M vet school was hiring then and paying salaries Dean Bradley couldn't match.

History: The first successful embryo transfer was performed in 1890 using rabbit embryos. The first bovine embryo was recovered by Hartman, Lewis, Miller and Swett in 1930 at the Carnegie Laboratory of Embryology in Baltimore. In the 1950s, embryo transfer technology in cattle expanded with the first successful transfer performed by Umbaugh and the first calf born through a joint effort by the USDA and the University of Wisconsin. Progress was slow until the 1970s, with many ideas ending in failure. As nonsurgical methods advanced through the efforts of Elsden, Hasler, Seidel, and others, the commercial use of embryo transfer exploded. In 2002, over 25,000 ET calves were registered in the United States.

Why perform embryo transfer: There are many reasons a producer might select embryo transfer for his/her particular operation. The first reason would probably be the potential for genetic improvement in the herd. Through artificial insemination, superior male genetics can be spread across a herd. With embryo transfer, superior female genetics can now be spread across a specific herd or even many herds. Superovulation and embryo transfer allows one particular female to produce many offspring in a given year and many more over her reproductive lifetime. Each of these offspring would potentially carry the superior traits of the mother, such as increased weight gain, improved carcass merit, or even increased milk production. Embryo transfer may also eliminate the stress of parturition on a desirable animal, thereby increasing her reproductive life span. Disease control, salvage of reproductive function, and potential twinning are a few of the other benefits of embryo transfer. Finally, the impact embryo transfer has had and will have on the research environment cannot be overlooked. Techniques such as gene insertion, embryo splitting, and pronuclear DNA injections would not be as feasible without embryo transfer technology.

The progress in ET has also changed the business of thoroughbred racing. Stallions could be bred almost daily; mares only yearly. With ET mares can now produce a number of foals—carried by donor mares—and even continue racing.

I asked René A. Carlson, DVM, AVMA President-Elect, for her thoughts, hopes, and desires for the veterinary profession. She responded:

> We are celebrating 250 years of veterinary medicine and all its contributions and changes over the years. This is the perfect time again to reassess this profession if we hope to retain the enormous pride we have, to provide the noble services we offer, and to continue to attract the amazing people who dream of becoming a veterinarian someday. I have complete faith that veterinary medicine will continue to be the most noble and rewarding profession into the future, but it won't be the veterinary profession of the past and it won't be without some bold changes.
>
> There are several initiatives this year from the Vision 20/20 Commission looking at governance of the AVMA and how it can continue to be of great service to veterinarians, the NAVMEC initiative looking at the future of veterinary medical education, task forces on updating the AVMA Strategic Plan, and one looking at how to better engage students and recent graduates into organized veterinary medicine, the National Academy of Sciences study on Needs for the Veterinary Workforce, and two different leadership training initiatives for up-and-coming AVMA members. There is a lot on the plate at the moment, which doesn't even include all the animal rights issues and international issues. We must to come up with a bold strategic plan to continue our meaningful and significant contributions to animal and human health for the next 100 years that provides relevant and competent services for a reasonable cost of education and appropriate financial reward.

"The State of the Art" keeps marching out in front of us. It boggles the mind to think of what the profession—indeed, society as a whole—will experience in the next 75 years. A friend once remarked, "Wouldn't it be wonderful to be 30 again?" "No," I responded, "Raising six kids—once—is enough for me." I'm happy to leave the future to the next generation. From what I've seen lately of their efforts all around the world, I'm positive they will be up to any task.

That's a Wrap!

"Wrap" is a phrase used by the director in the early days of the film industry to signal the end of filming. Nowadays, the call is more commonly, "That's a wrap!" Film makers have used this phrase since the 1920s when the filming is done and it needs to go into postproduction.

As this book goes into postproduction, it's appropriate to pause and reflect on my life's journey. One could call it Karma, Fate, or Luck. How else could one account for the good fortune that came my way over the last 82 years? Our family doctor, Lou Creighton, told me in the 1960s, "John, I'm going to tell you the secret of how to live a long life. Before you're born, be sure to pick grandparents who lived a long time." Genetics plays a major role in longevity. My maternal grandparents lived 83 and 88 years respectively. My paternal grandparents lived 63 and 91 years. The average life span in 1940 was 62 years, increasing to 67 years by 1950. Three of my forebears lived twenty years beyond their expected departure time.

Having "Type A" parents presents advantages and problems. Family discussions (arguments) around the dinner table were frequent and loud. Mom occasionally threw dishes at Dad. He was a good ducker. When the discussion got that heated, we three kids headed upstairs or out the door. I learned early to avoid confrontations. It took years of therapy to allow me to have a meaningful discussion without anger.

Birth order seems to affect who we become. As the second child and the oldest boy, my place in the family was complicated by separation from the family for a length of time in my youth. Each of the three kids—Marg, John, and Phil—became "only children" while spending months with relatives.

I know a number of couples made up of a fellow marrying the younger sister of a classmate. How fortunate to grow up with a similar background. Carol gave meaning, commitment, love, and joy to my life. We had very dissimilar upbringings but developed very like ideas on moral values. Our major family problems were disagreements on child rearing and money. Carol was a modified "clean freak." She would often do more than one clothes washing daily. Our babies slept right through vacuuming noise. Carol relaxed only a little as the kids kept coming. There wasn't enough time in the day to do all the household chores she deemed necessary. My theory was, "Do what you can, but the work will still be here tomorrow." Carol was the disciplinarian. I tended to tell her, "If they are not headed for jail, it couldn't be too bad." Each of our six children were unplanned and welcomed into our family. We rarely countermanded each other, trying to keep a united front.

Our family was fortunate to live from the '50s through the turn of the century—a time of almost unending prosperity. I can only imagine the heartache of modern families whose future is clouded by the housing collapse brought on by bankers on Wall Street gambling with "Other People's Money" and causing the greatest depression since the 1930s. Most people had little or no student loan debt we left college in the '50s. Nowadays, student debt approaching $100,000 is not uncommon.

I learned one lesson the hard way. I was ignorant of the common saying in real estate, "location, location, location." My animal hospital was located on a secondary road on the outskirts of Kenosha in 1956. It was in a beautiful oak forest, but hard to find, especially for newcomers to the community. In the early '60s, before the real estate boom, a one-acre property on the major highway leading into Kenosha from the just-finished interstate became available. The price of $10,000 was reasonable. I considered buying the land and either moving my hospital one half mile or building a new, modern animal hospital and remodeling the present structure into a residence. Norm Abplanalp even drew up plans for the switch. I guess I was too involved in our newly completed house to go ahead with the move. Over the next 20 to 30 years, three veterinarians have located on Highway 50, all very successful.

I had the thought of never retiring. Maybe I'd sell my practice to a younger vet and work a lot less and travel a lot more. Carol's back surgery and subsequent lameness changed our retirement plans. Sports were out of the question and traveling was curtailed. Our involvement in community activities in Peachtree City was similar to our time in Kenosha.

I've always admired individuals who responded to a need with action. Examples abound...

Greg Mortensen, Central Asia Institute, builds schools for girls in Afghanistan and Pakistan. His story is told in the best selling book, *Three Cups of Tea*. The *60 Minutes* investigation of

CAI revealed Greg to be a dedicated philanthropist but a poor business manager.

Jama Hedgecoth founded Noah's Arc near Atlanta to provide shelter for dozens of abused children and thousands of neglected wild and domestic animals. Her story is documented on pages 375–377 in this book.

Luma Mufleh founded Fugees Academy in Clarkson, Georgia, for displaced and orphaned kids from around the world with a common interest in football (soccer).

Stan Brock is the founder of the non-profit medical care organization, Remote Area Medical, that enlists thousands of volunteer medical professionals who provide medical care entirely free of charge to patients on a "first come, first served" basis. Most treatments are in the form of eye care, dental care, and general medical examinations. RAM veterinary care extends to companion animals. Stan has no money, no income, and no bank account. He spends 365 days a year at the charity events, sleeping on a small rolled-up mat on the floor and living on a diet made up entirely of porridge and fresh fruit.

Many other individuals are recognized on TV programs like *CNN Heroes 2012—Everyday People Changing the World.* I especially admire people who find a need and work to fulfill that need. It reminds me of the song we sang in the Quaker church seventy five years ago, "Brighten the Corner Where You Are." I've tried to do likewise, to look for a way to help my neighbor. I'm constantly amazed at how good it feels to give, especially of one's self. The idea of "pay it forward" is a good path to follow.

As Edward R. Morrow closed his TV newscasts 50 years ago, "Good Night and Good Luck."